D1263167

45.00

Speech-Language Pathology Desk Reference

Speech-Language Pathology Desk Reference

Ross J. Roeser, Ph.D.

Professor, Program in Communication Disorders
University of Texas at Dallas
Director, Callier Center for Communication Disorders/UT Dallas
and
Clinical Professor, Department of Otorhinolaryngology
University of Texas Southwestern Medical Center

Donise W. Pearson, M.S.

Clinical Manager of Speech-Language Pathology
Callier Center for Communication Disorders/UT Dallas
and
Faculty Associate, Program in Communication Disorders
University of Texas at Dallas

Emily A. Tobey, Ph.D.

Nelle C. Johnston Professor, Program in Communication Disorders
University of Texas at Dallas/Callier
Center for Communication Disorders

1998
Thieme
New York • Stuttgart

89705

Thieme New York
333 Seventh Avenue
New York, NY 10001

SPEECH-LANGUAGE PATHOLOGY DESK REFERENCE
Ross J. Roeser, Ph.D.
Donise W. Pearson, M.S.
Emily A. Tobey, Ph.D.

Library of Congress Cataloging-in-Publication Data

Roeser, Ross J.
    Speech-language pathology desk reference / by Ross J. Roeser,
Donise W. Pearson, Emily A. Tobey.
        p. cm.
    Includes index.
    ISBN 0-86577-696-2. — ISBN 3-13-110541-0
    1. Speech disorders—Handbooks, manuals, etc.   2. Speech therapy—
Handbooks, manuals, etc.   3. Audiology—Handbooks, manuals, etc.
I. Pearson, Donise W.   II. Tobey, Emily A.   III. Title.
    [DNLM: 1. Speech-Language Pathology—methods—handbooks.
2. Communicative Disorders—therapy—handbooks.   WL 39 R718s   1998]
RC423.R586   1998
616.85'5—dc21
DNLM/DLC
for Library of Congress   97-22115
                                                                     CIP

Copyright © 1998 by Thieme New York. This book, including all parts thereof, is legally
protected by copyright. Any use, exploitation or commercialization outside the narrow limits set by copyright legislation, without the publisher's consent, is illegal and liable to pros-
ecution. This applies in particular to photostat reproduction, copying, mimeographing or
duplication of any kind, translating, preparation of microfilms, and electronic data processing and storage.

Important Note: Medical knowledge is ever-changing. As new research and clinical experience broaden our knowledge, changes in treatment and drug therapy may be required. The
authors and editors of the material herein have consulted sources believed to be reliable in
their efforts to provide information that is complete and in accord with the standards accepted at the time of publication. However, in view of the possibility of human error by the
authors, editors, or publisher of the work herein, or changes in medical knowledge, neither
the authors, editors, publisher, nor any other party who has been involved in the preparation
of this work, warrants that the information contained herein is in every respect accurate or
complete, and they are not responsible for any errors or omissions or for the results obtained from use of such information. Readers are encouraged to confirm the information
contained herein with other sources. For example, readers are advised to check the product
information sheet included in the package of each drug they plan to administer to be certain
that the information contained in this publication is accurate and that changes have not been
made in the recommended dose or in the contraindications for administration. This recom-
mendation is of particular importance in connection with new or infrequently used drugs.
Some of the product names, patents, and registered designs referred to in this book are in fact
registered trademarks or proprietary names even though specific reference to this fact is not
always made in the text. Therefore, the appearance of a name without designation as proprietary is not to be construed as a representation by the publisher that it is in the public domain.

Printed in the United States of America

5 4 3 2 1

TNY ISBN 0-86577-696-2
GTV ISBN 3-13-110541-0

FONTBONNE LIBRARY

Ref
RC
423
.R586
1998

Contents

Expanded Contents

3 Phonology, Respiration, and Articulation–Adult • *161*

4 Child Language • *195*

5 Acquired Neurological Disorders • *251*

6 Fluency • *311*

7 Voice • *321*

Contents • **xv**

8 Oralfacial Structure and Function • 385

11 Audiology/Hearing Disorders • *451*

12 Professional Issues/Information • *487*

13 Periodicals and Professional Organizations • *497*

Index • *509*

Preface

Our aspiration in compiling the information in this book was to furnish clinicians and students with a wide range of relevant information in order to provide better treatment for individuals with communication disorders. As knowledge and information in speech-language pathology is expanding, it is becoming more and more difficult to keep up with it. It is our hope that the skills and knowledge of those professionals who read the material in this text will be enhanced.

Ross J. Roeser
Donise W. Pearson
Emily A. Tobey

Acknowledgments

This book could not have been written without the efforts of a host of people. Our deep gratitude goes first to Ms. Stacey Gurevitch, a speech-language pathology graduate student and our core worker. She had the seeming never-ending task of writing for and tracking permissions, scanning the material, and coordinating the necessary editing changes; she also did the majority of the computer work. We hope the experience she had in assisting us with this project will facilitate her in her professional career.

Others who assisted in this project were Ms. Linda Sensibaugh, administrative assistant to Dr. Roeser; Dr. Allen L. Clayton, Callier Librarian; Ms. Diana Roquillo, and Dr. Nathan Schwade, as well as graduate students in the Program in Communication Disorders at the Callier Center/University of Texas at Dallas, including Gretchen Gabbert, Rebecca Gordon, Julie Holton, Fereshteh Kunkel, Kelly Langston, Jay Perrin, and Angie Simpson.

Finally, to our colleagues whose materials appear in this book: Your willingness to allow publication of this material allows those who seek knowledge about speech, language, and hearing disorders and their treatment to be better informed and able to meet demanding individual professional goals.

Ross J. Roeser
Donise W. Pearson
Emily A. Tobey

1

Anatomy and Physiology

Mouth/Oral Cavity

The oral cavity is bounded anteriorly by the lips, posteriorly by the anterior faucial arch, inferiorly by the floor of the mouth, and superiorly by the hard and soft palates. It is continuous with the oropharynx through the anterior faucial arch (Fig. 1.1). The faucial arch and the base of the tongue form the *faucial isthmus*. The oral cavity is divided into two parts by the upper and lower alveolar process and the teeth: (1) the *vestibule of the mouth* lying between the lip and cheek on one side and the teeth and the alveolar process on the other; and (2) the *oral cavity proper*, limited externally by the alveolar process and the teeth.

The *vestibule of the mouth* communicates directly with the oral cavity proper on both sides, even when the teeth are in apposition, between the ascending ramus of the mandible and the last molar tooth. This is of practical importance (e.g., in intermaxillary wiring) because the patient can take a fluid diet making use of this communication, even when the teeth are fixed in occlusion.

The *tongue* fills the oral cavity almost completely when the mouth is closed. The presence of a slight negative pressure in the oral cavity ensures that the tongue adheres to the hard and soft palate, thus maintaining the closure of the mouth.

The following parts of the tongue are distinguished: the *tip,* the *margins,* the *body,* the *base,* the *dorsum,* and the *ventral surface* (Fig. 1.2).

The dorsum of the tongue is covered by a modified epithelium containing the filiform papillae at the tip, the fungiform papillae at the tip and margins, the foliate papillae on the posterolateral part of the tongue, and the vallate papillae on the dorsum. The boundary between the body of the tongue and the base of the tongue

1

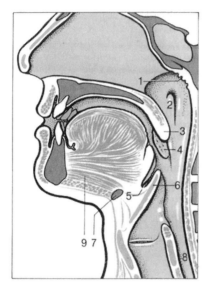

FIGURE 1.1. Anatomy of the mouth and pharynx.

1, roof of the nasopharynx; **2,** ostium of the eustachian tube; **3,** soft palate; **4,** palatal tonsil; **5,** vallecula; **6,** epiglottis; **7,** hyoid bone **8,** hypopharynx; **9,** floor of the mouth.

SOURCE: Becker W, Naumann HH, Pflatz CR: *Ear, Nose, and Throat Diseases,* p. 299. Thieme, New York, 1989.

is formed by the V-shaped *terminal sulcus,* whose central point is the foramen cecum, a remnant of the thyroglossal duct.

The base of the tongue contains the *lingual tonsil,* which may be the site of inflammation and abscess due to an impacted foreign body and which may also cause mechanical difficulty in swallowing when it is hypertrophic. The base of the

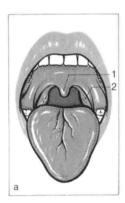
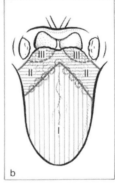
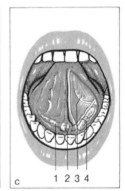

FIGURE 1.2. Tongue.

a. From above. **1,** uvula; **2,** palatine tonsils. **b.** Sensory innervation. **I,** lingual nerve with chorda tympani; **II,** glossopharyngeal nerve; **III,** vagus nerve. **c.** Lower surface of tongue and floor of the mouth. **1,** plica sublingualis; **2,** sublingual caruncle; **3,** lingual nerve; **4,** submandibular duct.

SOURCE: Becker W, Naumann HH, Pflatz CR: *Ear, Nose, and Throat Diseases,* p. 300. Thieme, New York, 1989.

tongue is limited inferiorly by the edge of the *epiglottis.* The two valleculae lie in the angle between the epiglottis and the base of the tongue. On occasion they may be difficult to inspect, and they may also be the site of cysts, foreign bodies, and malignant tumors. In supine, unconscious patients or patients under general anesthesia, the base of the tongue may fall backward to occlude the entrance to the larynx, and together with the epiglottis may lead to respiratory obstruction. This is prevented by pulling the tongue forward and by introduction of an oropharyngeal airway.

The arrangement of the musculature of the tongue provides it with extreme mobility. Two groups of muscles may be distinguished: (1) those without any bony attachments running free in the body of the tongue (i.e., the transverse, the superior, the inferior longitudinal muscles, and the vertical muscles); and (2) those muscles that are attached to fixed points (i.e., the styloglossus, the genioglossus, the hyoglossus, and the palatoglossus muscles [Fig. 1.3]).

The *floor of the mouth* is formed mainly by the mylohyoid muscle, which is stretched between the U-shaped mandible like a diaphragm and is inserted into the hyoid bone and the median raphe. On the *oral surface,* with the tip of the tongue elevated, the plica sublingualis with the sublingual caruncle may be found on both sides of the lingual frenulum (see Fig. 1.2c).

In the caruncle and the immediate neighborhood lie the efferent ducts of the submandibular gland, the submandibular duct (Wharton's duct), and the sublingual gland and sublingual duct (Bartholin's duct). The efferent duct of the parotid gland (Stensen's duct) opens into the cheek at the level of the second upper molar and that of the anterior lingual gland (Blandin's gland) in the region of the fimbriated fold on the ventral surface of the tongue (see Fig. 1.2c).

The *mandible* consists of two separate bones at birth, but these consolidate to form one bone within the first year of life. Figure 1.4a shows the most important anatomic details and the typical sites of fracture. The third branch of the trigeminal

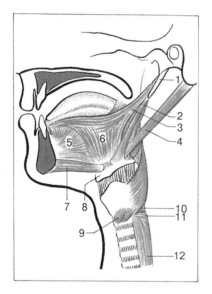

FIGURE 1.3. Muscles of the tongue and pharynx.

1, styloid process; **2,** stylohyoid muscle; **3,** styloglossus muscle; **4,** digastric muscle; **5,** genioglossus muscle; **6,** hyoglossus muscle; **7,** geniohyoid muscle; **8,** hyoid bone; **9,** cricothyroid muscle; **10,** Killian's triangle; **11,** inferior part of the cricopharyngeus; **12,** esophagus.

SOURCE: Becker W, Naumann HH, Pflatz CR: *Ear, Nose, and Throat Diseases,* p. 301. Thieme, New York, 1989.

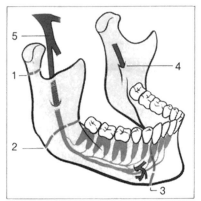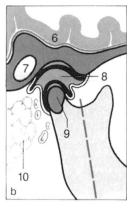

FIGURE 1.4.

a. Mandible with typical fracture lines. **1,** fracture of the neck; **2,** fracture of the angle of the jaw; **3,** fracture of the chin; **4,** mandibular foramen; **5,** mandibular nerve. **b.** Temporomandibular joint and surrounding structures. **6,** middle cranial fossa; **7,** external auditory meatus; **8,** articular disc; **9,** head of the mandible; **10,** parotid gland.

SOURCE: Becker W, Naumann HH, Pflatz CR: *Ear, Nose, and Throat Diseases,* p. 302. Thieme, New York, 1989.

nerve runs in the body of the mandible, together with the blood vessels that supply the lower teeth. The mandibular nerve enters the mandible at the mandibular foramen and leaves it at the mental foramen.

The *temporomandibular joint* is of great clinical interest because it may be involved in dental disease, in trauma of the facial skeleton and skull, in otologic diseases, and also generalized arthropathies. Furthermore, it may be the cause of headache in Costen's syndrome. Figure 1.4b shows the anatomic relationships. The proximity to the auditory meatus and mastoid, the lateral part of the base of the skull, the parotid gland, and the lateral wall of the oropharynx and nasopharynx should be noted.

The *epithelial lining of the oral cavity* consists of nonkeratinized, stratified, squamous epithelium, which is thickened in certain points such as the alveolar edges and hard palate, where it is united with the underlying periosteum to form a mucoperiosteum. Subepithelial collections of minor salivary glands are found all over the oral cavity, being more common at some parts than at others.

Vascular supply. The external carotid artery supplies the tongue via the lingual artery, the floor of the mouth via the sublingual artery, the cheek via the facial artery, and the palate via the ascending pharyngeal and descending palatine arteries. The latter arises from the internal maxillary artery. The *venous drainage* runs via the veins of the same names to the facial vein, the pterygoid venous plexus, and the internal jugular vein. There is also a connection to the cavernous sinuses via the pterygoid plexus.

The *lymph drains* via the regional submental, submandibular, and parotid nodes to the internal jugular chain. The lymph drainage of the base of the tongue and the floor of the mouth is to the same side *and* to the opposite side (Fig. 1.5). This fact is important in the formation of contralateral lymph node metastases.

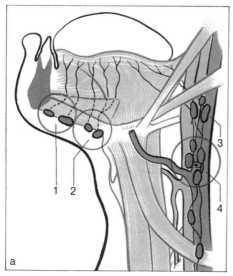
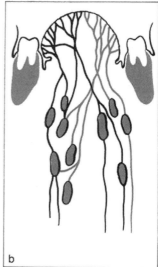

FIGURE 1.5. Lymph drainage of the tongue.
a. Groups of lymph nodes. **1,** submental; **2,** submandibular; **3,** upper deep cervical with lymph nodes at the superior venous angle (**4**). **b.** Contralateral lymphatic drainage of the tongue.
SOURCE: Becker W, Naumann HH, Pflatz CR: *Ear, Nose, and Throat Diseases,* p. 203. Thieme, New York, 1989.

Nerve supply. The *tongue* derives its *motor* supply from the hypoglossal nerve. Its *sensory* supply comes from the lingual nerve and the vagus nerve, which innervates the posterior part of the base of the tongue. Taste fibers come from the glossopharyngeal nerve to the base of the tongue and from the chorda tympani fibers of the VIIth cranial nerve accompanying the lingual nerve for the anterior two-thirds of the tongue (see Fig. 1.2a and 1.2b).

The *floor of the mouth* derives its *motor* supply from the mylohoid branch of the mandibular nerve and its *sensory* supply from the trigeminal nerve. Parasympathetic secretory fibers from the salivary glands are supplied from the chorda tympani and branches of the submandibular ganglion. Sympathetic fibers for blood vessels of the glands come from the carotid plexus.

The *masticatory muscles* derive their motor supply from the mandibular branch of the trigeminal nerve, but the buccinator muscle gets its supply from the facial nerve. The *teeth* of the upper jaw receive their sensory supply from the maxillary nerve and those of the lower jaw from the mandibular. These are both branches of the Vth cranial nerve.

The *temporomandibular joint* derives its nerve supply from the auriculotemporal branch of the mandibular nerve.

The *soft palate* derives its motor innervation from the glossopharyngeal, vagus, and trigeminal nerves, and probably the facial nerve also.

Naso-, Oro-, and Hypopharynx

The pharynx is a 12–13-cm-long muscular tube in the adult; it narrows from above downward, is covered with mucosa, and is divided into *three compartments,* each of which has an anterior opening (Fig. 1.6).

The *nasopharynx* is limited superiorly by the base of the skull, inferiorly by an imaginary plane through the soft palate, and it opens into the nasal cavity. The most important anatomic *structures* are as follows: anteriorly the choanae, superiorly the floor of the sphenoid sinus, posterosuperiorly the adenoid, laterally the pharyngeal ostium of the eustachian tube and the cartilaginous torus tubarius immediately posterior to which is Rosenmueller's fossa and the tubal tonsil, and anteriorly and inferiorly the soft palate. The embryonic *pharyngeal bursa* (Fig. 1.7) may persist in the posterior wall of the nasopharynx, causing chronic inflammation and retention of secretions. The posterior wall of the nasopharynx is separated from the spinal column by the tough prevertebral fascia that lies on the longus capitis muscles, the deep muscles of the neck, and the arch of the first cervical vertebra.

The shape and width of the nasopharynx show marked individual variation. The *epithelial lining* is respiratory ciliated and stratified squamous epithelium, with transitional epithelium at the junction with the oropharynx.

The *oropharynx* extends from the horizontal plane through the soft palate described above the superior edge of the epiglottis (Fig. 1.7) and is continuous with the oral cavity through the faucial isthmus. It contains the following important *structures:* the posterior wall, consisting of the prevertebral fascia and the bodies of the second and third cervical vertebrae; the lateral wall containing the palatine tonsil with the anterior and posterior faucial pillars; and the supratonsillar fossa lying above the tonsil between the anterior and posterior faucial arches.

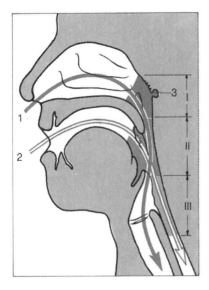

FIGURE 1.6. **Divisions of the pharynx.**
I, nasopharynx; **II,** oropharynx; **III,** hypopharynx. Crossing of the upper airway (**1**) and the upper food passage (**2**). Site of the pharyngeal bursa (**3**).
SOURCE: Becker W, Naumann HH, Pflatz CR: *Ear, Nose, and Throat Diseases,* p. 304. Thieme, New York, 1989.

The valleculae (see Fig. 1.1), the base of the tongue, the anterior surface of the soft palate, and the lingual surface of the epiglottis are usually described as being part of the oropharynx.

The *epithelial lining* consists of nonkeratinizing, stratified squamous epithelium.

The *hypopharynx* extends from the upper edge of the epiglottis superiorly to the inferior edge of the cricoid cartilage (see Fig. 1.6). It opens anteriorly into the larynx. On each side of the larynx lie the funnel-shaped piriform sinuses. Important anatomic *structures* and relations include on the anterior wall the marginal structures of the laryngeal inlet and the posterior surface of the larynx; on the lateral wall the inferior constrictor muscle and the piriform sinus, the latter being bounded medially by the aryepiglottic fold and laterally by the internal surface of the thyroid cartilage and the thyrohyoid membrane. Immediate relationships of the hypopharynx at the level of the larynx include the common carotid artery, the internal jugular vein, and the vagus nerve. Relations of the posterior wall, apart from the pharyngeal constrictor muscle, include the prevertebral fascia and the bodies of the third to the sixth cervical vertebrae. Inferiorly the hypopharynx opens into the esophagus, the boundary being the superior sphincter of the esophagus. The *epithelial lining* consists of nonkeratinized, stratified squamous epithelium.

The muscular tube of the entire pharynx consists of two layers with different functions:

1. A circular muscle layer consisting of the three pharyngeal constrictor muscles: the superior constrictor inserted into the base of the skull, the middle constrictor inserted into the hyoid bone, and the inferior constrictor inserted into the cricoid cartilage (see Figs. 1.3 and 1.7). Each of these funnel-shaped muscular segments is overlapped at its lower end by the segment below. All segments are inserted posteriorly into a tendinous median raphe.

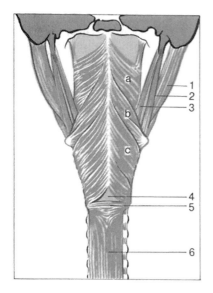

FIGURE 1.7. Pharyngeal musculature.

(**a**) superior constrictor, (**b**) middle constrictor, (**c**) inferior constrictor. **1,** digastric muscle; **2,** stylohyoid muscle; **3,** stylopharyngeus muscle; **4,** Killian's triangle; **5,** inferior part of the cricopharyngeus muscle; **6,** esophagus.

SOURCE: Becker W, Naumann HH, Pflatz CR: *Ear, Nose, and Throat Diseases,* p. 306. Thieme, New York, 1989.

The inferior constrictor muscle is of particular clinical importance. It is divided into a superior thyropharyngeal part and an inferior cricopharyngeal part. Figure 1.7 shows how the triangular dehiscence (*Killian's triangle*) is formed from the posterior wall of the hypopharynx between the superior oblique and the inferior horizontal fibers. A pharyngoesophageal pouch (Zencker's diverticulum) may develop at this weak point in the hypopharyngeal wall.

2. The raising and lowering of the pharynx is also achieved by three paired muscles radiating into the pharyngeal wall from outside. These are the stylopharyngeus, the salpingopharyngeus, and the palatopharyngeus muscles. The stylohyoid and styloglossus muscles are also responsible for elevation. A true longitudinal muscle does not occur in the pharynx and only begins at the mouth of the esophagus. The ability of the pharynx to slide over a distance of several centimeters is due to the existence of fascial spaces (parapharyngeal and retropharyngeal) filled with loose connective tissue. These tissue spaces are significant in the spread of infection.

Vascular supply of the pharynx. The *arterial supply* is provided by the ascending pharyngeal artery, the ascending palatine artery, the tonsillar branches of the facial artery, branches of the maxillary artery (i.e., the descending palatine artery), and branches of the lingual artery. All these arise from the external carotid artery. The *venous drainage* is via the facial vein and the pterygoid plexus to the internal jugular vein.

The *lymphatic drainage* is either via an inconstant retropharyngeal lymph node and then to the deep jugular lymph nodes or directly to the latter group. The inferior part of the pharynx also drains to the paratracheal lymph nodes, and thus gains a connection to the lymphatic system of the thorax.

Nerve supply of the pharynx. The individual pharyngeal muscles gain their motor supply from the glossopharyngeal, vagus, hypoglossal, and facial nerves. The nasopharynx derives its sensory nerve supply from the maxillary division of the trigeminal nerve, the oropharynx from the glossopharyngeal nerve, and the hypopharynx from the vagus nerve.

Lymphoepithelial System of the Pharynx

> **Note:** The term lymphoepithelial tissue is used to indicate a close symbiosis of epithelial and lymphatic cells on the surface of a mucosa.

The epithelial and subepithelial tissue is loosely arranged so that lymphatic cells can enter it in large numbers ("reticulated epithelium"). The reticulohistiocytic system (RHS), more commonly named reticuloendothelial systems (RES), with its storage cells is strongly represented in lymphoepithelial tissue. Figure 1.8 shows the principle of a lymphoepithelial unit. Solitary units of this type, solitary follicles, are found in all parts of the mucosa. The epithelium is also diffusely interspersed with lymphocytes.

A very pronounced collection of lymphoepithelial tissue, *Waldeyer's ring,* lies at the opening of the upper aerodigestive tracts. These *lymphoepithelial organs* are called *tonsils.* From above downward, the following may be distinguished:

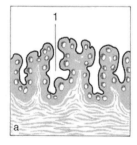

FIGURE 1.8. Lymphoepithelial tissue.
1, continuous squamous epithelium;
2, reticular epithelium; **3,** secondary nodes
with light centers and dark zone of small
lymphocytes; **4,** basic lymphoid tissue;
5, arterioles and venules; **6,** postcapillary
veins.

SOURCE: Becker W, Naumann HH, Pflatz
CR: *Ear, Nose, and Throat Diseases,*
p. 308. Thieme, New York, 1989.

1. The *pharyngeal tonsil,* the adenoids, which is single and lies on the roof and posterior wall of the nasopharynx.
2. The *tubal tonsil,* which is paired and lies around the ostium of the eustachian tube in Rosenmueller's fossa.
3. The paired *palatine tonsil,* lying between the anterior and posterior faucial pillars.
4. The *lingual tonsil,* which is single and lies in the base of the tongue. Less constant and obvious are:
5. The *tubopharyngeal plicae,* lateral bands, which run almost vertically at the junction of the lateral and posterior walls of the oro- and nasopharynx.
6. Lymphoepithelial collections in the laryngeal ventricle.

Unlike lymph nodes, lymphoepithelial organs possess only efferent lymph vessels and do *not* have afferent vessels. The difference in pathology and physiology of the individual collection of lymphoid tissue rests on their different structure. Figure 1.9a and 1.9b shows the structure of a *palatine tonsil* and of the *adenoids.*

The fine structure of a *tonsil* (see Figs. 1.3 and 1.9a and 1.9b) is in principle as follows: The soft tissue lamellae or septae arise from a basal connective tissue capsule. These serve as a supporting framework in which blood vessels, lymphatics,

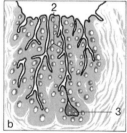

FIGURE 1.9. Diagram of (a) the nasopharyngeal tonsil, the adenoids and (b) the palatine tonsil.
1, tonsillar lacunae; **2,** tonsillar crypts; **3,** cryptic abscess.
SOURCE: Becker W, Naumann HH, Pflatz CR: *Ear, Nose, and Throat Diseases,* p. 308. Thieme, New York, 1989.

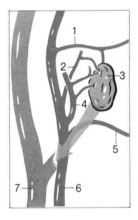

FIGURE 1.10. Vascular supply of the palatine tonsil.
1, internal maxillary artery with descending pharyngeal artery; **2,** ascending palatine artery; **3,** palatine tonsil; **4,** ascending pharyngeal artery; **5,** lingual artery; **6,** external carotid artery; **7,** internal jugular vein.
SOURCE: Becker W, Naumann HH, Pflatz CR: *Ear, Nose, and Throat Diseases,* p. 309. Thieme, New York, 1989.

and nerves run. This fan-shaped supporting framework considerably increases the active surface of the tonsil because it carries the actual lymphoepithelial parenchyma. It is estimated that the epithelial surface of one palatine tonsil amounts to 300 cm². In the *palatine tonsil,* the active surface is sunk within the mucosa, whereas in the *adenoids,* it projects above the surface. The broad, flat niches opening into the oral cavity caused by infolding are called *lacunae;* the branching clefts running throughout the entire substance of the tonsil are called *crypts.* The actual tonsil tissue consists of a collection of a very large number of the lymphoepithelial units described earlier (see Fig. 1.8). The crypts usually contain cell debris and round cells but may also contain bacteria and colonies of fungi, collections of pus, and encapsulated microabscesses.

The tonsils of Waldeyer's ring are present at the embryonal stage, but they only acquire their typical structure with secondary nodes in the postnatal period (i.e., after direct contact with environmental pathogens). They begin increasing rapidly in size between the first and the third year of life, with peaks in the third and seventh year. They involute slowly as of early puberty. Like the rest of the lymphatic system, they atrophy with increasing age.

The *arterial* blood supply of the pharyngeal tonsil is provided by various branches of the external carotid artery, including the ascending and descending pharyngeal artery, the ascending palatine, the lingual, and also possibly direct tonsillar branches (Fig. 1.10).

The *veins* of the pharyngeal tonsil usually drain via the palatal vein to the facial vein and from there to the jugulofacial venous angle of the internal jugular vein. There is also drainage via the pterygoid venous plexus to the internal jugular vein. This route provides a possible pathway of spread for infection from the tonsils to the cavernous sinus.

Physiological and Pathophysiological Principles

Several functional systems are collected in the mouth and pharynx, including the masticatory system, the swallowing apparatus, the taste organs, the lymphoepithelial ring, pregastric digestion, and articulation. Furthermore, the respiratory and digestive tracts cross in this area (see Fig. 1.6). This requires a reliable reflex protective system. An important prerequisite is a well-functioning autonomic and voluntary nerve supply to this region, and also a mucosa adapted to this double function. The mouth is only involved in respiration as a *supplementary measure:* Continuous mouth breathing causes considerable local damage and can also affect the entire body.

Eating, Preparation of Food, and Swallowing

Normal *feeding* requires a normal masticatory apparatus and teeth, masticatory muscles, and temporomandibular joint. The function of the cranial nerves must also be normal. The *preparation of the food* serves to reduce the size of the bolus of food by chewing and also to moisten the food with saliva, of which 1–1.5 liters are produced daily. The saliva lubricates the mucosa and makes the food capable of being swallowed. Furthermore, the enzymes contained in saliva prepare the food by partial chemical decomposition for further digestion in the gastrointestinal tract.

Satisfactory moistening of the mucosa of the oral cavity and pharynx by saliva is also necessary for normal speech and for normal taste.

The stages of the *swallowing act* are as follows:

1. Displacement of the food bolus posteriorly by pressure of the tongue on the hard palate and gliding deformation of the body of the tongue.
2. Stimulation of the swallowing reflex as soon as the bolus reaches the base of the tongue. All openings not connected to the digestive tract are closed off.
    a. The nasopharynx is closed off by posterosuperior elevation of the soft palate.
    b. The larynx is drawn upward and anteriorly under the base of the tongue by muscle traction. The epiglottis lies over the laryngeal inlet.
    c. Reflex closure of the vocal cords occurs in the same phase. The bolus of food slides past the laryngeal inlet through the two piriform sinuses.
    d. When the bolus enters the hypopharynx, the esophageal orifice opens. The bolus is further transported in the esophagus by serial contraction of the individual portions of the pharyngeal constrictor muscles.
    e. Autonomic peristalsis of the longitudinal and circular muscles then transports the bolus through the esophagus to the lower sphincter (the cardia) and to the stomach.

Primary, secondary, and tertiary peristalsis may be distinguished in the esophagus. Primary peristalsis is induced automatically by the swallowing act. Secondary peristalsis comes into effect when the esophageal wall is stretched by retention of food. Tertiary peristalsis is a concomitant symptom of an organic esophageal disorder (e.g., idiopathic esophageal spasm, presbyesophagus, etc.). The peristaltic wave does not move in this case but is stationary.

The nervous pathways of swallowing are as follows:

- Afferent pathways are supplied by the second division of the Vth, the IXth, and the Xth cranial nerves.
- The center is in the medulla oblongata.
- The efferent pathways are the Xth, IXth, and XIIth cranial nerves.
- The pharyngeal and esophageal phases are not under voluntary control.

Pathophysiological aspects. The closure of the laryngeal inlet by the epiglottis is not strictly necessary for normal swallowing. A patient whose epiglottis has been removed (e.g., in an operation for a tumor) usually learns to swallow without difficulty. However, the sensory nerve supply of the hypopharynx and the laryngeal inlet from the superior laryngeal branch of the vagus nerve must be intact, as well as the pharyngeal constrictor, for reflex protection of the laryngeal inlet. Increased tone or spasm of the cricopharyngeus is a common autonomic disorder (e.g., in the thyrotoxicosis or the Plummer–Vinson syndrome). This can be the cause of the *globus* symptom of discomfort on swallowing at the level of the cricoid cartilage, of true *dysphagia,* and possibly the development of a *hypopharyngeal diverticulum.*

Disturbances of swallowing may also occur in paralyses of one or more cranial nerves, especially the Xth, but also the IXth and the XIIth, which affect the tongue, the soft palate, or the pharyngeal musculature.

Immune-Specific Functions of Waldeyer's Ring

There is now doubt about the immune-specific function of the various lymphoepithelial organs in Waldeyer's ring and in the solitary nodes in the mucosa. Experimentally, it can be shown that appropriate foreign material (also antigenic substances) in the tonsillar crypts can penetrate the reticular epithelium to reach the tonsillar parenchyma. Cellular material, including lymphocytes, segmental nuclear leukocytes, and cell debris, on the other hand, are shed in relatively large amounts from the tonsillar parechyma and reticular epithelium into the lumen of the crypts and pass from here into the mouth. It is estimated that 100 million round cells are shed by *one* tonsil daily into the digestive tract in this way. The specific function of the round cells passing in this way from the tonsil into the cavity is not known with certainty. They are probably intended to protect the internal surface of the body. The lymphoepithelial organs also produce immunoactive lymphocytes of the B and T series, which are released into the general circulation of the blood and lymphatic vessels as from all other lymphatic organs.

The present knowledge of the *function of the tonsils* may be summarized as follows:

1. The tonsils ensure controlled and protected contact of the organism with the pathogenic and antigenic environment, serving the purpose of immunological surveillance. This allows adaptation to the environment, especially in children.
2. The tonsils produce lymphocytes.
3. The tonsils expose B and T lymphocytes to current antigens and are instrumental in the production of specific messenger lymphocytes and memory lymphocytes.
4. The tonsils produce specific antibodies after the production of the appropriate plasma cells. All types of immunoglobulins occur in tonsillar tissue.
5. The tonsils shed topical immune-stimulated lymphocytes for both humoral and cell-mediated immunity into the oral cavity and the digestive tract.
6. The tonsils are instrumental in the production and discharge of immunoactive lymphocytes into the blood and lymphatic circulation. The information from this part of the immune system (the spleen and the lymph nodes) provides information about the present antigen situation at the beginning of the internal surface of the body ("subclinical immunity").

Basic pathophysiology. The increase of the lymphoepithelial tissue during the early years of childhood development is explained by the immunobiological requirements. This increase of size is primarily only an expression of an active defensive function of the infantile organism to antigenic substances in the environment. *Tonsillar hyperplasia* at this period is therefore a welcome attribute and is in no way a demonstration of excess inflammation. Since the tonsils lie at a narrow point of the respiratory and digestive tract, the nasopharynx and the faucial isthmus, an increase of their volume *beyond a certain point* leads to increased narrowing of the diameter of this essential pathway, to the detriment of the rest of the body (Fig. 1.11a and 1.11b). Removal of the tonsils and adenoids in this circumstance is thus justified despite any possible immunological disadvantages. The *palatine tonsils alone* possess slitlike, branching, poorly drained *crypts* permeating their entire substance. As long as these clefts drain freely into the oral cavity, the function of the tonsil is not endangered. However, if the physiological content of the crypt stagnates due to anatomic or infective stenosis, an ideal culture medium is set up for microorganisms. Colonies of bacteria or fungi are established, leading to chronic suppuration (cryptitis), small abscesses in the crypts, and superficial ulceration of the surface of the crypts, that is, pathological anatomically speaking, a *chronic tonsillitis.* This is in no way related to the size of the tonsil. Figure 1.8 shows how the superficial tonsillar capillaries are unprotected and run close to the lumen of the crypt, allowing relatively unhindered access of infective or toxic contents to the general circulation.

Formation of Sound and Speech

The oral cavity and pharynx make an important contribution to the timbre of the speech and voice because of their action as a variable resonating space. Furthermore, the tongue, in conjunction with the palate, is necessary for the formation

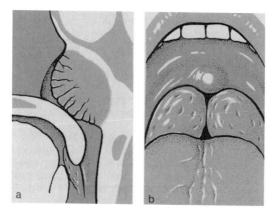

Figure 1.11. Obstruction of the nasopharynx by hypertrophied adenoid (a) and of the oropharynx by hypertrophied palatine tonsil (b).
Source: Becker W, Naumann HH, Pflatz CR: *Ear, Nose, and Throat Diseases,* p. 315. Thieme, New York, 1989.

of consonants and vowels. Despite that, experience of tumor surgery shows that large parts of the tongue may be removed, yet comprehensible speech is retained.

Larynx

Embryology

The *larynx* develops from a two-part angle: *The supraglottis develops from a buccopharyngeal bud, the glottis and subglottis from a tracheobronchial bud. This fact has clinical significance in the postnatal period. The nerves of the pharyngeal arches are branches of the vagus nerve.*

In the course of life, the larynx descends from about the level of the second vertebra at birth depending on sex to about the level of the fifth cervical vertebra in the adult.

Anatomy

The laryngeal skeleton consists of the thyroid, cricoid, and arytenoid cartilages, which are hyaline cartilage, the epiglottis, which is fibrous cartilage, and the fibroelastic accessory cartilages of Santorini and Wrisburg, which have no function.

Ossification of the thyroid cartilage begins at the time of puberty. Ossification of the cricoid and arytenoid cartilage follows somewhat later. The female larynx calcifies considerably later than that of the male. *The calcified parts of the laryngeal framework are often difficult to distinguish by radiography from bony foreign bodies.*

Internal and external ligaments and membranes unite the cartilages and stabilize the soft-tissue covering.

The laryngeal cavity is divided for clinical purposes into three compartments (Fig. 1.12 and Table 1.1):

- Supraglottis
- Glottis
- Subglottis

The *vocal cord* includes the vocal ligament, the vocalis muscle, and the mucosal covering (Fig. 1.13). The length of the vocal cord is 0.7 cm in the newborn, 1.6–2 cm in women, and 2–2.4 cm in men.

The *glottis* is formed by the edges of the true vocal cords. It is divided into an *intramembranous part* that lies between the paired vocal ligaments, and the *intracartilaginous part* that lies between the arytenoid cartilages of each side. The *transglottis space* is illustrated in Figure 1.12 and described in Table 1.1.

Note: Carcinoma occurs almost exclusively in the intermembranous part of the glottis, whereas intubation granuloma and contact ulcer caused by vocal abuse mainly affect the intercartilaginous part.

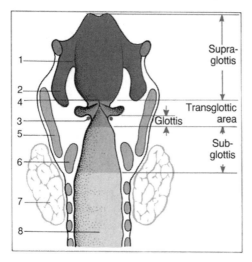

FIGURE 1.12. **Compartments of the larynx.**

1, aryepiglottic fold forming the boundary between the larynx and the hypopharynx; **2,** piriform sinus which belongs to the hypopharynx; **3,** vocal ligament; **4,** anterior commissure; **5,** thyroid cartilage; **6,** cricoid cartilage; **7,** thyroid gland; **8,** trachea.

SOURCE: Becker W, Naumann HH, Pflatz CR: *Ear, Nose, and Throat Diseases,* p. 387. Thieme, New York, 1989.

Superiorly, the larynx is limited by the free edge of the epiglottis, the aryepiglottic fold, and the interarytenoid notch. *Inferiorly,* the lower edge of the cricoid cartilage marks the junction with the trachea (see Fig. 1.12).

The *thyroid cartilage* is united by a joint to the *cricoid cartilage.* Rocking and slight gliding movements occur at this joint.

The *muscles, ligaments,* and *membranes* between the cartilages allow the functionally important movements between different parts of the larynx.

TABLE 1.1 **Classification and terminology of the laryngeal cavity.**

Supraglottic space	Epilarynx + vestibule = aditus
	Epilarynx = laryngeal surface of the epiglottis + aryepiglottic fold + arytenoid.
	Vestibule = the petiolus of the epiglottis + the vestibular folds + the ventricle as far as the upper surface of the vocal cords.
Glottic space	Vocal cords and 1 cm inferiorly
Subglottic space	Down to the lower border of the cricoid cartilage
"Transglottic space"	Glottis + ventricle + vestibular folds

SOURCE: Becker W, Naumann HH, Pflatz CR: *Ear, Nose, and Throat Diseases,* p. 387. Thieme, New York, 1989.

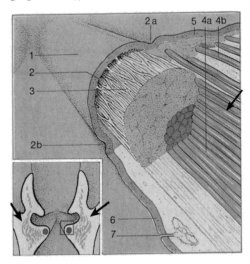

FIGURE 1.13. Frontal step section through the vocal cord.

The oblique three-dimensional section is through the glottis. The area indicated with arrows in the overview of the glottis in the inset on the lower left corresponds to the area indicated with arrows in the larger picture.

1, stratified squamous epithelium; **2,** Reinke's space: **2a,** superior arcuate line; **2b,** inferior arcuate line; **3,** vocal ligament; **4a,** medial part of the thyroarytenoid muscle, i.e., the vocalis muscle; **4b,** lateral part of the thyroarytenoid muscle; **5,** epithelium of Morgagni's space consisting of cylindrical ciliated epithelium; **6,** subglottic respiratory cylindrical ciliated epithelia zone; **7,** mucous gland. (Adapted from Lanz and Wachsmuth.)

SOURCE: Becker W, Naumann HH, Pflatz CR: *Ear, Nose, and Throat Diseases,* p. 388. Thieme, New York, 1989.

The *external ligaments and connective tissue membranes* anchor the larynx to the surrounding structures.

The most important membranes include the following:

- The thyrohyoid membrane has the opening for the superior laryngeal artery and vein and for the internal branch of the superior laryngeal nerve, which supplies sensation to the larynx above the vocal cords.
- The cricothyroid membrane is the point where the airway comes closest to the skin; it is the site of *laryngotomy.*
- The cricotracheal ligament provides attachment to the trachea.

The *internal ligaments and connective tissue membranes* (e.g., the conus elasticus and the thyroepiglottic ligament) connect the cartilaginous parts of the larynx to each other.

The *internal muscles and the one external muscle* act synergistically and antagonistically to control the functions of the larynx. They open and close the glottis and put the vocal cords under tension (Fig. 1.14).

This interplay explains the different positions of the vocal cords in paralysis of the recurrent laryngeal nerve or of the external branch of the superior laryngeal nerve (Table 1.2 and Color Plates 1 and 2).

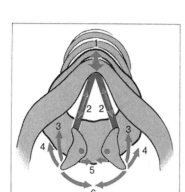

FIGURE 1.14. Directions of pull of laryngeal musculature.
1, the pull of the internal laryngeal muscles and the cricothyroid muscle [the anticus muscle]; **2,** medial part of the thyroarytenoid muscle (the vocalis muscle); **3,** lateral part of the thyroarytenoid muscle; **4,** lateral cricoarytenoid muscle (lateralis muscle); **5,** interarytenoid or transversus muscle; **6,** posterior cricoarytenoid muscle (posticus muscle).
SOURCE: Becker W, Naumann HH, Pflatz CR: *Ear, Nose, and Throat Diseases,* p. 389. Thieme, New York, 1989.

Note: There is only *one* muscle which opens the glottis, the "posticus." The muscles that close it are clearly in the majority. The ratio of their relative power is 1 : 3. Only the interarytenoid muscle with a pars obliqua and a part transversa is unpaired; all other muscles are paired (Color Plates 3, 4, & 5).

The *nerve supply* of the laryngeal musculature is provided by the external branch of the superior laryngeal nerve and by the recurrent laryngeal nerves that arise from the vagus nerve (see Fig. 1.21).

The *superior laryngeal nerve* divides into a *sensory internal branch,* which supplies the interior of the larynx down into the glottis, and an *external branch,* which provides the *motor supply* to the external cricothyroid muscle.

The *recurrent laryngeal nerve* provides *motor supply* to the *entire* ipsilateral *internal* laryngeal musculature and to the contralateral interarytenoid muscle. In addition, it provides *sensation* to the laryngeal mucosa *inferior* to the glottic cleft.

The left recurrent laryngeal nerve passes around the aortic arch to reach the larynx in the groove between the trachea and the esophagus. The right recurrent

TABLE 1.2. Functions of the laryngeal musculature.

Opening of the glottis, abduction of the vocal cords	Posterior cricoarytenoid muscle (posticus muscle)
Closure of the glottis, adduction of the vocal cords	Lateral cricoarytenoid muscle (lateralis muscle) Transverse arytenoid muscle (transversus muscle) Thyroarytenoid muscle, lateral part
Tension of the vocal cords	Cricothyroid muscle (anticus muscle) Thyroarytenoid muscle, medial part (vocalis muscle)

SOURCE: Becker W, Naumann HH, Pflatz CR: *Ear, Nose, and Throat Diseases,* p. 389. Thieme, New York, 1989.

laryngeal nerve passes around the subclavian artery and then runs superiorly in a groove between the trachea and esophagus.

Both recurrent laryngeal nerves enter the larynx at the inferior cornu of the thyroid cartilage. The relations of this nerve to the inferior thyroid artery and thyroid gland are important in surgical anatomy.

In the diagnosis of recurrent laryngeal paralysis, the cervical course of the nerve and possible intrathoracic and mediastinal disorders must be considered. Causes of recurrent paralysis include metastases, malignant lymphoma, malignant goiter, esophageal carcinoma, tuberculous lymphadenopathy, aortic aneurysm, and pulmonary hypertension.

The *blood supply of the larynx* is divided by the glottis into two areas.

The supraglottic blood supply from the superior laryngeal artery originates from the external carotid artery, whereas the subglottic vessels, the inferior laryngeal artery, derive from the thyrocervical trunk of the subclavian artery.

The *venous drainage* passes superiorly via the superior thyroid artery to the internal jugular vein and inferiorly via the inferior thyroid vein to the brachiocephalic vein.

The *lymphatic drainage* of the larynx is of great clinical importance. Here, again, the glottis forms the *embryological barrier between the superior and inferior lymphatic streams* (Fig. 1.15).

The *vocal cord,* consisting of elastic fibers, has *no lymphatic capillaries.* Sparse lymphatics begin only at the fibromuscular junction with the vocalis fold.

The *supraglottic space,* on the other hand, has a *rich lymphatic network.* A very dense and partly multilayered capillary network is to be found in the ventricular fold and the ventricle.

The *supraglottic* lymphatic pathway converges on the anterior insertion of the aryepiglottic fold and leaves in smaller collections of vessels along the neurovascular bundle of the larynx. Submucous and preepiglottic *horizontal anastomoses* are to be found in the midline of the larynx and are responsible for bilateral and contralateral metastases in carcinoma.

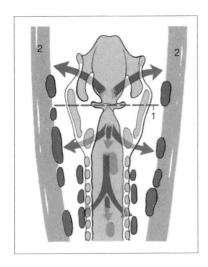

FIGURE 1.15. Glottic lymph barrier which produces a supraglottic and a subglottic lymph flow.

The first supraglottic lymph node stations are the inconstant prelaryngeal node and the upper deep cervical nodes. The first subglottic lymph node station is the pre- and paratracheal and lower deep jugular lymph nodes. **1,** glottic lymph barrier; **2,** internal jugular vein.

Source: Becker W, Naumann HH, Pflatz CR: *Ear, Nose, and Throat Diseases,* p. 391. Thieme, New York, 1989.

The *subglottic* capillary network is not as dense as the supraglottic network. Bilateral and contralateral invasion of the lymph nodes is again possible via the pre- and paratracheal lymph nodes. *The additional drainage to the peritracheal and mediastinal lymph nodes is of clinical importance.* The laryngeal lymph is ultimately collected into the superior and inferior deep cervical lymph nodes.

The *mucosal lining* of the larynx is adapted to its special position at the junction of the respiratory and digestive tracts. Stratified squamous epithelium, partially keratinized, covers the laryngeal surface of the epiglottis, the vestibular folds, the vestibule of the larynx, and the vocal cords. Ciliated columnar epithelium covers the remaining parts of the mucosal surface.

Reinke's space is a closed cleft beneath the epithelium of the vocal cord, with no glands or lymphatic capillaries. It is of clinical significance in *Reinke's edema* (see page 43 and Color Plate 6).

Physiology

The *sphincteric function* is the oldest phylogenetic function of the larynx (see Table 1.3).

Phonation. The tone, formed by the larynx, is modified by the movements of the pharynx, tongue, and lips to form speech.

Hoarseness is the result of noise formed by endolaryngeal turbulence of the airstream and irregularities of the normally periodic vibrations of the vocal cords. The phoniatrician distinguishes very slight, slight, moderate, and severe hoarseness. With increasing dysphonia, the harmonic part of the vocal sound decreases from the upper to the lower frequencies, and this can be measured by sonography. At the same time, the noise component becomes more marked. (Recording is not possible under controlled conditions using tape equipment.)

During respiration. The vocal cords are in the respiratory position (i.e., the glottis is open and under reflex control, which depends on gas exchange and acid–base balance).

Protection of the lower respiratory tract. The base of the tongue, the posterior pharyngeal wall, and the faucial pillars are involved in swallowing. The swallowing *reflex* transmitted in the glossopharyngeal nerve ensures *cessation of respiration* and contraction of the aryepiglottic folds, the vocal cords, and the vestibular folds, and tilting of the epiglottis by the thyroepiglottic muscle.

TABLE 1.3. Vital and communicative functions of the larynx.

Phonation		
Respiration		
Protection of the lower airway	Closure of the aditus Closure of the glottis }	on swallowing
	Reflex respiratory arrest	
	Cough reflex	
Fixation of the thorax aided by glottic closure		

SOURCE: Becker W, Naumann HH, Pflatz CR: *Ear, Nose, and Throat Diseases,* p. 391. Thieme, New York, 1989.

Simultaneously, the suprahyoid musculature contracts drawing the larynx anteriorly and superiorly by 2–3 cm.

Experience with surgical removal of the epiglottis shows that this structure is only of limited necessity for protection of the larynx. An intact sensory nerve supply to the mucosa of the laryngeal aditus from the internal branch of the superior laryngeal nerve is much more important. It controls reflex muscular contraction.

The *cough reflex* is stimulated by particles of food penetrating within the larynx. It consists of a deep reflex inspiration with the larynx open. The glottis closes with a rising intrathoracic pressure and then opens suddenly with an explosive expiratory stream, and the foreign body is coughed out.

Note: The larynx is the receptor field for other vasovagal reflexes. Mechanical irritation of the internal surface of the larynx can induce arrhythmia, bradycardia, and cardiac arrest. Satisfactory mucosal anesthesia must be ensured during endolaryngeal procedures. Particular care is necessary during obstruction by foreign bodies, and so on. The vagal reflex can be blocked by atropine and increased by opiates. Reflex irritability is increased in smokers.

Thoracic fixation. The respiratory system is closed off by the glottis to provide mechanical assistance during several bodily functions, notably coughing, defecation, micturition, vomiting, and parturition. Furthermore, the pectoral muscles are supplemented when doing chin-ups, while digging, and breathing during asthma attacks.

Methods of Investigation

These provide information about

- The position of the larynx and its relation to neighboring anatomic structures in the neck.
- The external and internal shape of the larynx.
- The type, site, and extent of lesions within and outside of the larynx.
- Functional disorders.

Inspection of the Larynx

Normally, the thyroid prominence can only be seen in men. It moves upward on swallowing; absence of this movement indicates fixation of the larynx by infection or tumor.

Indrawing of the suprasternal notch on inspiration combined with inspiratory stridor points to laryngotracheal obstruction by foreign body, tumor, edema, and so on.

Palpation

The laryngeal skeleton and neighboring structures are palpated during respiration and swallowing, paying attention to the following:

- The thyroid cartilage.
- The cricothyroid membrane and the cricoid cartilage.
- The carotid artery, with the carotid bulb, which must not be confused with neighboring cervical lymph nodes; the palpating finger picks up pulsations.
- The thyroid gland lying inferior and lateral to the thyroid and cricoid cartilages.
- The simultaneous movement of the larynx and thyroid gland on swallowing.

Indirect Laryngoscopy

The larynx is inspected by means of a mirror and the unaided eye or by a telescopic system.

The *technique of examination* is shown in Figures 1.16a–c and 1.17a–c. (See also Color Plates 1 and 2.) The tongue is grasped with the thumb and middle finger of the left hand, so that the thumb lies on the tongue. The index finger is used to push back the upper lip. The tongue must be drawn forward carefully to prevent damage to the frenulum by the lower teeth. The light from the mirror is directed toward the uvula. The laryngeal mirror is warmed on its glass surface, and its temperature is tested with the examiner's own hand. It is then introduced along the palate until it reaches the uvula.

Killian's position, in which the examiner sits in front of the standing patient, provides a better view of the *posterior commissure. Tuerck's* position, in which the examiner stands in front of the sitting patient, gives a better view of the *anterior commissure* (see Fig. 1.17b and 1.17c).

Stimulation of the base of the tongue and posterior pharyngeal wall is to be avoided because this can provoke the gag reflex. The posterior surface of the mirror is used to lift the uvula and push it upward and backward. The posterior part of the tongue, the pharynx, and part of the larynx are now visible in the mirror. The patient is asked to say "e" to bring the epiglottis into a more upright position and thus give a better view of the larynx. In a patient with a sensitive gag reflex, it may

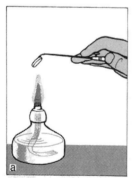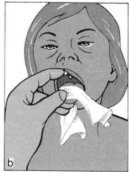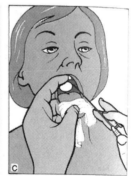

FIGURE 1.16. Indirect laryngoscopy.
SOURCE: Becker W, Naumann HH, Pflatz CR: *Ear, Nose, and Throat Diseases,* p. 394. Thieme, New York, 1989.

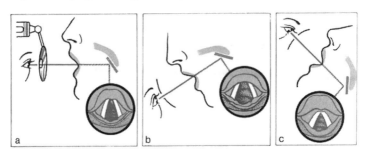

FIGURE 1.17. Indirect laryngoscopy.
(a) Normal direction of light and vision; **(b)** Killian's position producing a better view of the posterior commissure; **(c)** Tuerck's position which produces a better view of the anterior commissure.
SOURCE: Becker W, Naumann HH, Pflatz CR: *Ear, Nose, and Throat Diseases*, p. 394. Thieme, New York, 1989.

be necessary to spray the pharynx first with a topical anesthetic (e.g., Pontocaine) before this examination can be carried out (Fig. 1.18).

Telescopic Laryngoscopy

Telescopic laryngoscopies have become very useful in practice. These light, rigid endoscopes with wide-angle lenses supplement or may replace indirect laryngoscopy with the mirror.

The advantages of this procedure are that it provides variable magnification and a good view of hidden areas and that photographic documentation of conscious patients is possible.

> **Note:** Biopsies may be taken and polyps removed under indirect laryngoscopy using topic anesthesia applied by a cotton probe or spray (Fig. 1.18). However, microlaryngoscopy is preferable.

The larynx and the hypopharynx may be examined directly with a rigid laryngoscope supported via a lever arm on the patient's sternum. *Microlaryngoscopy* consists of the addition of the binocular operating microscope and a suitable set of instruments (Figs. 1.19 and 1.20) Anesthesia is achieved by intubation of endotracheal anesthesia or injection respiration without intubation. This procedure has been a considerable advance in endolaryngeal microsurgery. Microlaryngoscopy provides excellent illumination of the larynx, the upper trachea, and the hypopharynx, including all hidden areas. Some endolaryngeal procedures may also be carried out (Table 1.4).

The following features are looked for: the color of the mucosa; abnormal tissue; the appearance of local or diffuse lesions; smooth, rough, ulcerated, exophytic, etc.; the movement of the vocal cords; the lumen of the trachea; and the shape of the hypopharynx.

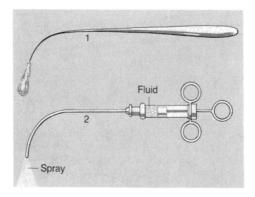

Figure 1.18. Instruments for mucosal anesthesia of the larynx.
1, curved metal cotton applicator; **2,** curved cannula.
Source: Becker W, Naumann HH, Pflatz CR: *Ear, Nose, and Throat Diseases,* p. 394.
Thieme, New York, 1989.

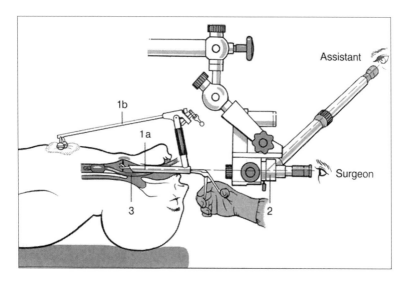

Figure 1.19. Microlaryngoscopy showing the laryngoscope.
(1a) introduced and held by a chest support and articulated lever arm **(1b)** supported on the
patient's sternum; **2,** operating microscope with assistant's eyepiece; **3,** endotracheal tube.
Source: Becker W, Naumann HH, Pflatz CR: *Ear, Nose, and Throat Diseases,* p. 396.
Thieme, New York, 1989.

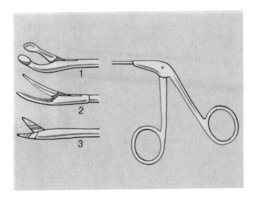

FIGURE 1.20. Typical instruments used in endolaryngeal microsurgery (magnified × 3).

1, double-cupped forceps; **2,** grasping forceps; **3,** scissors.

SOURCE: Becker W, Naumann HH, Pflatz CR: *Ear, Nose, and Throat Diseases,* p. 396. Thieme, New York, 1989.

Radiography

Plain views in the sagittal or lateral plane have limited value because of superimposition of the numerous soft-tissue and bony shadows. However, it is a relatively easy radiographic technique to augment.

Laryngography, in which the larynx and hypopharynx are coated with a contrast medium, provides information about the laryngeal surface and thus about the extent of the tumor.

Conventional tomograms and xerotomograms, particularly high-resolution computed tomography, provide accurate assessment of the site and extent of stenoses and tumors and the destruction of local, laryngeal, and neighboring structures. In the future, magnetic resonance imaging may well expand the diagnostic imaging capabilities in the head and neck.

TABLE 1.4. **Summary of areas to be examined on laryngoscopy.**

Oropharynx	Base of tongue, both valleculae, lingual surface of the epiglottis
Hypopharynx	Piriform sinus
Boundaries between the hypopharynx and the larynx	Glossoepiglottic and aryepiglottic folds
Larynx	Epiglottis, arytenoid cartilage, vestibular folds, vocal cords and ventricle
Subglottis	

SOURCE: Becker W, Naumann HH, Pflatz CR: *Ear, Nose, and Throat Diseases,* p. 395. Thieme, New York, 1989.

Special techniques include:

- *Stroboscopy*
- *High-frequency movies,* allowing scientific analysis of the laryngeal function, especially that of the vocal cords.
- *Electromyography*

Clinical Aspects

Congenital Anomalies

Congenital laryngeal anomalies appear clinically with three cardinal symptoms: *dyspnea, dysphonia, and dysphagia* (Table 1.5).

Laryngomalacia

Symptoms. Inspiratory stridor begins immediately or within the first few weeks postpartum, accompanied in severe cases by cyanosis. The symptoms worsen during feeding.

Pathogenesis. The cause lies in abnormal calcium metabolism, causing unusual weakness of the supraglottic laryngeal skeleton, particularly the epiglottis.

Diagnosis. This rests on direct laryngoscopy and bronchoscopy. The epiglottis is usually omega-shaped and soft, and folds over the laryngeal inlet on inspiration. The arytenoid eminences or aryepiglottic folds may be drawn in on inspiration. (Color Plate 7) The form and function of the vocal cords is normal.

Treatment. Treatment consists of careful observation of the child and reassurance of the parents. The cartilage becomes stiffer within the course of weeks or months, so that the symptoms slowly disappear. Feedings should be divided into fractions, with a pause after every two or three swallows. If necessary, tube feeding should be used. Tracheotomy is only exceptionally required, and severe temporary dyspnea may be managed by intubation.

Neurogenic Disorders

Symptoms. If unilateral, there is squealing and a weak cry. Bilateral lesions cause inspiratory stridor.

TABLE 1.5. Frequency of congenital laryngeal anomalies.

Laryngomalacia	About 75%
Neurological disorders	About 10%
	unilateral or bilateral recurrent nerve paralysis
Seldom	
Atresia and membranes	
Cysts and laryngoceles	
Subglottic stenoses	
Hemangioma	
Very rare	
Clefts	

SOURCE: Becker W, Naumann HH, Pflatz CR: *Ear, Nose, and Throat Diseases,* p. 398. Thieme, New York, 1989.

Pathogenesis. Some cases are idiopathic and some are due to congenital or cardiovascular anomalies or stretching of nerves during birth.

Diagnosis. This is made by direct laryngoscopy, which shows one or both vocal cords to be in the paramedian position. An intermediate position of the cords is considerably rarer.

Treatment. Unilateral lesions do not require treatment. A large proportion of recurrent paralyses recover spontaneously. Bilateral lesions initially require intubation and a later tracheotomy for persistent obstruction.

Atresias and Webs

Symptoms. cause powerful, useless attempts at respiration, cyanosis, and inability to cry immediately after birth, which leads rapidly to death. Webs cause respiratory obstruction of variable degrees.

Diagnosis. This is made by direct laryngoscopy, which shows an atresia or a (subtotal) web of the glottis.

Treatment. Asphyxia in severe cases of dyspnea is only prevented by endoscopic division of the web or tracheotomy in the immediate postpartum period. It may be repeated if necessary. It is said that endolaryngeal laser surgery provides better results.

Laryngoceles

Internal laryngoceles lie within the larynx in the vestibular fold (Color Plate 8).

External laryngoceles are a prolongation of the ventricle through the thyrohyoid membrane to form a palpable cystic mass in the neck.

Combinations of both forms and bilateral laryngoceles are rare.

Symptoms. Dyspnea and dysphonia are present.

Pathogenesis. This is a congenital or acquired expansion of the laryngeal saccule (i.e., a blind sac of the ventricle, filled with air or mucus).

Diagnosis. This is made by laryngoscopy, palpation, and tomography. The smooth swelling increases in size on puffing, straining, and on playing wind instruments.

Treatment. If severe dyspnea is not present, treatment is expectant. Later the sac may be exposed and removed via an external incision. Small internal laryngoceles may be removed endoscopically.

Subglottic Stenoses

Symptoms. Inspiratory and expiratory stridor are present but there is usually no abnormality of the voice. Recurrent pseudocroup may also occur.

Pathogenesis. The cause is usually an anomaly of the cricoid cartilage.

Diagnosis. This is made by direct laryngoscopy.

Treatment. Tracheotomy may be necessary in severe respiratory obstruction. The child is then observed until surgery becomes possible.

Hemangioma

Symptoms. These depend on the site; these tumors may cause hoarseness or respiratory obstruction. Spontaneous bleeding with aspiration of blood can lead to an acutely dangerous condition.

Diagnosis. Direct laryngoscopy provides the diagnosis.

Treatment. Occasionally, because of increase in respiratory obstruction or spontaneous bleeding, it may not be possible to wait for spontaneous regression of the hemangioma. In these cases, tracheotomy may be needed before surgery, which may include cryosurgery or laser surgery.

Functional Disorders

These are based on nervous, myogenic, articulation, or functional causes (e.g., laryngospasm). They are characterized by voice disorders such as dysphonia, aphonia, or dyspnea (see Table 1.6).

Dysphonia. Atypical vibrations of the vocal cords or abnormally increased or decreased passage of air through the glottis causes increased hoarseness rather than a clear tone. It is analyzed by endoscopy, stroboscopy, high-speed cinematography, and phoniatry.

Dyspnea. Audible stridor (shortness of breath, at times accompanied by cyanosis) occurs when the diameter of the respiratory tract is reduced by at least one-third. The anoxia can increase dramatically during physical exercise.

> **Note:** A 1-mm mucosal swelling in an infant narrows the lumen by more than 50%. Edema must be 3 mm thick in the adult to produce the same effect.

Neurogenic functional disorders in the cortical and subcortical areas mainly cause bilateral abnormalities of vocal cord movement. Bilateral, but more often unilateral, disorders of vocal cord function, usually combined with lesions of the vagus, glossopharyngeal, and hypoglossal nerves, are localized to the medulla oblongata. A combination of paralyses in older people occurring suddenly indicates cerebral ischemia or bleeding in the area of the brain stem. Ninety percent of *isolated defects* of the vagus nerve or its branches occur in the region between the nucleus ambiguous and the inferior ganglion centrally and the laryngeal musculature. Peripheral nerve lesions are to be expected in damage to the vagus nerve inferior to the inferior ganglion (Fig. 1.21).

The vocal cords take up different positions during function or in paralyses relative to the imaginary reference line of the sagittal glottic axis (Fig. 1.22).

Functional Positions

The median position is adopted in phonation (Color Plate 1). The lateral position of extreme abduction occurs on inspiration (Color Plate 2).

Vocal Cord Positions in the Most Common Pareses (see Fig. 1.22)

- Paramedian is seen in recurrent nerve paralysis, posticus paralysis.
- Intermediate is seen in complete paralysis of the superior and inferior laryngeal nerve, which thus paralyzes all internal and external laryngeal muscles.
- The cadaveric position is an incorrect term because it has no relationship to the vocal cord position in the corpse. It is rather an intermediate position similar to the position of the vocal cords in flaccid paralysis or in the end stage of a vocal cord paralysis, with bowing of the vocal cords due to disuse atrophy of the vocalis muscle and with the arytenoid cartilage tilted anteriorly.

Other anomalies of position combined with hyper- or hypokinetic dysphonia include

- *Internus weakness.* The glottic chink is elliptical on phonation due to absent tension of the vocalis muscle as a result of atrophy (e.g., in senile dysphonia).
- *Transversus weakness.* A triangular gap remains posteriorly on phonation.
- *Combinations of both forms of inadequate closure* may occur (Fig. 1.23a–c).

TABLE 1.6. Unilateral or bilateral recurrent nerve paralysis.

Causes	Details
Thyroidectomy	Most frequent cause of a laryngeal muscle paralysis
Malignant goiter	
Bronchial carcinoma	Particularly common in tumors arising from the upper and middle lobes and with involvement of the mediastinal lymph node metastases
Esophageal carcinoma	Particularly of the upper third
Mediastinal diseases	Lymphogranulomas, non-Hodgkin's lymphoma, metastases, mediastinitis
Aneurysms of the aorta or the subclavian artery	Congenital or syphilitic
Ductus operations	
Operations on the hypopharynx or the esophagus	Failure to display the course of the nerve during resection of the hypopharyngeal diverticulum
Cardiomegaly of various causes	May also occur in Ortner's syndrome
Pulmonary tuberculosis	
Pleural plaques	
Blunt or sharp cervical trauma	
Infective-toxic	Influenza; herpes zoster; rheumatism; syphilis; tissue toxins such as lead, arsenic, or organic solvents; streptomycin; quinine
Intubation anesthesia	Stretching of the recurrent nerve by incorrect position of the patient or pressure of the tube
Neurologic diseases	Wallenberg's syndrome, poliomyelitis, bulbar paralysis, multiple sclerosis, cerebral tumors
Idiopathic	It should be noted that a diagnosis of idiopathic recurrent nerve paralysis should only be made after all other causes have been excluded. In the great majority of these patients spontaneous recovery occurs within 2 to 3 months. After a longer period the chances of recovery become less.

SOURCE: Becker W, Naumann HH, Pflatz CR: *Ear, Nose, and Throat Diseases*, p. 401. Thieme, New York, 1989.

It is not always possible to predict the final position of the vocal cords after damage to the superior and recurrent laryngeal nerves because of partial recovery of residual function. Furthermore, atypical positions may be adopted because of fibrosis of the muscle or ankylosis of the arytenoid joint.

Recurrent Laryngeal Nerve Palsies (Unilateral or Bilateral)

All the internal laryngeal musculature is *paralyzed* on the affected side. Since the external cricothyroid muscle supplied by the external branch of the superior laryngeal nerve still puts the paralyzed vocal cord under tension, the *paramedian position* is adopted. In incomplete paralysis of the adductors, the single abductor of the vocal cords (the *posterior* cricoarytenoid muscle) is functionally predominant. This unilateral or bilateral form of paralysis is thus termed a *posticus paraly-*

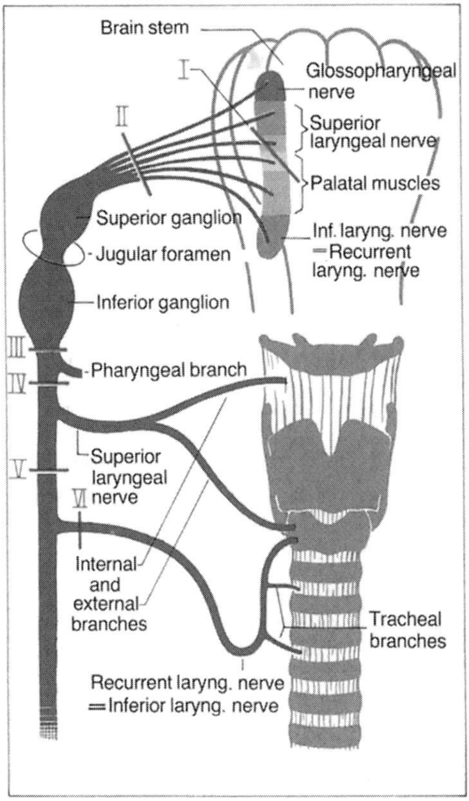

FIGURE 1.21. Vagus nerve and its branches with sites of possible lesions (I to VI) and effects on the larynx (modified from Burian et al.).

I. A lesion in the nucleus ambiguous produces paralysis in the intermediate or paramedian position.

II. Division of the roots of the vagus nerve causing several different types of paralysis: paramedian position, intermediate position, and simultaneous paralysis of the soft palate.

III. Loss of continuity in the jugular foramen or inferior ganglion causes paralysis of the superior laryngeal nerve and of the recurrent laryngeal nerve. The vocal cord is in the intermediate position, and the soft palate is paralyzed. Lesions in and around the jugular foramen may be accompanied by paralysis of the glossopharyngeal, accessory, and hypoglossal nerves.

IV. A lesion between the pharyngeal branches and the superior laryngeal nerve. The vocal cord is in the intermediate position and there is also loss of sensation.

V. Interruption of the vagus nerve at the superior laryngeal nerve caused a loss of tone of the cricothyroid muscle and loss of tension of the vocal cord.

VI. Division of the recurrent nerve causes a vocal cord paralysis in the paramedian position.

SOURCE: Becker W, Naumann HH, Pflatz CR: *Ear, Nose, and Throat Diseases*, p. 402. Thieme, New York, 1989.

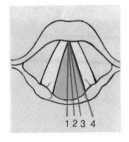

FIGURE 1.22. Positions of the vocal cord.
1, Median or phonatory position; **2,** paramedian position; **3,** intermediate position; **4,** lateral or respiratory position.
SOURCE: Becker W, Naumann HH, Pflatz CR: *Ear, Nose, and Throat Diseases,* p. 402. Thieme, New York, 1989.

nant. This unilateral or bilateral form of paralysis is thus termed a *posticus paralysis.* The stroboscope is very useful in long-term follow-up of vocal cord paralyses.

Unilateral Recurrent Nerve Paralysis

Symptoms. These include dysphonia in the acute phase, with later improvement in the voice. There is no appreciable respiratory obstruction except perhaps during severe physical activity. The patient can no longer sing.

Diagnosis. Laryngoscopy shows the vocal cord to be immobile in the paramedian position on one side. Thorough laryngological, neurological, and radiographic investigation is indicated, whose objective is shown in Table 1.6.

Treatment. If the causal disease cannot be treated satisfactorily, the patient is given speech therapy (electrotherapy) to achieve compensatory vocal cord closure by the action of the still-functioning vocal cord.

Bilateral Recurrent Paralysis

Symptoms. (1) Dyspnea occurs with the possibility of asphyxia due to narrowing of the glottic chink. Inspiratory stridor is particularly loud during sleep or physical activity. (2) Initially, there is *dysphonia* that lasts for a variable period, depending on the cause, and thereafter a weak, but only slightly hoarse voice. (3) Feeble cough is also symptomatic.

Pathogenesis. See Table 1.6.

Diagnosis. This is based on laryngoscopic findings. In bilateral paralysis, the vocal cords are in the paramedian position.

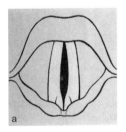
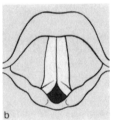
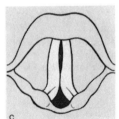

FIGURE 1.23. Myogenic abnormalities of position of the vocal cords.
(a) weakness of the internus muscle, **(b)** weakness of the transversus muscle, **(c)** combined type.
SOURCE: Becker W, Naumann HH, Pflatz CR: *Ear, Nose, and Throat Diseases,* p. 403. Thieme, New York, 1989.

Treatment

1. Relief of the airway takes first priority. Immediate tracheotomy is often necessary. The patient can later be provided with a *speaking valve* (tracheotomy inner tube).

2. If spontaneous remission does not occur, an operation to widen the glottis is indicated, at the earliest 10–12 months later, if the patient wishes to be rid of his speaking valve.

Principles of surgery. An arytenoidectomy is carried out, and one of the paralyzed vocal cords is moved laterally or superolaterally. The operation is done endoscopically with a CO_2 laser (Fig. 1.24a–c).
Speech therapy is used to supplement the operation.

> **Note:** The wider the glottic opening after the operation, the more unsatisfactory is the voice.

Unilateral or Bilateral Paralysis of the Superior Laryngeal Nerve

Symptoms. These include aspiration of food and drink, loss of power of the voice, and inability to sing in the higher part of the range, particularly in a bilateral paralysis. Breathing is scarcely affected.

Pathogenesis. The paralysis affects the function of the cricothyroid muscle as well as the sensory nerve supply to the supraglottic part of the larynx. The paralysis is due to mechanical lesions of the nerve, particularly after thyroid gland operations, tumors, and viral infections.

Diagnosis. Laryngoscopy shows that the tension of the vocal cords is reduced so that the glottis does not close completely on phonation. In unilateral paralysis, the ipsilateral vocal cord is often shortened and lies lower than the nonparalyzed side.

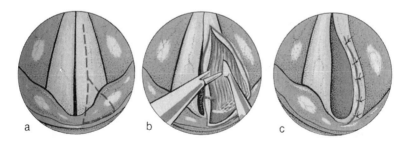

a   b   c

FIGURE 1.24. Endoscopic operations, to widen the glottis.
a. Arytenoidectomy and laterofixation of the vocal cord. The incision is shown by a dotted line. **b.** The arytenoid cartilage is removed and the vocalis muscle is grasped with a forceps. It is then dissected free with a round knife from the muscles. **c.** The vocal cord is then displaced laterally and sutured.

Source: Becker W, Naumann HH, Pflatz CR: *Ear, Nose, and Throat Diseases,* p. 405. Thieme, New York, 1989.

Treatment. Corticosteroids should be tried and speech therapy prescribed.

Combined Lesions of the Laryngeal Nerve

Included are lesions of the superior laryngeal and recurrent laryngeal nerves (see Fig. 1.21).

Symptoms. Unilateral paralysis includes dysphonia and breathy voice due to air loss. The healthy vocal cord compensates later. Aspiration occurs because of absence of the sensory protection. In *bilateral paralysis,* there is dysphonia or aphonia, and almost always good respiration at rest. There is also aspiration and a marked feeling of shortage of breath during bodily exertion.

Pathogenesis. The basic cause is central or peripheral damage to the vagus nerve, causing a flaccid paralysis with immobility of the affected vocal cord in the intermediate position. There is bilateral flaccid paralysis with bilateral lesions (see Fig. 1.21).

Diagnosis. Laryngoscopy shows one or both of the vocal cords to be bowed and paralyzed in the intermediate position.

Treatment. It is seldom possible to treat the cause of this paralysis, and the mainstay of treatment is speech therapy.

> **Note:** If speech therapy for a unilateral atrophic vocal cord paralysis does not succeed in producing compensation by movement of the healthy vocal cord across the midline, the volume of the affected side of the larynx may be supplemented to produce a satisfactory voice by injection of the affected vocal cord with Teflon paste or by subperichondrial implantation of autologous cartilage.

Neuralgia of the Superior Laryngeal Nerve

This is one of the localized or mononeural pain syndromes of the head and neck, such as trigeminal neuralgia or occipital neuralgia.

Symptoms. These include episodic, stabbing pain usually on one side, localized to the upper part of the thyroid cartilage, the angle of the jaw, or the lower part of the ear. Pain or pressure is experienced at the level of the greater cornu of the hyoid or in the region of the thyrohyoid membrane.

Pathogenesis. The cause is unknown. The disease occurs between the 40th and 60th years of life. The trigger zone lies in the piriform sinus and is set off by swallowing, speaking, and coughing.

Treatment. Repeated anesthetic block of the superior laryngeal nerve should be tried. The site of injunction lies between the greater cornu of the thyroid and the superior cornu of the thyroid cartilage (Fig. 1.25). Medical treatment with carbamazepine (Tegretol) may also be tried.

Traumatology

The function of the larynx may be affected by vocal abuse, intubation injury, external trauma, chemical toxins, and foreign bodies.

The symptoms are dictated by the abnormal laryngeal function and include voice disorders, respiratory obstruction, coughing, and surgical emphysema of the neck.

The appropriate endoscopic and radiological procedures must be used to diagnose and localize the lesion.

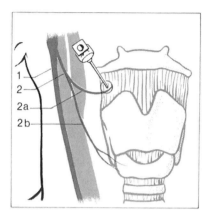

FIGURE 1.25. Infiltration anesthesia of the superior laryngeal nerve.
1, Vagus nerve; **2,** superior laryngeal nerve. **(2a)** Internal branch; **(2b)** external branch.
SOURCE: Becker W, Naumann HH, Pflatz CR: *Ear, Nose, and Throat Diseases,* p. 406. Thieme, New York, 1989.

Vocal Abuse

Acute

Symptoms. These include dysphonia, or even aphonia, and pain on speaking.

Pathogenesis. This is caused by extreme overuse of the voice in sporting spectators, politicians, market traders, and disco habitues.

Diagnosis. Indirect or direct laryngoscopy that shows hyperemia or swelling of the vocal cords and subepithelial bleeding.

Treatment. Strict voice rest and inhalations are required. If polyps form, they are removed by microlaryngoscopy.

Chronic

Symptoms. The voice is hoarse and croaking, or disappears under stress. Singing is difficult or impossible.

Pathogenesis. Screamer's or singer's nodules develop because of chronic overuse or misuse of the voice.

Screamer's nodules occur in children and are frequent in mothers of large families and in teachers who must talk a lot.

Singer's nodes are due to unsatisfactory singing technique.

Diagnosis. Direct or indirect laryngoscopy shows the nodules on the typical site at the junction between the anterior and middle third of the vocal cords, which is the point of maximal amplitude of the vibrations of the vocal cords. They are usually bilateral (Color Plate 3).

Treatment. Once the nodules progress beyond a certain size, they become fibrotic, and voice rest and speech therapy are no longer successful. Most patients then require endolaryngeal microsurgery with postoperative speech therapy.

Contact Ulcer

Symptoms. These include dysphonia and pain in the larynx on speaking.

Pathogenesis. The history almost always shows misuse of the voice (e.g., in stock exchange workers, and market and fairground workers). These patients are also often smokers. Vocal abuse causes the arytenoid cartilages to impinge sharply against each other.

Diagnosis. Indirect or direct laryngoscopy typically shows a hollow depression, with a pronounced border over the vocal process on one side and a reactive pachydermia on the other side (Color Plate 5).

Differential diagnosis. This includes ulceration or granulation due to intubation, tumors, and tuberculosis.

Treatment. The patients are usually hyperactive and do not persist with voice rest or speech therapy. The edges of the defect and the contralateral thickening are removed by microsurgery, but there is a marked tendency to recurrence.

Intubation Injury

Acute

Symptoms. Immediately or shortly after removal of the tube, patients complain of dysphonia, attacks of coughing, and hemoptysis. They also have pain in the larynx and neck.

Pathogenesis. Injury is caused by repeated or incorrect intubation, intermittent positive-pressure respiration, a protruding guide wire, a wrong-sized tube, insufficient relaxation, overextension, and pressure of the tube cuff. These factors lead to a myogenic or neurological paralysis. Drying of the mucosa due to the premedication facilitates mucosal injury. Laryngeal complications may be expected in adults after less than 48 hours of intubation, whereas in young children, the average time interval for the onset of mucosal injuries is between 3 and 7 days.

Diagnosis. Laryngoscopy shows a subepithelial hematoma, superficial and deep mucosal injuries, and rarely a tear of the vocal cord or subluxation of the arytenoid cartilage. An intubation granuloma is usually bilateral and lies on the vocal process (Color Plate 4).

Treatment. A hematoma or a superficial mucosal lesion can heal spontaneously within a few days. Pressure paralysis of the recurrent laryngeal nerve is also capable of spontaneous resolution, but tears of the vocal cord or subluxation of the arytenoid cartilage require surgery.

Chronic

Symptoms. Dysphonia or laryngeal dyspnea develop 2–8 weeks after intubation anesthesia or prolonged intubation.

Pathogenesis. Incorrect intubation, a tube that is too large or too rigid, incorrect (endolaryngeal or subglottic) position of the cuff, or prolonged intubation can all cause damage. The general condition of the patient, including factors such as shock, retching, and vomiting, are additional factors.

> **Note:** The early lesions, including endolaryngeal or subglottic hyperemia and edema, ischemic mucosal defects with fibrinous membrane, necrosis, and ulceration lead to late injuries. The latter include ulceration, granulation, perichondritis, cartilaginous necrosis, synechiae, and strictures.

Diagnosis. This is made by laryngoscopy, tomography, and pulmonary function studies.

Treatment. Granulomas are removed by endolaryngeal microsurgery or laser. Postoperative speech therapy is indicated, but there is a tendency for recurrence (see below).

Laryngotracheal Stenoses and Synechiae

These often require several operations over a long period. The operations include excision or splitting of the scar tissue, and, if necessary, of the cricoid cartilage, with mucosal or cartilaginous grafts. A stent must be worn in the reconstructed larynx for several weeks until the patency of the lumen is assured (Fig. 1.26a and 1.26b).

External Trauma

Blunt and penetrating injuries, and open and closed injuries, occur and must be diagnosed.

Symptoms. These include immediate or increasing dyspnea, even complete respiratory obstruction due to hematoma, edema, and dislocation of cartilage fragments, bleeding, and dysphonia. Dysphagia and pain occur when the esophagus is affected.

Pathogenesis. These injuries are particularly common in traffic accidents, especially due to impact with the steering wheel and dashboard (Fig. 1.26a–c). Other causes include athletic injuries, karate blows, fighting, and attempted strangulation. In addition to the direct trauma resulting in subluxation and disruption of the laryngeal framework, the blow may force the larynx against the vertebral column, causing endolaryngeal mucosal tears and vertical, horizontal, or combined fractures. Subluxation of the larynx from the trachea can occur. Perforations or contusions in the neighboring hypopharynx and upper esophagus lead to tracheoesophageal or laryngoesophageal fistulas. The neighboring nerves and vessels may also be injured (Fig. 1.27 and Color Plate 9).

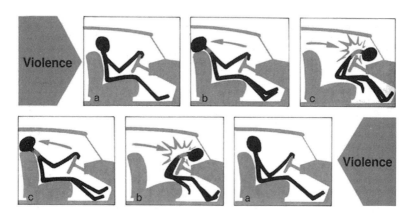

FIGURE 1.26. Laryngeal trauma due to a traffic accident with frontal collision.
SOURCE: Becker W, Naumann HH, Pflatz CR: *Ear, Nose, and Throat Diseases,* p. 410. Thieme, New York, 1989.

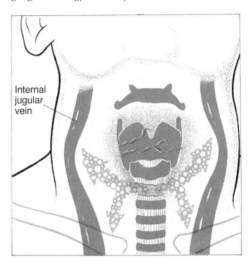

FIGURE 1.27. **Laryngeal trauma showing transverse laryngeal fracture and tear of the trachea, escape of air into the surrounding tissues, and congestion due to compression of the large cervical veins caused by hematoma, edema, and surgical emphysema.**
SOURCE: Becker W, Naumann HH, Pflatz CR: *Ear, Nose, and Throat Diseases*, p. 410. Thieme, New York, 1989.

TABLE 1.7. **Type and treatment of laryngeal trauma.**

Type of Injury	Treatment
BASIC PRINCIPLE IS TO SECURE A FREE AIRWAY	
Hematoma and edema. Small tears of the mucosa.	Voice rest, inhalation, steroids, tracheotomy if necessary
Extensive soft tissue injuries of the neck, exposed cartilage with otherwise intact or easily reconstructable laryngeal skeleton	Open exploration and reconstruction. A silicone keel should always be used in the anterior commissure to prevent scars.
Loss of thyroid cartilage and mucosa	Mucosal grafts and stenting of the inside of the larynx
Laryngeal fractures, vertical or horizontal	Suturing of the fragments with or without stenting
Laryngotracheal subluxation	End-to-end anastomosis of the stumps
Late stenosis	Open exploration, excision of scar, mucosal and cartilaginous grafts and stenting

SOURCE: Becker W, Naumann HH, Pflatz CR: *Ear, Nose, and Throat Diseases*, p. 411. Thieme, New York, 1989.

Diagnosis. Inspection, palpation, and laryngoscopy demonstrate fractures, crepitation, or displacement of laryngeal fragments and surgical emphysema of the neck. Tomography and pulmonary function tests should also be carried out.

Treatment. Preservation of the airway is the most important measure, if necessary by bronchoscopy, tracheotomy, or intubation (see Table 1.14). Emergency bronchoscopy may be used with bronchoscopes of the appropriate size. Distressing attacks of coughing are suppressed by codeine preparations. Some patients require admission to the intensive care unit (e.g., for treatment of shock, for infusions, or transfusions, etc.). Further procedures are shown in Table 1.7.

Inhalational Trauma by Chemical Toxins

Symptoms. Acute symptoms include severe attacks of coughing, a feeling or burning and asphyxia, and epiphora. *Chronic* symptoms include hoarseness, a feeling of dryness, clearing the throat, and coughing attacks.

Pathogenesis. The cause is escaping gases or steam after explosions of industrial chemicals and the effect of smoke in fires. The most common chronic toxin is inhalation of tobacco smoke.

Diagnosis. Laryngoscopy shows redness, mucosal maceration, and edema.

Treatment. Voice rest, giving up smoking, humidification of the air, corticosteroids for edema, inhalation therapy, and laryngoscopic follow-up are indicated.

Foreign Bodies

Symptoms. The initial symptoms are attacks of coughing, stabbing pains in the larynx, and dysphagia, which occur during eating. Dyspnea may occur especially because of the tendency of the infant's mucosa to produce edema. Large, especially vegetable foreign bodies, may cause asphyxia due to their swelling properties.

Pathogenesis. Laryngeal foreign bodies are rarer than tracheal or bronchial foreign bodies. Sharp-edged, pointed, or large foreign bodies may remain impacted within the larynx. The danger of foreign-body aspiration is particularly great in sudden fright, laughing, or absence of the sensory innervation of the larynx.

Diagnosis. This is made by indirect laryngoscopy. Laryngotracheobronchoscopy should also be carried out in all suspected cases. Edema may overlie an impacted foreign body. Only radiopaque, especially metallic, foreign bodies can be recognized easily by radiography.

Treatment. The foreign body is removed carefully using the rigid endoscope, taking care to preserve the mucosa. A tracheotomy may be necessary before the removal of large, impacted foreign bodies in the larynx with associated edema.

A laryngeal foreign body may occasionally be coughed out, but it is more often aspirated into the tracheobronchial tree.

Course. The mucosa tend to produce reactive edema, particularly in children. Steroids are then indicated and precautions taken for emergency tracheostomy should severe dyspnea develop.

Inflammation

Acute Laryngitis

Symptoms. These include hoarseness, aphonia, pain in the larynx, and coughing attacks. In children, there is a danger of airway obstruction. Acute laryngitis is usually due to ascending or descending infections from other parts of the airway.

Pathogenesis. The cause is viral or bacterial infection, although thermal, allergic, or inhaled chemical toxins may occasionally be responsible.

Diagnosis. Laryngoscopy shows the vocal cords to be red and swollen. Depending on the underlying disease, the neighboring pharyngeal or tracheal mucosa may also be inflamed.

Treatment. Since viral infections are often followed by secondary bacterial infection, antibiotics are indicated. Steroids are also indicated for marked edema. General measures include fluids by mouth, aspirin, and stem inhalation.

> **Note:** Oil-containing inhalations should not be used. Only aerosols of a particle size of 30 (+20) mm precipitate in the larynx.

Voice rest is indicated, and smoking should be forbidden. Chemicals such as certain dyestuffs or artificial products and allergic toxins such as hair sprays, shellfish, and crustaceans should be eliminated.

> **Note:** If the symptoms do not improve considerably or resolve within 3 weeks, telescopic or microlaryngoscopy is indicated to exclude other laryngeal diseases. Ulceration, proliferation, and exudate are not typical of uncomplicated nonspecific laryngitis, and specific diseases, premalignant lesions, and tumors must be excluded.

Croup Syndrome

Diphtheritic croup, beginning with laryngeal membranes and obstruction, is presently rare. However, occasionally endemic foci still persist in Western Europe.

Diphtheritic laryngitis, with greyish-white membranes occurring in isolation, is becoming less and less common. It is more commonly combined with lesions of the oropharynx. Tracheotomy is required for increasing dyspnea.

The term *pseudocroup* includes a group of acute laryngotracheal diseases mainly affecting children.

Acute Subglottic Laryngitis

Symptoms. There is a previous common cold followed by dry, barking cough, rapidly becoming worse, hoarseness and inspiratory, expiratory, or mixed stridor, leading to severe respiratory obstruction depending on swelling of the mucosa and site. There is indrawing of the suprasternal notch and intercostal spaces on inspiration, cyanosis, perioral pallor, and worsening of the symptoms due to a fear of asphyxia in children.

Pathogenesis. This is a very serious acute disease of early infancy, most common between the first and fifth years of life. In a short time, life-threatening narrowing of the relatively narrow child's airway due to inflammatory mucosal swelling of the conus elasticus in the subglottic space or, in a descending infection, of the tracheobronchial tree, can develop. The disease is basically due to a viral infection with accompanying secondary bacterial infection. Cool, damp, and foggy autumn and winter weather appears to increase the morbidity. *However, recurrent infections in the nasopharynx and nasal obstruction due to chronically in-*

flamed hypertrophied adenoids and tonsils are important in the etiology. Whether air pollution plays an important role in the pathogenesis of this disease remains uncertain.

Diagnosis. The clinical picture is usually very typical. Laryngoscopy shows glottic mucosal edema or crust formation.

Treatment. Mild cases, assessed on the degree of respiratory obstruction, may be managed by the family practitioner or pediatrician. Reliable observation must be provided to ensure that the effect of treatment is monitored (Table 1.8).

If these measures fail and there is increasing dyspnea, the child must be admitted to the hospital as an emergency, there to be treated with oxygen therapy and endotracheal intubation, and depending on the degree of dyspnea and the results of blood gas analysis. Tracheostomy is carried out for severe obstruction and when there is a progressive sicca-type crust formation.

Acute Epiglottitis

Symptoms. These include severe pain on swallowing, so that food is refused, which may lead to dehydration and the possibility of circulatory collapse. Inspiratory stridor usually forces the patient to sit upright in bed. The speech is thick, and the temperature is elevated.

Pathogenesis. The disease is sometimes caused by mucosal damage by swallowing sharp-edged food, allowing entry of pathogenic organisms. The disease mainly affects children up to the 10th year of life, and adults and older children are only rarely affected.

Diagnosis. The diagnosis is *epiglottis acutissima* if the course is particularly fulminant. Laryngoscopy or examination with a tongue depressor shows a thick, swollen, red epiglottis rim (Color Plate 10). A lateral radiograph shows the cherry-shaped epiglottic swelling.

Differential diagnosis. Pseudocroup may also be caused by congenital anomalies, impacted foreign bodies, angioneurotic edema of the larynx, hypocalcemic laryngospasm, tumors, and infected epiglottic cysts.

Treatment. The child is admitted to hospital and treated with intravenous steroids and broad-spectrum antibiotics in high doses, also intravenously. The airway is ensured by nasotracheal intubation for life-threatening dyspnea. Tracheostomy is now rarely required because of the usually short course of the illness.

TABLE 1.8. **Treatment of acute subglottic laryngitis.**

BASIC PRINCIPLE: RELIEF OF BOTH OBSTRUCTION AND DISTRESSING COUGH
WHICH IMPEDES CIRCULATION

Sedation of child (avoid respiratory depressive drugs)
Steroids
Antibiotics to prevent secondary infection
Administration of fluids
Croup tent

SOURCE: Becker W, Naumann HH, Pflatz CR: *Ear, Nose, and Throat Diseases,* p. 414. Thieme, New York, 1989.

> **Note:** In patients with respiratory obstruction, particularly children, diagnostic procedures may lead to complete obstruction. Preparations for intubation or tracheotomy must therefore be made *before* the investigation. The patient should be referred to a hospital if the diagnosis of epiglottitis is suspected.

Prognosis and course. The disease usually improves rapidly within a few days. Possible complications include epiglottic abscess and perichondritis.

Chronic Laryngitis

Chronic, nonspecific laryngitis must be distinguished from the group of specific forms such as tuberculosis, amyloid, and so on. Chronic, nonspecific laryngitis requires assessment and treatment by the otolaryngologist.

Chronic Nonspecific Laryngitis

Symptoms. These persist for weeks or months, in contrast to those of acute laryngitis. They include hoarseness, deepening of the voice, and sometimes a dry cough. The voice is less able to withstand stress, there is a globus sensation in the larynx, a feeling of a need to clear the throat, but little or no pain.

Pathogenesis. This disease is mainly due to exogenous toxins such as cigarette smoke, occupational air pollution, and climatic influences. Another cause is vocal abuse in bartenders, construction workers, long-distance truck drivers, and professional speakers. Nasal obstruction is also an important factor in pathogenesis.

> **Note:** Laryngopathia gravidarum, due to vocal cord edema with dysphonia and deepening of the voice, is sometimes observed in the second half of pregnancy. The hoarseness almost always resolves spontaneously after delivery.

The administration of male sex hormones and anabolic steroids causes voice change in women, including deepening of the tone, disorders of the singing voice, and reduction of the carrying power of the speaking voice. These disorders persist because of the virilization of the laryngeal structures.

Diagnosis. Laryngoscopy shows the vocal cords to be thick and red, with rough edges (Color Plate 11). There is tenacious mucus, and the rest of the laryngeal mucosa often shows similar appearance.

Treatment. The duration of treatment is protracted. Elimination of exogenous toxins such as tobacco is the mainstay of treatment. Voice rest is prescribed and, if necessary, a deviated nasal septum is corrected to restore normal nasal respiration. Antibiotics are given for accompanying inflammation, and a short course of steroids, saline inhalations, and mucolytic agents are given.

> **Note:** Regular laryngoscopic checkups are advisable in chronic laryngitis because of the possibility of dysplasia. Microlaryngoscopy and biopsy should be performed in every doubtful case. This is the only method of early detection of malignancy.

Specific Forms of Chronic Laryngitis

Laryngeal Tuberculosis

Symptoms. These include hoarseness and cough persisting for several months and pain on swallowing, radiating to the ear.

Pathogenesis. Tuberculous laryngitis is almost always secondary to active pulmonary tuberculosis. The infection is transmitted to the larynx by bacillae contained in the sputum. The posterior part of the larynx, the interarytenoid area, and the epiglottis are those most commonly affected. There is a danger of perichondritis. Monocorditis may also be caused by a miliary tuberculous deposit.

Diagnosis. Microlaryngoscopy in fresh cases initially shows reddish-brown submucous nodules that are partly confluent. Later ulcerations or granulations develop. *Monocorditis* is characterized by redness and thickening, occasionally with small ulcerations of *one* vocal cord. Other investigations include histology, culture, radiography, and examination by an internist.

Differential diagnosis. This includes vasomotor monocorditis, nonspecific chronic laryngitis, and carcinoma.

Treatment. Antituberculous treatment is given in cooperation with a chest physician. Pain is treated by blocking the superior laryngeal nerve (Fig. 1.25). The patient must be isolated, and contacts are investigated. *The disease is reportable.*

Course and prognosis. Laryngeal tuberculosis is infectious. Mucosal lesions often heal with no permanent effects on laryngeal function, but if the tuberculosis has affected the laryngeal cartilaginous framework, defects arise during healing. The prognosis currently is good.

Laryngeal Sarcoid

Laryngeal sarcoid as an extrapulmonary manifestation is nowadays rare. Dysphonia and a globus sensation are caused by sarcoid deposits in the larynx.

Biopsy, if necessary combined with prescalene lymph-node biopsy, is necessary to establish the diagnosis.

In contrast to tuberculosis, the epithelioid cell nodules do not caseate or ulcerate. Radiography is a supplementary investigation. The disease is treated by an internist.

Laryngeal Syphilis

Isolated laryngeal syphilis is unusual, and it is much more often a manifestation of oropharyngeal syphilis in the secondary, generalized stage of the disease.

Mucous placques or hazy, smoke-colored mucosal lesions occur in the larynx, similar to those of syphilitic pharyngitis. The patient is also hoarse. *The disease is reportable.*

Respiratory obstruction only occurs in the presence of marked mucosal swelling. The cartilage is destroyed in a gumma in stage III. The differential diagnosis from carcinoma is difficult to make.

Scleroma of the Larynx

Pale-red swellings and granulations with crusts develop mainly in the subglottic space. Subglottic, laryngeal, and intratracheal stenoses occur in Stage III, causing hoarseness, cough, and increasing stridor.

Diagnosis. This is established by microlaryngoscopy, histopathology, and culture.

Treatment. Tracheotomy followed by appropriate operative treatment of laryngotracheal stenosis is necessary for respiratory stridor.

Pemphigus Vulgaris and Pemphigoid Vesicles

Both affect the epiglottis preferentially and are often incidental findings. The vesicles are usually painless, but may occasionally cause a globus sensation and can lead to stenosis.

Generalized Rheumatoid Arthritis

The *cricoarytenoid joint* is often affected, causing hoarseness, stridor, and pain on swallowing radiating to the ear.

Laryngeal Amyloid

Tumorous, polypoid lesions covered by smooth mucosa and pale-waxy in appearance may develop in the larynx in this dysproteinemia. The sites of predilection are the vocal cords and the subglottic space. Surgical removal is required for severe hoarseness and respiratory obstruction.

Laryngeal Perichondritis

Symptoms. These include pain in the larynx, increasing on swallowing or external pressure, hoarseness, and dyspnea.

Pathogenesis. Surgical and accidental trauma, infiltration of the cartilage by tumor, and infection (e.g., tuberculosis, and irradiation) can all be causes. Provided that the cartilage is not invaded by tumor, it usually tolerates radiation up to 6000 rads. The usual clinical problem is chondroradioneurosis with inflammation of the overlying mucosa.

Diagnosis and findings. The laryngoscopic picture of radiogenic pallid mucosal edema, particularly on the epiglottis and the arytenoid cartilages is, together with the history, very typical. There are intra- and extralaryngeal swelling, fistulae, and sequestration of necrotic bits of cartilage.

Treatment. Sequestrated or exposed cartilage must be removed. Broad-spectrum antibiotics are given in high doses combined with steroids.

Note: Radiation edema is very difficult to treat and often disguises persistent or recurrent tumor.

Benign Tumors

Vocal Cord Polyps

Symptoms. These include hoarseness, aphonia, and attacks of coughing. Dyspnea occurs with large polyps. If the polyp has a pedicle and is floating between the cords, the voice may return to normal for short intervals.

Pathogenesis. This is the most common benign tumor of the vocal cords, mainly affecting men between 30 and 50 years of age. It is often initiated by agents causing laryngeal inflammation. Hyperkinetic voice disorders and vocal abuse are important.

Diagnosis. Laryngoscopy (Color Plate 12) shows the polyp usually lying on the free edge of the vocal cord, either on a pedicle or sessile. It is seroedematous and occasionally hemorrhagic. Older polyps appear firm due to fibrosis and thickening of the overlying epithelium.

Treatment. The polyp is removed by endolaryngeal microsurgery, with preservation of the vocal ligament and vocalis muscle. Patients are advised to rest the voice until the defect epithelializes.

If endotracheal anesthesia is contraindicated, the polyp may be removed by direct or indirect laryngoscopy after premedication to inhibit reflexes and topical anesthesia.

Note: The polyp should always be examined histologically to establish the diagnosis.

Reinke's Edema

Symptoms. These include hoarseness and deepening of the voice, or diplophonia. Stridor may occur, particularly on exertion, if the edema is marked.

Pathogenesis. The edema is almost always bilateral and broad-based. It develops in Reinke's space. The edema usually affects professional speakers who speak a great deal and smokers.

Diagnosis. Laryngoscopy shows a bilateral, broad-based edematous mass on the vocal cords (Color Plate 6).

Treatment. The mucosa is removed by decortication or stripping with microsurgery, preserving the vocalis muscle (Fig. 1.28). If the anterior commissure is involved, the cords must be stripped in two separate sittings to prevent adhesions anteriorly (CO_2-Laser).

Papillomas

Symptoms. Depending on the site and extent of the lesions, these include hoarseness that is often severe and respiratory obstruction.

Pathogenesis. This disease has etiological and morphological similarities to the common wart that occurs on the skin. A viral cause has been suggested. Some juvenile papillomas resolve spontaneously about the time of puberty due to hormonal influences. Many adult patients have suffered papillomas since early childhood.

Diagnosis. This is made by direct laryngoscopy and histological examination. Papillomas may be pedicled, solitary, or widespread. Their surface is pale yellow to red, granular, villous, and often has a *rasberry appearance.*

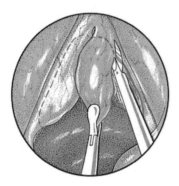

FIGURE 1.28. Decortication of the vocal cords for Reinke's edema. The dotted line shows the limits of excision. The anterior commissure is spared because of the danger of web formation.
SOURCE: Becker W, Naumann HH, Pflatz CR: *Ear, Nose, and Throat Diseases*, p. 419. Thieme, New York, 1989.

Other areas of papillomatosis may lie in the oropharynx and the subglottic space (Color Plate 13).

Treatment. Spontaneous regression rarely occurs. The effects of immunological and antiviral treatment and vaccines have not been reproducible. *Today, there is no alternative to surgery.* Microsurgery is being progressively replaced by the laser. The problem of surgery is the marked tendency of papilloma to recur, the appearance of new foci, and the interference with the function of the vocal cords, caused by defects and scars due to repeated operations.

Note: Papillomas in adults tend to undergo malignant degeneration.

Retention Cysts

These are glazed, white, or occasionally blue cysts derived from mucosal glands. They are localized to the vestibular fold, the ventricle, the epiglottis, the aeryepiglottic folds, and the vallecula.

Small cysts are sometimes found accidentally; larger cysts can cause a globus sensation, dysphonia, and dyspnea.

Treatment. Treatment is removal by microsurgery.

Chondromas

Symptoms. These include hoarseness, dyspnea, dysphagia, or globus, depending on the site.

Pathogenesis. The tumors grow slowly and often arise from the cricoid cartilage.

Diagnosis. Laryngoscopy usually shows a subglottic tumor covered with smooth mucosa. The tumor is sometimes palpable externally. Tomography demonstrates the site and extent of the tumor.

Treatment. Surgery is performed, depending on the symptoms. Chondromas are radioresistant.

Leukoplakia, Dysplasia, and Carcinoma in Situ of the Laryngeal Mucosa

Leukoplakia is a clinical term covering lesions of various different histological grades. A leukoplakic lesion may be premalignant and therefore requires histological investigation.

The following grades may be distinguished:

- Grade I: *Simple dysplasia,* that is, an epithelial hyperplasia without nuclear atypia, without disturbances of maturation or stratification of the squamous epithelium. This is a clinically benign disease.

- Grade II: *Middle-grade epithelial dysplasia* with basal-cell hyperplasia, loss of basal-cell polarity, moderate cell polymorphism, slightly increased mitotic rate, and occasionally dyskeratosis. This is to be regarded clinically as a premalignant lesion.

- Grade III: *High-grade dysplasia* with basal-cell hyperplasia, loss of basal-cell polarity, cell polymorphism, increased mitotic rate, numerous dyskeratoses, and abnormalities of epithelial stratification. Transition to carcinoma in situ is shown by intensification of high-grade dysplasia, loss of epithelial stratification, but no invasion of the stroma. Carcinoma in situ may be a *forerunner* of carcinoma, an intraepithelial offshoot, or an isolated satellite focus.

Note: Many squamous-cell carcinomas of the larynx arise from a precancerous change with a varied length of history and may be diagnosed at this stage by the appropriate steps. Complete removal in the preinvasive stage not only establishes the diagnosis but is also the definitive treatment. A smaller number of carcinomas arise without a preexisting, precancerous epithelial lesion. The carcinoma arises from basal cells, which immediately invade deeply. These cases are termed *microcarcinomas,* or microinvasive carcinomas.

Symptoms. These include hoarseness, feeling of a foreign body in the throat, and a desire to clear the throat.

Pathogenesis. This includes exogenous toxins (e.g., smoking and irradiation).

Diagnosis. Microlaryngoscopy shows the mucosa of the larynx or the vocal cords to be rough, thickened, occasionally deepened by scar tissue, and occasionally altered in color.

Treatment. The histological classification determines the type and extent of treatment. Lesions confined entirely to the vocal cords are treated by decortication (i.e., removal of the epithelium of the vocal cord by microlaryngoscopy). Obvious etiological agents should be eliminated.

Malignant Tumors

Laryngeal Carcinomas

Laryngeal carcinoma forms about 45% of carcinomas of the head and neck. It is most common between the ages of 45 and 75 years. At the present time, men are 10 times more frequently affected than women, although in the last few decades, the number of female patients in Europe and the United States has increased due to increased incidence of smoking in women.

Symptoms. Hoarseness is the first and main symptom when the tumor affects the glottis. Further symptoms, which may occur alone or in combination depending upon site and extent, include a feeling of a foreign body, clearing the throat, pain in the throat or referred elsewhere, dyspnea, dysphagia, cough, and hemoptysis. Regional lymph node metastases may also occur.

Note: Hoarseness persisting for more than 2–3 weeks must always be investigated by a specialist; omission of this step is dangerous.

Pathogenesis. Invasive carcinoma may develop from epithelial dysplasia, especially from carcinoma in situ. More than 90% of laryngeal carcinomas are keratinizing or nonkeratinizing squamous-cell carcinomas. Unusual forms include verrucous carcinoma, adenocarcinoma, carcinosarcoma, fibrosarcoma, and chondrosarcoma.

Most patients with squamous carcinoma of the larynx were or are heavy cigarette smokers and, in addition, often heavy drinkers. Chronic exposure to irritation with heavy metals such as chromium, nickel, uranium, or asbestos, and irradiation are rare causes.

There are racial differences in the frequency of site distribution within the larynx. For example, supraglottic carcinoma is commoner in Spain and in parts of South America than in Germany.

Laryngeal carcinoma infiltrates locally in the mucosa and beneath the mucosa, and metastasizes via the lymphatics and the bloodstream. The limits of vascular spread are embryologically determined (Fig. 1.15). Thus, supraglottic carcinomas usually remain confined to the supraglottic space and spread anteriorly into the preepiglottic space, whereas glottic carcinomas seldom spread into the supraglottic area but rather into the subglottic space. A *transglottic carcinoma* is a glottic carcinoma involving the ventricle and the vestibular folds in which the site of origin can no longer be recognized. *The characteristics of the intralaryngeal lymphatics influence the frequency of regional lymph-node metastases.* Other factors influencing the frequency of metastases are the duration of the symptoms, the histological differentiation, and the size and site of the tumor. Lymph-node metastases at the time of presentation are very rare in carcinoma of the vocal cord, but are found in about 20% of the subglottic carcinomas, about 40% of supraglottic carcinomas, and in about 40% of transglottic carcinomas.

Contralateral metastases are unusual in unilateral glottic tumors. *Bilateral metastases* become more common if the carcinoma crosses the midline (e.g., at the anterior or posterior commissure or in the trachea), or if the tumor arises primarily in the supraglottic space.

Distant hematogenous metastases are relatively unusual in laryngeal carcinoma at the time the patient is first seen. *Second primary carcinomas* of the respiratory and digestive tracts also occur.

Diagnosis. The clinical diagnosis rests initially on the findings of indirect laryngoscopy and telescopic laryngoscopy. The site and extent of the tumor and the mobility of the vocal cord must be assessed (Table 1.9). It is very important to carry out microlaryngoscopy (Figs. 1.19 and 1.20). This allows accurate evaluation of the site and extent of the tumor, provides a view of hidden angles, such as the ventricle and the piriform sinus, and allows assessment of the superficial characteristics such as nodular, exophytic, granulomatous, ulcerating, and so on (Color Plates 14, 15, 16, 17).

Differential diagnosis. This includes chronic laryngitis and its specific forms, and benign laryngeal tumors.

Treatment. If untreated, laryngeal carcinoma leads to death within an average of 12 months by asphyxia, bleeding, metastases, infection or chachexia. The existence of cardiovascular or pulmonary diseases and diabetes mellitus determines

TABLE 1.9. **Classification and involvement of laryngeal carcinomas according to the tumor, node, metastases (TNM) system.**

Glottis (65%)		
	T_{is} =	preinvasive carcinoma, carcinoma in situ
	T_1 =	tumor confined to the glottis with normal cord movement
		T_{1a} = one cord
		T_{1b} = both cords
	T_2 =	cord tumor with extension subglottically or supraglottically with normal or slightly impaired cord mobility (see Color Plate 14)
	T_3 =	tumor confined to the larynx with fixation of one or both cords (see Color Plate 15)
	T_4 =	tumor extending beyond the larynx, e.g., extending into the thyroid cartilage, piriform sinus, postcricoid region or into adjacent skin

Subglottis (5%)		
	T_{is} =	preinvasive carcinoma, carcinoma in situ
	T_1 =	tumor of the subglottic region with normal cord mobility
		T_{1a} = one side subglottis
		T_{1b} = both subglottic areas
	T_2 =	tumor of the subglottic region with extension to one or both cords
	T_3 =	tumor confined to the larynx with fixation of one or both cords
	T_4 =	tumor extending beyond the larynx, e.g. into the postcricoid region, trachea or skin

Supraglottis (30%)		
	T_{is} =	preinvasive carcinoma, carcinoma in situ
	T_1 =	tumor confined to the supraglottic area with normal cord mobility
		T_{1a} = tumor confined to the laryngeal surface of the epiglottis, one aryepiglottic fold, one ventricle, or one false cord
		T_{1b} = tumor of epiglottis with involvement of one ventricle or false cord
	T_2 =	tumor of the epiglottis, ventricle or false cord extending to the cord without fixation
	T_3 =	tumor confined to the larynx with vocal cord fixation and destruction or other signs of deep infiltration
	T_4 =	tumor extending beyond the limits of the larynx with involvement of the piriform sinus, postcricoid region, vallecula or tongue base

SOURCE: Becker W, Naumann HH, Pflatz CR: *Ear, Nose, and Throat Diseases,* p. 423. Thieme, New York, 1989.

the course of treatment and the course of the disease. The indications for *radiotherapy* or *surgery* for laryngeal carcinomas vary depending on the site and stage of the tumor. They are often used in combination. *Chemotherapy* alone has so far proved to be useless for this type of tumor. *Radiotherapy achieves similar results to surgery for $T_1 N_0$ glottic tumors and for some $T_2 N_0$ tumors. However, the* danger of a radiation-induced carcinoma after a latent period of several years must be borne in mind in young patients. Radiotherapy must also be used for patients with inoperable tumors or those unwilling to undergo surgery. Extension of a laryngeal carcinoma to the hypopharynx may also be an indication for radiotherapy because even the most extensive surgery does not produce a 5-year survival rate better than 20%.

For all other sites and stages of tumor, especially if lymph-node metastases are present, surgery is clearly superior to radiotherapy.

Both methods of treatment may be combined (e.g., pre- or postoperative radiotherapy or sandwich radiotherapy). This latter form of treatment gives the best result for selected patients in advanced stages.

Complications after radiotherapy include persistent edema, which makes it difficult to assess the local appearances and detect a recurrence. The edema is usually due to chonroradionecrosis leading to cartilaginous necrosis, which may require laryngectomy. Other complications include dysphagia, ageusia, xerostomia and the sicca syndrome, recurrent tumor, or lymph-node metastases. If surgery must be undertaken after a full course of radiotherapy, the wound healing and prognosis are considerably worse.

Surgical Procedures for Laryngeal Carcinoma

1. *Microsurgical decortication of the vocal cord* is indicated for severe dysplasia and some carcinomas in situ.

2. *Cordectomy* is indicated for a vocal-cord carcinoma with a mobile vocal cord ($T_1 N_0, T_2 N_0$).

Principle of the operation (Fig. 1.29a–c). The thyroid cartilage is split by a thyrotomy, the affected vocal cord is excised, and the thyroid cartilage is closed again. The breathing is normal after this operation. The voice is rough or hoarse postoperatively but may return to normal after several months as scar tissue forms a pseudocord.

1. *Vertical or horizontal partial laryngectomies* are used for carcinomas for which a cordectomy is not suitable because of the extent or site of the tumor, but for which total laryngectomy is not necessary. Partial laryngectomies *preserve the vocal function and a normal airway.* The prerequisites for success are careful assessment and good surgical judgment to ensure that the tumor is removed completely.

Vertical partial laryngectomy. Principle of the operation (Fig. 1.30a and 1.30b). Several methods are available, but the principle common to all of them is that a wide vertical segment of the thyroid cartilage and, occasionally the cricoid cartilage, is removed, together with the laryngeal soft tissues and the tumor. A *hemilaryngectomy,* removal of half of the larynx, may be carried out for a tumor limited strictly to one side.

Horizontal partial laryngectomy. Principle of the operation (Fig. 1.31a and 1.31b). The supraglottic space is completely removed, with retention of the vocal cords and the arytenoid cartilage.

After a partial resection, the functional results are good, and the airway is normal as is the vocal function, but the latter depends on the type of resection, the results of which are variable. The patient may have temporary difficulty in swallowing, which may persist in elderly patients. There is a danger of recurrence at the excisional margins if the tumor was incorrectly evaluated preoperatively, or if the technique was inadequate.

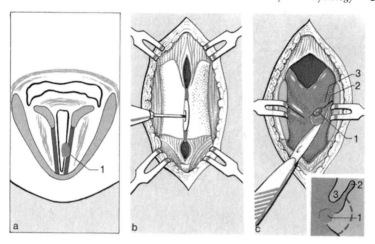

FIGURE 1.29. Cordectomy.

a. Carcinoma in the center of the vocal cord. **b.** Thyrotomy: division of the thyroid carti-lage with a rotating saw. In the diagram the incision into the conus elasticus and into the superior thyrohyoid membrane has already been undertaken. **c.** Excision of the affected part of the vocal cord with a good margin. **1,** Vocal cord with tumor; **2,** ventricle; **3,** vestibular fold.

SOURCE: Becker W, Naumann HH, Pflatz CR: *Ear, Nose, and Throat Diseases,* p. 425. Thieme, New York, 1989.

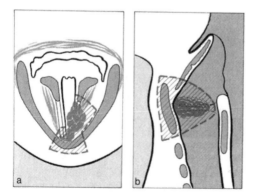

FIGURE 1.30. Vertical frontolateral partial resection. The area to be resected is shown in red, and the limits of resection by the dashed line.

SOURCE: Becker W, Naumann HH, Pflatz CR: *Ear, Nose, and Throat Diseases,* p. 425. Thieme, New York, 1989.

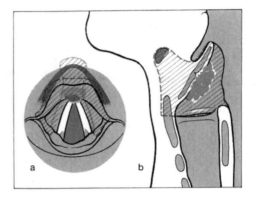

FIGURE 1.31. Horizontal supraglottic partial resection.
The area to be resected is shaded, and the limits of resection are shown by the dashed line.
The **dotted** line indicates the area to be resected not clinically visible by laryngoscopy.
SOURCE: Becker W, Naumann HH, Pflatz CR: *Ear, Nose, and Throat Diseases*, p. 426.
Thieme, New York, 1989.

2. *Total laryngectomy* may on occasion be combined with removal of the hypopharynx. This technique is indicated for tumors that cannot be removed by cordectomy or partial laryngectomy, and for tumors that have spread to neighboring structures such as the tongue, the hypopharynx, the thyroid gland, and the trachea. Total laryngectomy is also indicated for tumors that have recurred after radiotherapy or partial procedures.

Operative technique (Figs. 1.32–1.35). The entire larynx is removed from the base of the tongue to the trachea, if necessary, with removal of parts of the tongue, the pharynx, the trachea, and the thyroid gland. If part of the tongue or the pharynx is removed, reconstructive procedures must be undertaken at the same time. After this operation, *breathing* is only possible via the tracheostomy. *Swallowing* is normal once the wound has healed, and *voice* is produced either by esophageal speech, creation of a neoglottis, or by means of an external electronic larynx.

Complications after laryngectomy include pharyngocutaneous fistula and recurrent tracheobronchitis.

> **Note:** Removal of the primary tumor by a partial or total laryngectomy should be combined with a therapeutic neck dissection en bloc if lymph-node metastases are present (see Fig. 1.36). If there is a known high risk of lymphatic metastases for a tumor at a particular site, many surgeons carry out an *elective neck dissection,* even if lymph-node metastases cannot be palpated. The results of treatment are summarized in Table 1.10.

Rehabilitation of the Laryngectomee.

1. Voice and speech
   a. Eighty-five percent of laryngectomees can learn esophageal speech under the direction of a speech therapist. The esophagus is used as the air source and the mouth of the esophagus as the pseudoglottis.

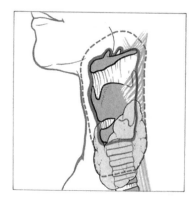

FIGURE 1.32. Area resected in laryngectomy.

The boundaries to be resected may be extended for involvement of the tongue, the hypopharynx, the upper trachea, and the thyroid gland (shown by the dashed line).

SOURCE: Becker W, Naumann HH, Pflatz CR: *Ear, Nose, and Throat Diseases,* p. 426. Thieme, New York, 1989.

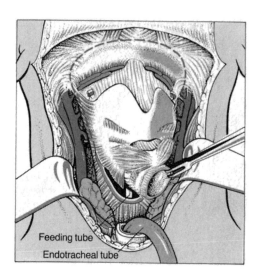

Feeding tube
Endotracheal tube

FIGURE 1.33. Laryngectomy.

A U-shaped incision is made and the skin-platysma flap turned superiorly over the chin. The larynx together with the hyoid bone (dashed line above) is freed from its connection with the surrounding soft tissue and from the trachea and is divided from the trachea inferiorly. It is also divided from the esophagus below and the hypopharynx. The excision may also proceed from above downward. The feeding tube can be seen in the open hypopharynx. The thyroid gland, which is divided and sutured laterally, can be recognized in the lower part of the diagram.

SOURCE: Becker W, Naumann HH, Pflatz CR: *Ear, Nose, and Throat Diseases,* p. 427. Thieme, New York, 1989.

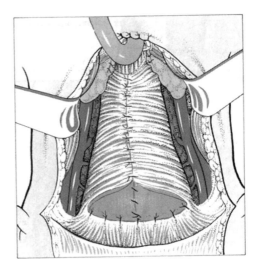

FIGURE 1.34. Situation after removal of the larynx and closure of the pharyngeal mucosa in layers.
SOURCE: Becker W, Naumann HH, Pflatz CR: *Ear, Nose, and Throat Diseases,* p. 427. Thieme, New York, 1989.

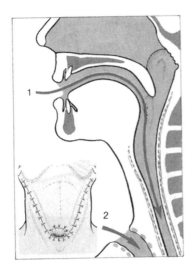

FIGURE 1.35. Appearance after conclusion of laryngectomy.

The replaced U-shaped skin flap covers the newly repaired pharynx. The T-shaped pharyngeal suture line is shown by the dotted line in the left inset. **1,** Food passage reconstructed. Normal swallowing may be resumed after healing. **2,** Tracheostomy for a new airway.

SOURCE: Becker W, Naumann HH, Pflatz CR: *Ear, Nose, and Throat Diseases,* p. 428. Thieme, New York, 1989.

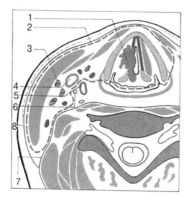

FIGURE 1.36. Laryngectomy with radical neck dissection.

The area to be resected is shown by the dashed line. **1,** Larynx with the tumor; **2,** superficial cervical fascia which coincides with the limits of radical neck dissection; **3,** cervical lymph nodes; **4,** internal jugular vein; **5,** carotid artery; **6,** vagus nerve; **7,** deep cervical fascia; **8,** platysma.

SOURCE: Becker W, Naumann HH, Pflatz CR: *Ear, Nose, and Throat Diseases,* p. 428. Thieme, New York, 1989.

b. An alternative is surgical creation of a fistula between the tracheal stump and the pharynx or esophagus, the neoglottis procedure, with or without a supplementary mechanical device. At the moment, these procedures have numerous functional disadvantages.

c. An electronic device may be used to produce sound. This device delivers externally produced vibrations to the pharyngeal wall or the floor of the mouth.

2. Tracheostomy

a. Since it is possible to breathe only via the tracheostomy, problems arise during showering, bathing, and swimming. However, these can be overcome by a device like a snorkel.

b. Once the tracheostomy has stabilized, it is usually unnecessary to use a tracheostomy tube. If the tracheostomy tends to stenose, a short, individually fitted stoma button may be used, or it may be necessary to widen the stoma surgically.

TABLE 1.10. Five-year survival in laryngeal carcinoma*

Type of tumor	%	Treatment
GLOTTIC CARCINOMA		
T_1N_0	> 90	Surgery or radiotherapy
T_2N_0	70–80	Surgery or radiotherapy
T_3	60–70	Surgery or combined surgery and radiotherapy
T_4	< 50	Surgery or combined surgery and radiotherapy
SUPRAGLOTTIC CARCINOMA		
T_1 and T_2	80	Surgery or combined surgery and radiotherapy
T_3 and T_4	50–60	Surgery or combined surgery and radiotherapy
SUBGLOTTIC CARCINOMA	< 40	Surgery or combined surgery and radiotherapy
TRANSGLOTTIC CARCINOMA	< 50	Surgery or combined surgery and radiotherapy

SOURCE: Becker W, Naumann HH, Pflatz CR: *Ear, Nose, and Throat Diseases,* p. 429. Thieme, New York, 1989.

*The presence of a regional *lymph node metastasis* reduces the above figures *considerably.* If the nodes are fixed the survival rate is markedly reduced.

   c. There is often a tendency to develop tracheitis with crusts, particularly in the spring and autumn, because of the absence of the air-conditioning mechanism of the nose. Treatment is described under "Trachea."

3. Social Reintegration
     The patient and his relatives need thorough instructions before the operation about future functional defects. Medical and psychological training is necessary after the operation. It is advisable that the patient join a laryngectomee club.

Hypopharynx

The most important diseases are foreign bodies (Color Plate 18), pulsion diverticulum (Color Plate 19), and *carcinoma* (Color Plate 17).

Hypopharyngeal Carcinoma
The TNM classification distinguishes three regions (see Fig. 1.37):

- Piriform sinus
- Posterior pharyngeal wall
- Postcricoid region (Color Plate 20)

The T staging is as follows:

- T1 is a tumor that is confined to one region.
- T2 is a tumor that involves two regions.
- T3 is a tumor that extends beyond the borders of the hypopharynx, larynx, esophagus, and cervical soft tissues.

Symptoms. In more than 40% of cases, the patient presents because of lymph-node metastases. The typical site is at the angle of the jaw under the sternocleidomastoid muscle. The patient has also dysphagia and pain irradiating to the ear. Hoarseness and difficulty in breathing occur when the tumor extends to the larynx or paralyzes the recurrent laryngeal nerve. Oral fetor and bloodstained sputum also may occur.

Pathogenesis. The previous term of extrinsic laryngeal carcinoma is no longer tenable on anatomical or clinical grounds.

   In recent years, the peak age of incidence has fallen because of alcohol and nicotine abuse. The ratio of men to women in Germany is now 4 : 1. In the Scandinavian countries, the tumor occurs more frequently in women, especially postcricoid carcinoma. The disease is said to be related to the Plummer–Vinson syndrome. About 50% of patients have T3 N1–2 tumors when first seen. Carcinomas of the posterolateral pharyngeal wall and of the postcricoid region have a particularly high rate of metastases, often bilateral in the latter lesions. Distant metastases at the time of diagnosis are found in 10% of cases in the lung, liver, and skeleton, and in as many as 80% of patients at autopsy. Virtually all tumors are poorly differentiated carcinomas.

   Order of frequency of hypopharyngeal carcinoma. Tumors of the piriform sinus are the most common followed by lesions of the posterior pharyngeal wall. Postcricoid tumors are rare (Fig. 1.37).

   Diagnosis. The early symptoms of interference with swallowing and cervical-lymph-node metastases are often misinterpreted by both the patient and the doctor, so that diagnosis is delayed. The time interval between the early symptoms

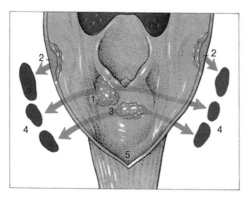

FIGURE 1.37. The sites of carcinomas of the hypopharynx (1, 2, 3) and pathways of lymphatic metastases. The hypopharynx has been opened posteriorly. The esophageal orifice (5) lies inferiorly.

1, Piriform sinus; **2,** posterior pharyngeal wall; **3,** postcricoid region; **4,** chain of deep cervical nodes along internal jugular vein.

SOURCE: Becker W, Naumann HH, Pflatz CR: *Ear, Nose, and Throat Diseases,* p. 431. Thieme, New York, 1989.

and the first examination by a specialist is further increased by the difficulty of examining the hypopharynx with the mirror. Microlaryngoscopy should always be carried out if a hypopharyngeal carcinoma is suspected. The tumor may be ulcerating or exophytic in type, often surrounded by edema and covered with retained saliva and food remnants.

Note: Cervical-lymph-node metastases with an unknown primary tumor require special investigation of the hypopharynx.

Treatment. Surgery is only justifiable in a limited number of patients, depending on the site and extent of the tumor and the presence of lymphatic or bloodborne metastases. If surgery is possible, it consists of pharyngectomy, or pharyngolaryngectomy, if the larynx is involved.

A neck dissection is indicated on one or both sides because of the very high rate of metastases to the cervical lymph nodes. Reconstruction of the pharynx and upper esophagus by musculocutaneous flaps from the neck or chest wall is often necessary.

All therapeutic measures are limited by the usually advanced stage of the disease and the associated poor general condition of the patient. In early stages, surgery supplemented by radiotherapy achieves a 5-year survival rate of 20–30%. In stage T3 with cervical-lymph-node metastases, the 5-year survival rate for surgery or radiotherapy is less than 20%.

Tracheobronchial Tree

Study of the tracheobronchial system is common to several disciplines. The trachea is largely localized to the neck and is a continuation of the larynx, so that diseases of one organ often affect the other. Endoscopic diagnosis and treatment (bronchoscopy) was developed by ear, nose, and throat surgeons and is still practiced by them, although other specialists in bronchial diseases, such as chest physicians and thoracic surgeons, practice diagnostic bronchoscopy.

Applied Anatomy and Physiology

Basic Anatomy

The *trachea* is attached to the cricoid cartilage, which is the most narrow rigid element of the airway and moves in response to movements of the floor of the mouth and the cervical muscles. It is 10–13 cm long in the adult, and its lumen is held open by 16–20 horseshoe-shaped cartilaginous rings. The posterior part of the tube is formed by the membranous part that lies in contact with the anterior esophageal wall.

The carina (i.e., the origin of the two main bronchi) lies at the level of the sixth thoracic vertebra. It has an angle of 55 degrees open inferiorly. The right main bronchus lies at an angle of about 17 degrees to the midline and the left bronchus at an angle of about 35 degrees (Fig. 1.38).

The *bronchial tree* has an extra- and intrapulmonary course. The horseshoe-shaped cartilaginous rings of the bronchial wall gradually become complete rings,

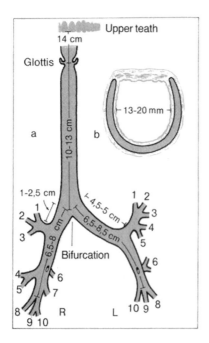

FIGURE 1.38. Tracheobronchial tree (a) and cross-section of the trachea (b).

Nomenclature of the segmental bronchi. **Right. 1,** Apical; **2,** posterior; **3,** anterior; **4,** lateral; **5,** medial; **6,** apical; **7,** cardiac; **8,** anterobasal; **9,** laterobasal; **10,** posterobasal (1 +2 +3 = the upper lobe; 4 + 5 = the middle lobe; 6 + 7 + 8 + 9 + 10 = the lower lobe). **Left. 1,** Apical; **2,** posterior; **3,** anterior; **4,** superior; **5,** inferior; **6,** apical; **8,** anterobasal; **9,** laterobasal; **10,** posterobasal. (1 + 2 + 3 + [4 + 5 = lingula] = upper lobe; 6 + 8 + 9 + 10 = lower lobe).

SOURCE: Becker W, Naumann HH, Pflatz CR: *Ear, Nose, and Throat Diseases,* p. 433. Thieme, New York, 1989.

encircling the bronchus fully in the more peripheral parts. The bronchioles do not possess cartilaginous elements in the wall but only a spiral muscle. Changes in the lumen are produced by the bronchial musculature and additionally in the middle and small bronchi by the bronchial veins.

The trachea and bronchi are lined by respiratory mucosa, which becomes flatter toward the periphery and passes into a single layer of cubical epithelium in the bronchioles.

Vascular supply. The trachea is mainly supplied by the inferior thyroid artery, but there are also connections with the superior thyroid artery. The bronchi and the carina derive their blood supply directly from the aorta through bronchial arteries. There are numerous anastomoses with the pulmonary arteries for the lung tissue.

Lymphatic drainage. The trachea mainly drains to the lymphatic network of the neck but also connects with the thoracic lymphatic system, which is important in the spread of metastases.

Nerve supply. This is provided by the vagus nerve and the sympathetic trunk. The anatomy of the central parts of the bronchial tree is shown in Figure 1.38.

Basic Physiology

The mucociliary apparatus works in the direction of the larynx. Warming, humidification, and cleaning of the inspired air begin in the nose and are completed in the lower airway, so that under normal anatomic conditions, the intratracheal air temperature is maintained between 36 degrees at an external temperature above 0°C, and 27°C at an external temperature of −15°C. These temperatures are considerably lower during mouth breathing. The relative humidity of the intratracheal air is 99% in normal breathing but considerably lower during mouth breathing.

Methods of Investigation

Bronchoscopy

Two methods of bronchoscopy are available.

1. The *rigid endoscope* (Fig. 1.39a–d) is historically the older method. It remains in universal use, is more productive, and has the greatest number of indications.
2. The *flexible fiberscope* (Fig. 1.40) is preferred in some special circumstances. Both methods supplement each other.

Rigid bronchoscopes are tubes of different caliber with a proximal cold light source as well as distal and combined illumination systems (see Fig. 1.39a–d). Since bronchoscopy is usually carried out under general anesthesia, the bronchoscope has a direct connection to the anesthetic apparatus, *respiration bronchoscope,* so that it acts like an elongated, rigid anesthetic tube. These bronchoscopes may be combined with instruments for aspiration, lavage for cytological diagnosis, swabs for culture, aspiration biopsy, peribronchial needle biopsy, injection, curettage, biopsy, and foreign-body extraction. They may also be used in combination with catheters for bronchography or catheter aspiration biopsy and with telescopes of various angles. The simultaneous combination of bronchoscopy and radiographic screening is especially useful for an aspiration biopsy, manipulation of a catheter, and the extraction of a foreign body, which is a common indication for bronchoscopy, especially in children.

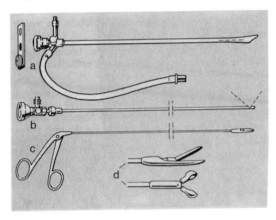

FIGURE 1.39. Rigid bronchoscope.
a. Bronchoscope with anesthetic attachment, light carrier, and interchangeable window.
b. Bronchoscopic telescope. **c.** Instrument for endoscopy used with different attachments (**d**).
SOURCE: Becker W, Naumann HH, Pflatz CR: *Ear, Nose, and Throat Diseases,* p. 434.
Thieme, New York, 1989.

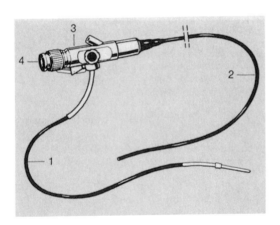

FIGURE 1.40. Flexible fiberoptic bronchoscope.
1, cold light cable; **2,** flexible fiberglass telescope; **3,** handlegrip with control; **4,** telescope.
SOURCE: Becker W, Naumann HH, Pflatz CR: *Ear, Nose, and Throat Diseases,* p. 435.
Thieme, New York, 1989.

The laser may be used via a rigid endoscope for a relatively bloodless removal of benign tumors. The rigid bronchoscope may also be used for photographic, movie, and television documentation.

Indications for the use of the rigid bronchoscope are given in Table 1.11.

TABLE 1.11. Indications for bronchoscopy.

Bronchoscopy with rigid tube

As a therapeutic measure:
- Emergency bronchoscopy as a temporary measure in sudden obstructive respiratory insufficiency
- Removal of tracheal or bronchial foreign bodies
- Arrest of bleeding in the trachea or bronchi
- Removal of retained secretions in obstructive disease of the lung or trachea
- Aspiration of tuberculous lymph nodes at the carina and of lung abscess
- To allow the use of the laser to remove a benign endotracheal or endobronchial tumor or a cicatricial membrane

As a diagnostic procedure in:
- Tracheal and bronchial stenoses
- Suspicion of a tracheal tumor or a tumor in the surrounding tissue. The elasticity of the tracheal wall and its mobility should be assessed.
- Suspicion of a bronchial tumor
- Unexplained persistent attacks of coughing and wheezing
- Hemoptysis of uncertain cause
- Suspicion of tracheal or bronchial trauma
- Transtracheal or transbronchial aspiration of a lymph node or a central tumor
- To allow a specimen to be taken for biopsy
- Bronchial lavage
- Brochiectasis or bronchography (currently rarely indicated)

Advantages: Very versatile procedure, which allows endoscopic overview, can also be used in bleeding and in the extraction of a foreign body. It gives an excellent visualization.

Disadvantages: Technically difficult in the presence of abnormal anatomy such as kyphoscoliosis. Limited access to the periphery and more discomfort to the patient than the fiberoptic bronchoscope.

Bronchoscopy with a flexible endoscope

Used as a *diagnostic measure* in:
- Suspicion of peripheral bronchial tumors, i.e., distal to the segmental ostia
- Hemoptysis of uncertain cause after the bleeding has stopped
- Undiagnosed disorders of the lung parenchyma
- Pleural effusion of uncertain cause
- Unresolved pneumonia, interstitial pneumopathy
- Middle lobe syndrome

Advantages: This endoscope can be introduced far into the periphery as far as the fifth-generation bronchi. It therefore complements the rigid endoscope. It can also be used with local anesthesia which is less troublesome to the patient.

Disadvantages: It has a very narrow working radius and cannot be used for large foreign bodies or in the presence of bleeding, atelectasis, or respiratory failure. The image obtained is not as good as with a rigid endoscope.

SOURCE: Becker W, Naumann HH, Pflatz CR: *Ear, Nose, and Throat Diseases,* p. 436. Thieme, New York, 1989.

Flexible bronchoscopes (see Fig. 1.40) have a diameter of 4–5 mm and are thinner than rigid bronchoscopes. Their distal end can be controlled externally, so that they can be introduced into lobe bronchi, segmental bronchi, and even into the segmental bronchi. The instrument may be introduced via the nose or the mouth, or a tracheostomy, if one is present. A flexible telescope may be combined with a fine, flexible excision forceps, and this instrument may also be used in combination with simultaneous radiographic monitoring.

Flexible bronchoscopy may be carried out under local anesthesia, with the patient sitting, or lying under general anesthesia. In the latter case, the endoscope is introduced through the endotracheal tube. Indications are shown in Table 1.11.

Clinical Aspects

Stenoses

Acute and chronic stenoses must be distinguished depending on the site of origin in the trachea or bronchi. Furthermore, stenoses originating within the wall of the trachea, *intramural,* or outside it, *extramural,* may be distinguished, as may those affecting the internal lining, *endoluminal.* Finally, there are those that affect the mucosa and the supporting elements of the wall, *compression stenoses and tracheomalacia* (Fig. 1.41a–c).

Tracheal stenoses usually require urgent treatment because there is no possibility of compensation, and the consequence is the danger of asphyxia.

Acute Stenoses

Symptoms. The main symptom is inspiratory stridor, in addition accompanied by restlessness, coughing, attacks, a fear of dying, cyanosis, and choking (Tables 1.12 and 1.13).

Pathogenesis. The cause is sudden narrowing of the tracheal lumen by more than 50% by blunt trauma, an aspirated foreign body, edema, swelling, bleeding, infection, crusts, and so on.

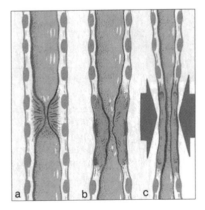

FIGURE 1.41. Typical tracheal stenoses.

(a) of the internal lining alone, (b) affecting all elements of the wall, (c) tracheomalacia, compression stenosis.

SOURCE: Becker W, Naumann HH, Pflatz CR: *Ear, Nose, and Throat Diseases,* p. 437. Thieme, New York, 1989.

Diagnosis. The considerable inspiratory and often expiratory stridor also indicates an urgent situation. The history usually indicates the cause. The level of the obstruction may be localized by auscultation. Bronchoscopy is carried out using the rigid bronchoscope, with preparations for immediate tracheostomy. Radiographs are taken only if delay carries no risk.

Differential diagnosis. This includes laryngeal stenoses, bronchial stenoses lying near the carina, pulmonary emboli and edema, and an asthmatic attack, which does not cause *inspiratory* stridor (see Tables 1.12 and 1.13).

Treatment. Rigid bronchoscopy is performed and, if necessary, tracheotomy with respiration is assured by leaving the bronchoscope in place. Foreign bodies are extracted if present.

TABLE 1.12. Inspiratory stridor.

Site of the Stenosis	Disease	Details
Oro- and hypopharynx	Diphtheria	Typical local findings, including a membrane
	Peritonsillar abscess	Swelling of Waldeyer's ring, pain on swallowing, trismus
	Retropharyngeal abscess	Swelling of the posterior pharyngeal wall
	Angioneurotic edema	Typical local findings, sudden onset
	Posterior displacement of the tongue in unconscious patients	
	Abscess of the base of tongue	Marked dysphagia, thick speech
	Lingual thyroid	Thick speech, long history
	Benign and malignant tumors	Fetor, typical local findings, possibly pain and bleeding in malignant tumors
Larynx	Congenital stridor	Indrawing of the epiglottis on
	Epiglottitis and epiglottic abscess	inspiration, congenital webs or flaccid epiglottis. Occurs in early infancy (see Table 1.5)
	Glottic edema	Typical local findings
		Typical laryngoscopic findings
	Vocal cord paralysis	Bilateral abductor paralysis
	Laryngeal spasm	Sudden life-threatening symptom, history often shows a previous tendency to glottic spasm
	Pseudocroup (subglottic laryngitis)	Typical laryngeal findings, affects small children
	Laryngeal diphtheria	Typical laryngoscopic findings (membrane)
	Foreign body	History, attacks of coughing, variable symptoms

(continued)

TABLE 1.12. (*continued*)

Site of the Stenosis	Disease	Details
Larynx (cont.)	Benign tumors such as cysts and celes	Usually slowly worsening symptoms
	Malignant tumors	Hoarseness, gradually worsening symptoms, pain, possibly hemoptysis
	Results of trauma	History
Trachea and bronchial tree	Tracheitis or bronchitis with stenosis or crusts	History of infection, possibly history of an operation on the trachea
	Foreign body	History
	External compression, e.g., by goiter or bleeding into a goiter	Gradually increasing symptoms; in addition, symptoms of disease of neighboring organs
	Tracheomalacia	History of goiter or trauma
	Cicatricial stenosis	History shows trauma or intubation
	Traumatic tracheal subluxation	History
	Intratracheal tumor or bronchial tumors lying close to the carina	Long history, tomograms, endoscopic findings
	Complications during and after tracheostomy	See p. 71

Initial diagnostic measures include:
1. History
2. Examination with a tongue depressor
3. Indirect laryngoscopy
4. Direct endoscopy of the larynx, trachea, and bronchi
5. Radiography
If sufficient time is available, (5) is carried out before (4).

SOURCE: Becker W, Naumann HH, Pflatz CR: *Ear, Nose, and Throat Diseases*, p. 438–439. Thieme, New York, 1989.

Chronic Stenoses

Symptoms. The history shows a long period of increasing dyspnea, at times previous attacks of dyspnea, and weak voice. The degree of severity of the respiratory obstruction often depends on the position of the head. In acute exacerbations, the cause of the respiratory obstruction is usually already known because of previous diagnostic measures. The head is held forward with the chin downward. The patient prefers to have the body upright.

Pathogenesis includes trauma, scarring due to injury, incorrect or prolonged intubation causing injury to the tracheal wall (Fig. 1.42), incorrect tracheotomy (Fig. 1.42), intratracheal tumors, goiter, malignant thyroid, bronchial and esophageal tumors, lymphadenopathies, tracheomalacia, tracheopathia, chondro-osteo-

TABLE 1.13. Dyspnea.

Type	Characteristic Symptoms
Obstructive respiratory insufficiency	Inspiratory stridor. If the stenosis lies distal to the bifurcation there may also be an expiratory stridor. Indrawing of the suprasternal notch, and the supraclavicular and intercostal areas on inspiration Restlessness, anxiety, loss of orientation, loss of consciousness, increased pulse rate Respiratory rate usually slowed. Inspiration longer than expiration Auscultation shows the stridor to be loudest over the stenosed area. A slapping noise is heard with mobile foreign bodies. Skin color initially pale, later cyanosed Tiredness, increasing exhaustion, anxious facies
Restrictive respiratory insufficiency, e.g. pneumonia, pneumothorax and pleuritis	Respiratory rate increased, shallow superficial breathing, vital capacity restricted Both inspiration and expiration shortened Additional abnormal findings in the lung or pleura Patient prefers to lie flat
Bronchial asthma	Respiratory rate decreased, typical wheezing noise or rhonchi noise on expiration Expiration clearly longer than inspiration Leaning on the arms on breathing to supplement the auxiliary muscles of respiration Typical findings on auscultation over the lung Shortage of breath in paroxysmal attacks
Cardiac respiratory insufficiency	Respiratory rate increased No stridor, free air passage Skin pale or cyanotic, blue lips, the patient is sweaty The patient prefers to sit upright Attacks of shortness of breath at night, cardiac asthma Additional abnormal findings in the heart and the circulation
Extrathoracic respiratory insufficiency, e.g. in central respiratory paralysis, diabetes, uremic coma, conditions of increased oxygen requirement, etc.	Irregular gasping or periodic respiration Increasing disturbance of consciousness and loss of consciousness. Stridor may also occur if the tongue is allowed to fall backward.
Psychogenic respiratory insufficiency	Respiratory rate increased, hyperventilation syndrome No stridor, possibly sighing respiration Well-perfused skin and mucosa

SOURCE: Becker W, Naumann HH, Pflatz CR: *Ear, Nose, and Throat Diseases,* p. 440. Thieme, New York, 1989.

plastica, (Color Plate 21) tuberculosis, syphilis, scleroma, nonspecific infection, radiotherapy, and mediastinal causes such as dermoid cysts, emphysema, tumors, abscess, and aortic aneurysm.

Diagnosis is made by radiography of the chest, tomography of the trachea in two planes, and during attempts at sucking and straining, thyroid scans, pulmonary function tests, bronchoscopy, and biopsy.

Differential diagnosis is shown in Tables 1.12 and 1.13 and Figure 1.42.

Treatment is always by surgery but varies depending on the cause.

1. *Tracheopexy* consists of holding open the tracheal lumen using retaining loop structures (e.g., in tracheomalacia) due to goiter (see Fig. 1.41).

Principle of the operation. Several techniques are used:
   a. Introduction of loop sutures (e.g., after thyroidectomy) into the weakened wall of the trachea and anchoring the loop to structures close to the trachea such as the muscles, the clavicle, and so on.
   b. Stiffening of the collapsed trachea with gold, tantalum, or synthetic rings (Fig. 1.43).

2. *Tracheal resection* with end-to-end anastomosis for scars, strictures, and tracheal trauma is used for severe destruction of *all* elements of the tracheal wall (Fig. 1.44a and 1.44b).

Principle of the operation. The diseased segment is resected and the stumps are anastomosed end-to-end. Resection of more than 4 cm requires division of the strap muscles above or below the hyoid (supra- or subhyoid mobilization of the larynx). Mobilization of the roots of the lung may also be needed.

3. *Partial tracheoplasty,* with or without a previous *open gutter,* is used for stenoses affecting only the inner lining of the trachea or for relatively circumscribed defects of the entire wall.

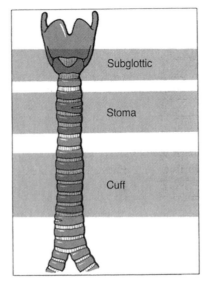

FIGURE 1.42. Typical locations of laryngotracheal stenoses.

(**1**) *Subglottic:* affecting the cricoid cartilage or the first tracheal rings as a result of prolonged or incorrect intubation, incorrect tracheostomy, or trauma. (**2**) *Stomal:* as a result of a tracheostomy, an incorrectly carried out tracheostomy, tracheomalacia, or scar tissue. (**3**) *Cuff:* in the lower two thirds of the trachea due to prolonged intubation or excessive pressure on the tracheal wall during inflation of the tube.

SOURCE: Becker W, Naumann HH, Pflatz CR: *Ear, Nose, and Throat Diseases,* p. 441. Thieme, New York, 1989.

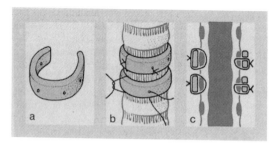

FIGURE 1.43. Tracheopexy using extratracheal synthetic ring.
(a) Synthetic ring, (b) two rings in position, (c) fixation of the ring to the tracheal wall by sutures.
SOURCE: Becker W, Naumann HH, Pflatz CR: *Ear, Nose, and Throat Diseases,* p. 442. Thieme, New York, 1989.

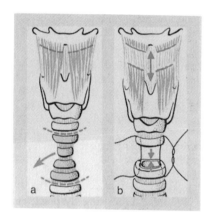

FIGURE 1.44. Horizontal resection of the trachea and end-to-end anastomosis.
a. Resection of the stenosed area and incision for subhyoid laryngeal mobilization.
b. End-to-end anastomosis of the tracheal stumps by laryngeal mobilization.
SOURCE: Becker W, Naumann HH, Pflatz CR: *Ear, Nose, and Throat Diseases,* p. 442. Thieme, New York, 1989.

Figure 1.45a–c shows the principle of the operation. The stenosed segment is removed and the defect is covered with pedicled or free graft of cartilage and skin. Healing is achieved either by forming an open gutter, which is closed secondarily, or by the use of a synthetic prosthesis with the trachea closed (Fig. 1.46a and 1.46b).

4. *Endoscopic removal* is used for stenoses, webs, diaphragms, and small benign tumors.

The technique is as follows: The stenosed area is divided through a rigid bronchoscope using fine instruments or the laser without tracheotomy, provided that the stenosis is not too extensive and does not affect the cartilaginous rings.

Organic bronchial stenoses are, at this time, only rarely an indication for *therapeutic* bronchoscopy, although it is possible that the laser may change this.

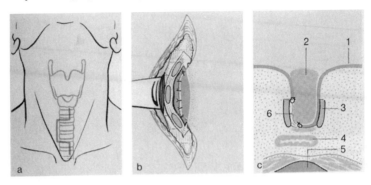

FIGURE 1.45. Partial tracheoplasty.

(a) incision of the overlying skin, (b) turning in of the soft tissue zone into the defect in the tracheal wall, (c) situation after reconstruction of the wall. **1,** External cervical skin; **2,** synthetic obturator to stabilize the new tracheal lumen; **3,** lateral portions of the tracheal cartilage after median tracheofissure and excision of the stenosis; **4,** esophagus; **5,** vertebra; **6,** half-portion of the tracheal wall with healthy mucosal lining.

SOURCE: Becker W, Naumann HH, Pflatz CR: *Ear, Nose, and Throat Diseases,* p. 443. Thieme, New York, 1989.

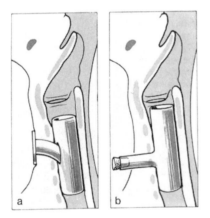

FIGURE 1.46. Tracheal endoprosthesis for stabilization of the reconstructed segment of the trachea.

(a) A hollow synthetic prosthesis combined with a tracheostomy tube, (b) Montgomery's silicone T tube.

SOURCE: Becker W, Naumann HH, Pflatz CR: *Ear, Nose, and Throat Diseases,* p. 443. Thieme, New York, 1989.

Tracheotomy, Laryngology, and Intubation

Indications: Tracheotomy, laryngotomy, and intubation are life-saving measures that must often be carried out as emergency procedures. Table 1.14 summarizes the indications for tracheotomy. Tracheotomy reduces the dead space by 70–100 ml.

Depending on the site of tracheal entry (Fig. 1.47), tracheotomy may be divided into *high* access, above the thyroid isthmus, *middle* access, after division of the isthmus, and *low* access, below the isthmus. In urgent cases a high tracheotomy is usually carried out, although a low tracheotomy is usually carried out in

TABLE 1.14. Indications for tracheotomy and endotracheal intubation.

Tracheotomy

A. Mechanical airway obstruction due to
- Tumors affecting the pharynx, larynx, trachea, or esophagus
- Congenital anomalies of the upper respiratory or digestive tract
- Trauma of the larynx or trachea
- Bilateral recurrent nerve paralysis
- Trauma of the facial skeleton with soft tissue swelling or fractures, especially in the mandible
- Aspiration of a foreign body
- Inflammation causing edema of the larynx, trachea, tongue and pharynx

B. Obstruction of the airway by secretions or inadequate respiration, or both
- Retention of secretions and ineffective coughing and self during or after
   1. Thoracic or abdominal surgery
   2. Bronchopneumonia
   3. Vomiting or aspiration of stomach contents
   4. Burns of the face, neck, or respiratory tract
   5. Precoma and coma due to diabetes, liver disease, or renal insufficiency

- Alveolar respiratory insufficiency during or after
   1. Drug intoxication and poisoning
   2. Blunt thoracic trauma with fractures of the ribs
   3. Paralysis of the respiratory musculature
   4. Chronic obstructive lung diseases, such as emphysema, chronic bronchitis, bronchiectasis, asthma, and atelectasis

- Retention of secretions with alveolar respiratory insufficiency in
   1. Central nervous diseases such as a stroke, encephalitis, poliomyelitis, and tetanus
   2. Eclampsia
   3. Severe trauma to the head, neck, and thorax
   4. Postoperative neurosurgical coma
   5. Air or fat embolus

Intubation

Short-term intubation (i.e., less than 48 hours)
- For respiration of patients under muscle relaxants, e.g. intubation anesthesia
- In acute obstructive respiratory insufficiency whose cause can probably be relieved within 24–48 hours by minor operative procedures or anti-inflammatory measures such as steroids and antibiotics or which can be relieved in a short period by assisted respiration, assisted respiration as a temporary *emergency measure*
- If a tracheotomy is impossible or contraindicated

Long-term intubation, i.e., for several days or weeks
Long-term intubation should not be undertaken *in adults* because of the great danger of resulting scar tissue stenosis in the larynx or trachea. Also modern forms of tubes and cuffed tubes do not reliably prevent the development of stenosis which may only become manifest several months later. Patients with infections of the airway, those taking steroids, those with hypotension, or those under the influence of intoxicants are particularly at risk.

On the other hand, in *small children* prolonged intubation using the correct technique (transnasal-endotracheal) and inert soft materials often produces fewer complications than a tracheotomy.

SOURCE: Becker W, Naumann HH, Pflatz CR: *Ear, Nose, and Throat Diseases,* p. 444–445. Thieme, New York, 1989.

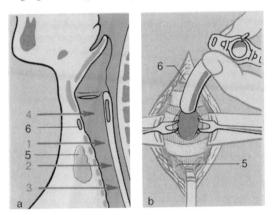

FIGURE 1.47.

a. Operative access for tracheotomy or laryngotomy. **1,** High tracheotomy; **2,** middle tracheotomy; **3,** low tracheotomy; **4,** laryngotomy; **5,** thyroid gland; **6,** cricoid cartilage. **b.** Introduction of a tracheostomy tube into the stoma.

SOURCE: Becker W, Naumann HH, Pfaltz CR: *Ear, Nose, and Throat Diseases,* p. 446. Thieme, New York, 1989.

children. If the isthmus is in the normal position and there is enough time, a middle tracheotomy is preferred because of the lower complication rate.

Principle of the operation. The operation may be carried out under intubation anesthesia using an endotracheal tube or the rigid bronchoscope, or under local anesthesia. A collar incision is made halfway between the suprasternal notch and the superior border of the thyroid cartilage, or a median vertical incision may be used. The trachea is dissected out in the midline, and a window is then created through one or two rings (see Fig. 1.47b). Hemostasis must be secured because of the danger of aspiration of blood. A tracheotomy tube of suitable size is introduced, and the wound is closed as far as possible.

Complications. Intraoperative complications include massive hemorrhage especially by venous congestion or by goiters or tumors overlying the trachea. *Damage to the cricoid cartilage* causes a cricoid stenosis. For this reason, the first tracheal ring should not be included in the tracheostomy if at all possible. *Damage to the pleura* causes pneumothorax, which is more likely if the pleura lies higher than normal. Other complications include recurrent nerve paralysis and *sudden cardiac arrest,* or vasovagal collapse.

Postoperative complications include *secondary hemorrhage* with aspiration of blood from the wound into the trachea, *hemorrhage due to erosion* external to the trachea because of a poorly fitted tube, and *false position of the tube* outside the trachea. In children, the tube may be coughed out if it is not fixed securely. Other complications include emphysema, tracheal stenosis, tracheitis, cervical cellulitis, mediastinitis, pneumonia, lung abscess, esophagotracheal fistula, and difficult decannulation.

Figure 1.48 shows several different types of tracheostomy tubes.

Initially a silver tube is suitable. It has an inner tube that can be removed easily for cleaning and can then be replaced (Fig. 1.48).

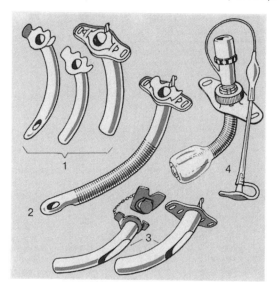

FIGURE 1.48. Various types of tracheostomy tubes.
1, Metal cannula with introducing tube, inner tube, and outer tube; **2,** lobster tail tube; **3,** tube with speaking valve; **4,** inflatable tube with cuff.
SOURCE: Becker W, Naumann HH, Pfaltz CR: *Ear, Nose, and Throat Diseases,* p. 447. Thieme, New York, 1989.

A cuffed tube is used if there is danger of aspiration of blood or secretion. The site of the cuff must be changed, and correct cuff pressure must be used to prevent pressure necrosis of the tracheal wall (Fig. 1.48).

Special tubes include the *lobster tail* tube, which is a flexible elongated tube for use in rigid, curved stenoses. Its disadvantage is that it has no inner tube, and there is therefore the danger of obstruction by crusts, blood clots, or tumors (Fig. 1.48).

A *speaking valve* allows inspiration via the tracheostomy while the expiratory system passes through the larynx (Fig. 1.48).

Plastic tubes are made of several different materials. Their *advantage* is their light weight; their *disadvantage* is that they are easily compressible if the tracheal stenosis tends to increase.

In addition, rigid plastic tubes may be made individually for specific circumstances.

Laryngotomy

This is an emergency procedure. It must be revised as rapidly as possible by a regular tracheostomy because of the danger of laryngeal stenosis.

Principle of the operation (Fig. 1.49). A skin incision is made just superior to the prominent arch of the cricoid cartilage with the head extended. At this point the cricothyroid ligament lies superficially under the skin, and there are no large vessels at this site. The membrane is exposed and a horizontal incision is made in

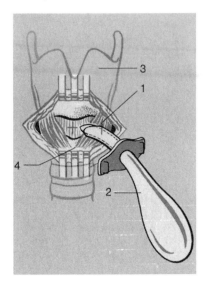

FIGURE 1.49. Laryngotomy.

1, Short cannula mounted over a trocar; **2,** trocar with handle; **3,** thyroid gland; **4,** cricoid cartilage. The cross shows the point at which the conus elasticus is opened.

SOURCE: Becker W, Naumann HH, Pfaltz CR: *Ear, Nose, and Throat Diseases,* p. 448. Thieme, New York, 1989.

it. The incision is held open with a tube or a spreading instrument. A special laryngotomy tube is shown in Figure 1.49.

Note: Laryngotomy should not be carried out if intubation, emergency bronchoscopy, or tracheotomy are feasible. If delay would be life-threatening, laryngotomy can be carried out, if necessary even with a penknife. The incision can then be held open with a piece of rubber tube or other suitable utensil. A definitive tracheotomy must then be carried out as rapidly as possible.

Emergency bronchoscopy is described on page 57 and Figure 1.39a–d.

Intubation. The indications are shown in Table 1.14.

Technique (Fig. 1.50a and 1.50b). Intubation may be carried out *without* anesthesia in patients who are already deeply unconscious; otherwise, a short intravenous anesthetic relaxant is used. The operator must be able to ventilate the patient with a mask, which should be available. The operator must have sufficient practical experience in intubation.

Intubation technique. (1) The position of the patient must be such that the head and neck are mobile and accessible. (2) The blade is introduced and the glottis exposed. (3) The tube, stiffened with a guide wire, is introduced into the trachea through the glottis *under direct vision.* (4) The tube is secured, and the guide wire is withdrawn. Correct positioning of the tube is assessed by the air flow. The tube is connected to a respiratory and fixed with adhesive plaster.

Increasing respiratory obstruction due to tracheal stenosis may not manifest itself for several months.

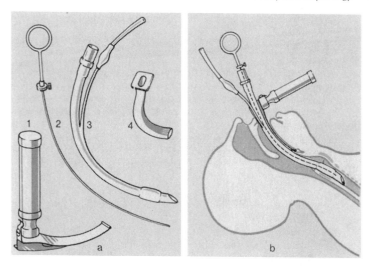

FIGURE 1.50. Intubation.
a. Necessary instruments. **1,** McIntosh laryngoscope; **2,** stylette; **3,** tube with cuff; **4,** Guedel tube. **b.** Introduction of the tube.
SOURCE: Becker W, Naumann HH, Pfaltz CR: *Ear, Nose, and Throat Diseases,* p. 449. Thieme, New York, 1989.

> **Note:** An indwelling tube to provide assisted respiration (e.g., in the intensive care unit or after cervical injuries, etc.) should not be retained for longer than 24–48 h and certainly for no more than 72 h. Otherwise, there is a danger of scar tissue stenosis of the trachea. If assisted respiration is needed for longer periods, the tube should be replaced by a tracheotomy. Infants are an exception because experience has shown that a soft transnasal tube carries less risk than a tracheotomy.

Fast-acting medication to relieve swelling (i.e., in pseudocroup in a child) includes corticosteroids, calcium (and possibly 40% dextrose) dosed according to age, successively intravenously.

Practical Points for the Nursing Care of a Tracheostomy Patient

1. The tube must be cleaned daily or even more often when there are profuse secretions or crusts. Sterile suction catheters must be used, and the hands must be washed.

2. The secretion must be aspirated from the trachea several times daily.

3. The tube must not be left out of the trachea for too long in a recent tracheostomy because it is then difficult to reintroduce. A rubber catheter of a caliber smaller than the lumen of the tracheostomy tube should be available, which can be

inserted into the tracheal lumen and used as a guide over which the tracheostomy tube can be reinserted.

4. Humidification, inhalation, and mucolytic agents should be used to prevent formation of crusts.

5. Five percent saline inhalation solution is used to loosen and remove crusts. This can be achieved by the installation of several drops of 1–2% saline solution with a pipette into the tracheostomy or instillation of several drops of olive oil. Calcium iodate in a 10% solution may be given by mouth in a dose of one tablespoon several times a day.

6. Spring and autumn are particularly dangerous for patients with a tracheostomy because of the increased tendency to tracheitis and tracheobronchitis.

7. A heat and moisture exchanger ("artificial nose") may be attached to the opening of the tracheostomy.

8. The skin around the tracheostomy may be covered with zinc paste if the patient develops dermatitis. Once the acute phase has healed, bland fatty ointments or skin oil are used.

9. Difficulty in breathing through the tracheostomy may be due to the following causes: (a) incorrect reintroduction of the cannula; (b) crusts at the distal end of the tube in the trachea or in the tube itself; (c) granulations of the trachea at the end of the tube; (d) false position of the tube; (e) a tube of wrong shape or width for the individual trachea; (f) stenosis of the tracheobronchial tree beyond the tracheostomy.

10. Bleeding in a tracheostomy may have the following causes: (1) tracheitis; (2) granulations in the trachea; (3) erosive hemorrhage from the brachiocephalic trunk or other vessels surrounding the trachea (e.g., due to a decubitus ulcer caused by the end of the tube); (4) bleeding from a tumor.

Note: Immediate expert advice and assistance should be sought for difficulty in breathing or bloodstained tracheal secretion.

Difficult decannulation. Decannulation may be impossible due to incorrect technique or care of the tracheostomy. Factors include injury to the first tracheal ring or cricoid arch leading to perichondritis of the cricoid cartilage; a hole in the tracheal wall that is too small or too large; granulations around the orifice; tracheomalacia; and extratracheal causes such as goiter or tumor. In these cases, the cause of the stenosis must be dealt with first by reconstruction procedures on the trachea or larynx (see p. 64) or by dealing with the extratracheal cause as appropriate (e.g., by thyroidectomy).

Foreign Bodies

Foreign bodies in the trachea and bronchi usually occur in children, with about 80% occurring between the first and third year of life. Typical foreign bodies include peanuts, nails, needles, buttons, coins, balls, peas, and bits of eggshell.

Symptoms. The main symptoms are episodes of coughing, intermittent or continuous dyspnea, cyanosis, pain, and intermittent hoarseness. Total occlusion of the airway causes sudden death. There may also be apparently symptom-free intervals of days to weeks.

Site. This depends on the size and shape of the foreign body. The most common site is the right main bronchus because of its straighter angle or origin from the trachea. If the foreign body is retained for a longer period, the following occur depending on the type of foreign body and duration: accumulation of secretions; tracheitis or bronchitis with edema, swelling, and granulations; bleeding and bloodstained secretions; inspiratory and expiratory valvular stenoses; partial obstruction of the lower airway or emphysema; atelectasis or overinflation of the poststenotic part of the lung.

Pathogenesis. The cause is usually aspiration. Rare causes include broncholiths (i.e., calcification of retained sputum), rupture of tuberculous lymphadenopathy into the trachea, and ascarides.

Diagnosis. The history shows that the symptoms are of sudden onset, often coinciding with eating. Percussion shows a dampened or hyperresonant note. Auscultation reveals a hissing stenotic noise at the level of the foreign body and bronchi. If the bronchus is occluded, there is cessation of respiratory sounds and delayed movement of one half of the thorax on respiration. *Radiography* includes chest views, tomograms, and bronchography. Holzknecht's symptom consists of oscillation of the mediastinum in bronchial stenosis. Bronchoscopy is the most important therapeutic procedure.

Differential diagnosis. This includes diphtheria, pseudocroup, laryngeal spasm, whooping cough, bronchial asthma, intraluminal tumors, pulmonary tuberculosis, pneumonia, and laryngeal stenosis. Marked up and down movements of the larynx are absent on *tracheal stenoses.*

Treatment. Endoscopy is performed and the foreign body is extracted.

Trauma

Trauma is due to stabbing and gunshot injuries, blunt and penetrating traffic accidents, and injuries to the neck and thorax.

Symptoms. These are always variable. The history indicates the cause.

The main symptoms are dyspnea or danger of suffocation, hemoptysis, escape of air from an unusual site, surgical emphysema, pneumothorax, tension pneumothorax, and atelectasis.

Pathologic anatomy includes rupture of the trachea or bronchi, damage to the great vessels, infection of surrounding structures, and mediastinitis.

Diagnosis. This is made by auscultation, chest radiographs, tomograms, and bronchoscopy.

Treatment. Ruptures or tears of the trachea or main bronchi should be treated as rapidly as possible by exploration of the area, *immediate* suture and introduction of an internal prosthesis, or anastomosis. Peripheral bronchial rupture is treatment by lobectomy. Scar tissue stenosis is described on p. 62.

Tracheoesophageal fistula is dealt with by separation of the two tubes and reconstruction (see p. 65 and Fig. 1.45a–c).

Infections

Tracheitis

Acute tracheitis is often due to spread of a laryngitis or bronchitis, but it may also occur primarily and is usually viral in origin. Chronic tracheitis may occur in chronic inflammation of associated organs such as the sinuses, larynx, and bronchi, and in bronchiectasis. It may also be due to unfavorable climatic and occupational environment, neoplasms, and pulmonary cavities.

Symptoms. These include coughing, retrosternal pain, increased purulent or nonpurulent sputum, occasionally mixed with blood, and mild dyspnea. By itself this disease is not a life-threatening condition and there is no fever.

Treatment. This is the same as for laryngitis (see p. 40).

Acute Laryngotracheobronchitis in Children, Subglottic Laryngitis, Croup

This occurs in infants and young children up to about the age of 3 years. It is a life-threatening disease with a barking cough, stridor, indrawing of the suprasternal notch and of the intercostal spaces, cyanosis, and a moderate fever.

Pathogenesis. Infection by viruses or bacteria produces a serious inflammation of the mucosa of the middle and lower airway with edema, tenacious secretions, and formation of crusts. There is cardiac and circulatory insufficiency and danger of atelectasis or suffocation.

Differential diagnosis. These include epiglottitis and diphteria.

Treatment. Therapy consist of inhalation of oxygen, steroids, humidification of the air, and antibiotics. When severe respiratory obstruction occurs, nasotracheal intubation or tracheotomy are necessary. Sedatives are contraindicated!

Diphtheritis Tracheitis

Main symptoms. The typical signs of diphtheria are found in the larynx or the pharynx. Bits of membrane formed from secretions on the mucosal surface are expectorated.

Treatment. High-dose penicillin and antitoxic serum are given, and tracheotomy is performed if indicated.

Tracheitis Sicca

This usually accompanies rhinitis or laryngitis sicca (sicca syndrome). Dry crusts are coughed out, and there is an audible wheeze.

Treatment. This includes removal of the crusts, liquefying the secretions, inhalation, and humidification of the air.

Rare forms of tracheitis include tuberculosis, sarcoid, stage II and III syphilis, and scleroma

Congenital and Hereditary Anomalies

These include accessory bronchi opening into the trachea, megatrachea, megabronchi, and congenital stenoses of the trachea and bronchi.

Bronchiectases (Cylindrical or Saccular)

This is congenital or acquired, usually affecting the lower lobes on the right more often than the left. *Congenital* forms are due to weakness of the wall of the bronchi or mucoviscidosis. *Acquired* forms are due to bronchitis, emphysema, chronic obstructive bronchitis, and secondary bronchial stenosis. *Kartagener's triad* consist of bronchiectasis, sinusitis, and/or nasal polypi, and situs inversus.

Symptoms. The main symptom is chronic coughing and profuse sputum. Examination demonstrates finger clubbing. Tomograms of the chest and bronchography are carried out.

For further details, see textbooks on internal medicine and pulmonary diseases.

Tumors

Benign tumors of the trachea are very rare and include adenomas (common in the *bronchi*), fibromas, lipomas, chondromas, amyloid tumors, neurinomas, hemangiomas, papillomas (usually accompanied by papillomas of the larynx), and pleomorphic adenomas. An added lesion is an intratracheal goiter, which is thyroid tissue growing into the trachea, usually the posterior wall.

Main symptoms. These include coughing attacks, increasing dyspnea, and occasionally hemoptysis. Pains in the chest, wheezing, and expectoration are less common.

Treatment. The tumor is endoscopically removed, using the laser if possible. Otherwise, the tracheobronchial tree must be opened by the cervical or thoracic route.

Malignant Tracheal Tumors

Adenoid Cystic Carcinoma

This is relatively common in the trachea, where it grows slowly especially along nerve sheaths. It extends very aggressively and tends to produce hematogenous and lymphatic metastases.

Treatment. Extensive surgery is required.

Note. Vague terms such as "semimalignant" or "facultative malignancy" can be fatal for the patient. These terms depend on morphological appearances and not on the clinical course. Adenoid cystic carcinoma must *always* be treated as an extremely aggressive malignant.

Carcinoma

A tumor arising in the *trachea* is relatively unusual. More often the tumor extends from a neighboring organ such as the larynx, esophagus, bronchus, mediastinum, or thyroid gland. The lower half of the trachea is the more common site.

Morphology. Squamous and adenocarcinoma have a roughly equal frequency, and both metastasize frequently.

Main symptoms. These include cough, increasing dyspnea, hemoptysis, and dysphagia. Dysphonia or aphonia occur if the recurrent laryngeal nerve is invaded.

Diagnosis. This rests on radiographs of the chest, tomograms of the trachea, bronchoscopy, which is mandatory, and biopsy.

Treatment. Tumors of the cervical trachea are treated, if possible, by resection and neck dissection. Tracheostomy and later reconstruction may be indicated. Otherwise the patient is irradiated. The long-term prognosis is poor whatever the type of therapy.

Bronchial Carcinoma (Color Plate 22)

About 80% of the lesions occur in men, most commonly between the ages of 50 and 70 years.

Main symptoms. In the early phases the symptoms may be slight. They include attacks of coughing, pains in the chest, difficulty in breathing, sputum, hemoptysis, a feeling of being unwell, loss of weight, and atypical and recurrent infections of the airway with fever, pneumonia, and dyspnea.

Diagnostic procedures. These include chest radiographs, tomograms, bronchoscopy, biopsy, and cytology. Bronchography, possibly needle biopsy, pulmonary function tests, and exploratory thoracotomy are indicated depending on the individual lesion.

Diagnostic and therapeutic details are included in texts on internal medicine and pulmonary surgery.

Congenital Anomalies of the Mouth and Pharynx

Congenital anomalies of the tongue such as cleft tongue, microglossia, aglossia, congenital stenosis of the junction between the nasopharynx and the oropharynx, or stenosis at the junction of the hypopharynx and the esophagus are rare. Macroglossia is much more common and is treated by surgery. Ankyloglossia is caused by a frenulum that is too short; it is corrected by a Z-plasty.

Clefts of the Lip, Jaw, and Palate

One in a thousand members of the White races suffer a congenital cleft of the lip, upper jaw, or palate; the incidence is considerably lower in the Black races, but higher in the Mongolian races. Clefts of the lip, upper jaw, and palate are more common in boys, whereas pure cleft palates are more common in girls. The following types may be distinguished: *cleft lip* (hare lip), *cleft lip and upper jaw, and cleft palate,* and these may be unilateral, bilateral, incomplete, or complete. Complete *clefts of the lip, upper jaw, and palate* may occur. Total cleft, if bilateral, causes the so-called wolf's nose (Fig. 1.51a–c).

Symptoms. The appearances are typical. In infants, there is considerable difficulty in nursing because it is not possible to close the lips and shut off the palate. Food escapes through the nose, and the child tends to aspirate milk into the trachea.

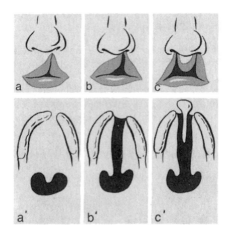

Figure 1.51. Typical cleft formations.
(a) Cleft lip; **(b)** cleft lip and upper jaw; **(c)** bilateral cleft of lip, upper jaw, and palate; **(a′)** cleft upper jaw; **(b′)** cleft upper jaw and palate; **(c′)** bilateral cleft of lip, upper jaw, and palate.
Source: Becker W, Naumann HH, Pfaltz CR: *Ear, Nose, and Throat Diseases,* p. 372. Thieme, New York, 1989.

Infections of the upper and lower airways occur due to disordered swallowing and respiratory physiology. Abnormal tubal function leads to serous otitis media, chronic otitis media, and conductive deafness. The speech is affected with rhinolalia aperta, lisping, abnormal articulation, and velopharyngeal insufficiency. There are anomalies of occlusion and position of the teeth. The nose is almost always involved in clefts of the lips and palate.

Pathogenesis. The cause is probably multifactorial. Embryonic damage is caused by hypoxia, embryopathy, virus infections of the mother, toxins, and genetic lesions. There is familial clustering that is irregularly dominant.

Diagnosis. This is made from the typical facial appearance and examination with the laryngeal mirror.

A *submucous cleft palate* is often overlooked. The clue is a *slight* speech disorder. It is diagnosed by palpation, which shows a bony dehiscence under an intact palatal mucosa.

Complete assessment requires the combined efforts of an ear, nose, and throat surgeon with training in plastic surgery, a phoniatrician, a dentist, an oral surgeon, and an orthodontist, so that all the important aspects and defects may be detected and a common plan of treatment decided upon.

Treatment. Operative treatment is multilayered closure of the defect to form a solid floor of the nose and to correct the nasal deformity. Often many corrective operations and orthodontic and phoniatric assessments and treatments are necessary depending on the type and extent of the defect.

Time Schedule for Correction of Clefts

Cleft lips are corrected between the fourth and sixth (-eighth) months of life by a cheiloplasty with final correction between the fourteenth and sixteenth years of life if necessary.

Cleft lip and maxilla are corrected between the fourth and sixth (-8th) months of life by an operation on the lip and nostril. Final correction may be carried out between the fourteenth and sixteenth years of life. Orthodontic measures begin as necessary from the fifth year of life.

Cleft lip, maxilla, and palate are corrected between the fourth and sixth (-8th) months of life by primary veloplasty and cheiloplasty. The remaining cleft is closed between the twelfth and fourteenth years of life, and a final correction of lip and nose is carried out around the age of 16 years. Speech therapy begins at the age of 4 years, and orthodontic management with an obturator for the remaining cleft from the age of 6 years.

Cleft palate is treated between the fifth and eighth months of life by a primary veloplasty. Speech therapy begins at 4 years, and orthodontic management with an obturator for the remaining cleft from the age of 6 years. The remaining cleft is closed between the twelfth and fourteenth years of life.

Plastic Procedures to Improve Speech

Plastic closure of the cleft is intended to improve the speech and articulation and is successful in about 70% of cases. Tissue available for the repair may be inadequate so that *velopharyngeal insufficiency* persists in some cases and further procedures are necessary. Several reconstructive procedures are available to narrow the pharynx. The principle of a pharyngoplasty is to return the function of the short, immobile insufficient soft palate to as near normal as possible.

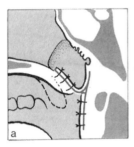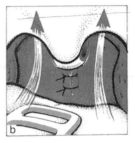

FIGURE 1.52. Pharyngoplasty.
(a) Principle of bridging by a flap pedicled above, (b) view from the mouth.
SOURCE: Becker W, Naumann HH, Pfaltz CR: *Ear, Nose, and Throat Diseases*, p. 374.
Thieme, New York, 1989.

1. Pharyngoplasty is performed with formation of a velopharyngeal flap (Fig. 1.52a and 1.52b). The soft palate is brought into contact with the posterior pharyngeal wall by a soft tissue flap (the Schoenborn–Rosenthal or Sanvenero– Rosselli method).
2. Protrusion of the posterior wall of the pharynx by implantation of autogenous or synthetic material is done to supplement Passavant's bar and to form a mucosal bolster.
3. Posterior displacement, push back, of the soft palate is performed.

Esophagus

Applied Anatomy

The esophagus begins at the level of the lower border of the cricoid cartilage, at the level of the 6th cervical vertebra, and ends at the cardia, which lies at the level of the 11th thoracic vertebra. The opening of the esophagus in the adult lies about 15 cm from the upper incisor teeth and the cardia at about (35 to) 41 cm. The entire length of the esophagus is thus approximately 26 cm.

The wall of the esophagus is capable of expanding and contracting, and is resistant to considerable mechanical stress. The internal lining is of stratified, nonkeratinized squamous epithelium. The external longitudinal musculature and internal circular muscle layer form separate layers of the wall (Fig. 1.53b). There are also muscle fibers running spirally.

The *esophageal musculature* is striated in the upper third, consists of mixed smooth muscle fibers and striated fibers in the middle third, and is almost exclusively smooth muscle in the lower third.

The esophagus has *three physiological sphincters* (Fig. 1.53a):

1. The *upper* is the opening of the esophagus formed by the cricopharyngeus muscle.
2. The *middle* is caused by the crossing of the esophagus by the aortic arch and the left main bronchus. This lies at 27 cm from the incisor teeth in the adult.
3. The *lower* lies at the level of the esophageal hiatus, the cardia.

There are *cervical and thoracic* portions of the esophagus.

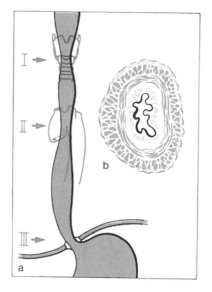

FIGURE 1.53. Esophagus.
a. With the zones of physiologic narrowing, I to III. **b.** Cross-section through the esophageal wall.
SOURCE: Becker W, Naumann HH, Pfaltz CR: *Ear, Nose, and Throat Diseases,* p. 455. Thieme, New York, 1989.

The *blood supply* is segmental as is the lymphatic drainage.

Innervation is mixed somatic from the IXth and Xth cranial nerves and autonomic from the sympathetic nervous system.

Physiology and Pathophysiology

The esophagus possesses its own active motility and also a passive mobility due to respiration and to movement of the neighboring great vessels and the heart. The *act of swallowing* may be divided into an *oral phase,* which is under voluntary control, and a *pharyngeal and esophageal phase.* The latter are under reflex control depending on stimulation of the posterior pharyngeal wall and can be recognized by the elevation of the larynx.

The entrances of the esophagus and the cardia are usually closed. The entrance of the esophagus opens during swallowing, and the cardia opens in response to the oncoming peristaltic wave.

The sphincteric and transport functions can be investigated by the following: radiography with contrast medium, roentgenkymography and manometry (intraluminal measurement of pressure in the esophagus).

Disorders of peristalsis and tone are possible in the following: (1) mechanical obstruction and narrowing, and (2) paralysis of the muscles or nerves.

In *presbyesophagus,* there is a disorder of coordination of the various phases of motility, with increased tertiary contractions and atonic phases. This causes prolonged transit time of food.

Clinical Examination

Inspection and palpation of the external part of the neck shows redness, swelling, tenderness (e.g., over the carotid sheath), venous congestion, and lymphadenopathy. The course of the esophagus should be auscultated. A complete mirror examination of the nose and throat should be carried out; cranial nerve paralyses, particularly of the IXth, Xth, and XIIth cranial nerves, should be looked for, and the pharynx and larynx should be examined.

Respiration

The Lungs

The primary task of the lungs is *respiration*. In addition, they play a role in *metabolism*. They convert, for example, angiotensin I to angiotensin II and remove certain substances (e.g., serotonin) from the circulation. Furthermore, the pulmonary circulation *buffers* the *blood volume* and traps small blood clots (emboli) before they can cause damage in the arterial pathways (heart, brain).

Functions of Respiration

Respiration in its narrowest sense, that is, "external" respiration, is *gaseous exchange* between organism and environment ("internal respiration" =oxidation of nutrients). In contrast to unicellular organisms, if O_2 and CO_2 between cell and environment are sufficiently short, the multicellular human organism requires a special convective transport system for gaseous exchange, that is, the respiratory tract and the circulatory system.

O_2 in the air that is inspired in the course of respiratory movements reaches the *alveoli* of the lungs (*ventilation*), where it diffuses into the blood. The O_2 is transported in the blood to the tissues, where it diffuses to the mitochondria inside the cells. The CO_2 formed here moves in the reverse direction. The respiratory gases are thus alternately transported by *convection* over long distances (ventilation, circulation) and by *diffusion* across thin, limiting membranes (gas/fluid in the alveoli, blood/tissue at the periphery).

About 300 million thin-walled vesicles, the *alveoli* (diameter of about 0.3 mm) form the endings of the terminal branches of the bronchial tree. They are enmeshed in a dense network of *pulmonary capillaries*. The total surface area of the alveoli is about 100 m$_2$. Here, owing to the enormous area, gaseous exchange can take place by diffusion; that is, CO_2 diffuses into the alveoli, and O_2 diffuses out of the alveoli into the blood of the pulmonary capillaries. In this way, the oxygen-deficient ("venous") blood in the pulmonary artery is "arterialized" and, via the left ventricle, once again reaches the periphery.

When the blood is at rest, the heart pumps about 5 l/min blood (*cardiac output*) through the lung and subsequently through the systemic circulation. With this blood flow, roughly 0.3 l/min O_2 are conveyed at rest, from lungs to the periphery (*oxygen consumption* V O_2) and approximately 0.25 l/min CO_2 in the reverse direction (V CO_2). (These are *net values,* i.e., the difference between l/min transported in the arteries and in the veins.)

In order to bring this volume of O_2 from the environment into the alveoli, and to expire the CO_2, a *total ventilation* (V$_T$) of about *7.5 l/min* is necessary. This is achieved by breathing in and out a *tidal volume* (T$_V$) of roughly *0.5 l* about *15 min* (*respiratory frequency f*). Aveolar ventilation (V$_A$) is smaller than T$_V$ because dead space ventilation (V$_D$) makes up a significant fraction of V$_T$.

In a mixture of gases, the *partial pressure* of each gas (the pressure that each gas exerts) equals the total pressure of the gas mixture times the relative fraction (fractional "concentration" F) of the individual gas. The partial pressure of the individual gases adds up to the total gas pressure (*Dalton's law*). At sea level, air has a mean barometric pressure of 101.3 kPa (= 760 mmHg).

Composition of Dry Air

Gas	F (1/1)	P at sea level	
		(kPa)	(mmHg)
O_2	0.209	21.17	158.8
CO_2	0.0003	0.03	0.23
N_2 + inert gases	0.791	80.1	601
Dry air	1.0	101.3	760

During its passage through the respiratory channels (mouth, nose, throat, bronchial system), the inhaled air becomes totally saturated with *water* so that the PH_2O rises to the constant value (at 37°C) of 6.37 kPa (47 mmHG). This causes a drop in the PO_2 from about 21.2 kPa (= 159 mmHg) to 19.9 kPa (149 mmHg), and a corresponding drop in the PN_2. The partial pressures in the alveoli, arterial, and venous blood, and in the expired air, are shown in Figure 1.54.

Respiratory Mechanics

The *driving force for ventilation* is the pressure difference between the atmosphere and the *intrapulmonic pressure* in the alveoli (Ppul, see Fig. 1.56). For inspiration, Ppul must be below the external atmospheric pressure (negative), for expiration it must be above positive (Fig. 1.56). These pressure gradients are established when the lung volume is increased on inspiration and decreased on expiration by action of the diaphragm and thorax (Fig. 1.55).

Inspiration is an *active* process. Muscular contraction increases the volume of the chest, the lungs inflate, and Ppul falls so that air flows into the lungs. At the end of quiet inspiration, the lungs and chest recoil to the positions they occupied at the beginning of inspiration. Thus, quiet expiration is largely a *passive* process.

Respiratory muscles. The *diaphragm* exerts a direct influence on lung volume by contracting (inspiration) and relaxing (expiration). It accounts for 75% of the volume change in quiet inspiration. It moves much as 7 cm on deep inspiration. More indirect influences on inspiration are exerted when the thorax enlarges by contraction of the *scalene* and *external intercostal muscles* and other accessory muscles. The diaphragm or the external intercostal muscles alone can maintain adequate ventilation at rest.

Expiration occurs chiefly by passive recoil. It can be assisted by contraction of the *abdominal muscles,* which increase intra-abdominal pressure, pushing the relaxed diaphragm toward the chest cavity, and by contraction of the *internal intercostal muscles.*

The external intercostal muscles run downward and forward from rib to rib (Fig. 1.55). The attachment of the muscle to the upper rib (B) is closer to the pivot point (A) than the attachment to the lower rib (C′) and to its joint (A′); the lower rib has a longer lever arm (A′−C′ > A −B). Therefore, when the external intercostal muscles contract, they *elevate* the lower rib, which pivots on its joint at the vertebra. This action pushes the sternum outward and increases the anteroposterior diameter of the rib cage. The internal intercostal muscles are oppositely oriented (Fig. 1.55), and their contraction causes the ribs to pivot in the opposite direction.

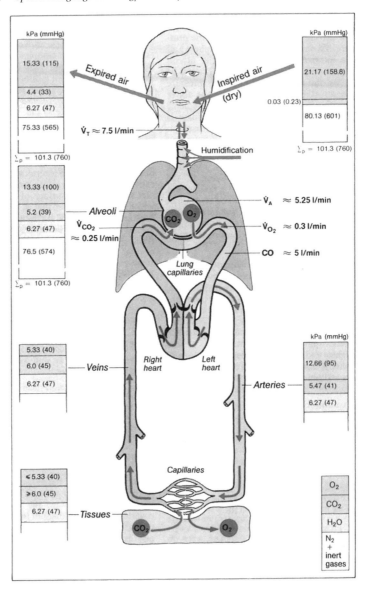

FIGURE 1.54. Respiration

SOURCE: Despopoulos A, Silbernagl S: *Color Atlas of Physiology,* 4th ed., p. 79. New York, Thieme, 1991.

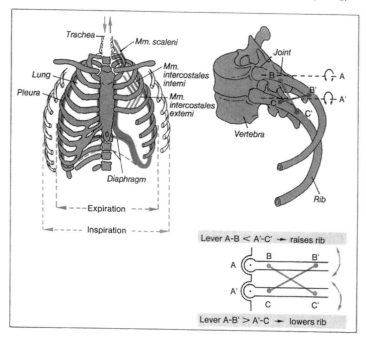

FIGURE 1.55. Respiratory musculature.
SOURCE: Despopoulos A, Silbernagl S: *Color Atlas of Physiology,* 4th ed., p. 81. Thieme, New York, 1991.

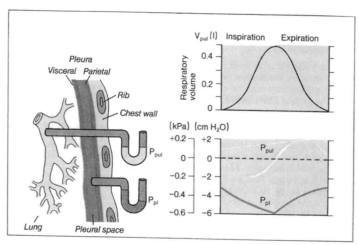

FIGURE 1.56. Intrapleural and intrapulmonary pressures.
SOURCE: Despopoulos A, Silbernagl S: *Color Atlas of Physiology,* 4th ed., p. 81. Thieme, New York, 1991.

In order for the movement of the thorax and diaphragm to help in ventilation, the lungs must follow these movements without, however, being completely fixed to thorax and diaphragm. This is made possible by the presence of a thin layer of fluid between two layers of the *pleura,* one of which covers the lungs (pleura pulmonalis), while the other covers the surrounding organs (*pleura parietalis*).

In their natural position, the lungs tend to "shrink" due to their elasticity and the surface tension of the alveoli. Because the fluid in the pleural space cannot expand, the lungs therefore remain in contact with the inner surface of the thorax, which results in suction, that is, to a negative pressure relative to the surroundings (*intrapleural pressure* or *intrathoracic pressure [Ppl]*; see Fig. 1.56). When the thorax expands during inspiration, the suction becomes stronger, decreasing again at expiration (Fig. 1.56). Only in forced respiration, assisted by the expiratory muscles, can Ppl become positive.

Cleansing of the Inspired Air

Many dirt particles in the inspired air are caught by the *mucus* covering the nasal and pharyngeal cavities, as well as the trachea and the bronchial tree.

In the *bronchial tree* (more than 20 successive branchings), the total cross-sectional area of a set of branches is greater than that of the respective stems from which it arises. Therefore, the air flow produced by the changes in Ppul comes to a stop in the terminal branches of the bronchioles and with it any remaining particles of dust from the outside air. (O_2 and CO_2 cover the remaining few mm to or from the alveoli by diffusion.)

In the bronchial tree, the particles are either phagocytosed on the spot or are returned toward the glottis by the *cilia* of the tracheobronchial epithelium (*mucociliar escalator*). Celia beat 12–20 times/s and propel the mucous film at a speed of about 1 cm/min. Mucus is produced at a rate of 10–100 ml/day, depending on local irritants (e.g., smoke) and on vagal stimulation. The mucus is usually swallowed and its fluid resorbed in the gastrointestinal tract.

Artificial Respiration

Artificial respiration is necessary when spontaneous ventilation is insufficient or fails completely. In these cases, artificial respiration should always be attempted, because the heart continues to function even after respiratory stimuli have ceased. Lack of oxygenation for seconds causes loss of consciousness and for only a few minutes causes irreversible damage to the central nervous system and death.

Mouth-to-mouth respiration is an emergency measure until spontaneous respiration can be restored (Fig. 1.57). In all attempts at artificial respiration, the air passage should be cleared. The subject is turned onto the back with the nose held closed. The first-aid assistant blows into the subject's mouth. This process raises the Ppul (Fig. 1.56) above atmospheric pressure and inflates both the lungs and the chest. Breaking the mouth-to-mouth contact allows expiration as the chest collapses passively by elastic recoil. Pressure applied to the chest can increase the rate and completeness of expiration. The helper inspires fresh air and repeats the cycle about 15 times/min. The O_2 content of the helper's expired air (FEO_2) provides the patient with adequate O_2. The *success of artificial respiration* can be recognized by a change in the patient's skin color from blue (cyanotic) to pink.

A similar principle is involved in *mechanical positive-pressure respiration* that is employed (during narcosis) in operations in which the patient's respiratory musculature is deliberately paralyzed (curare-like substances). Air is blown in

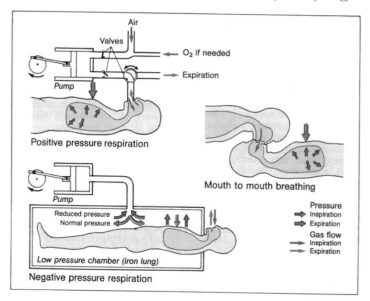

FIGURE 1.57. Artificial respiration.
SOURCE: Despopoulos A, Silbernagl S: *Color Atlas of Physiology,* 4th ed., p. 83. Thieme, New York, 1991.

(inspiration) by a pump (Fig. 1.57 left). The expiration and inspiration pathways in the machine must be well separated (control valve, Fig. 1.57 top), because the dead space would otherwise be too large. This kind of artificial respiration can be performed with a constant volume (*volume controlled*) or at a constant pressure (*pressure controlled*). Each method has its advantages and disadvantages, but in either case, respiration must be continuously monitored (i.e., concentration of expired gases, blood-gas composition, etc.).

The conventional respirator used for the treatment of chronic respiratory insufficiency, as may occur after bulbar poliomyelitis, is the "iron lung" (Fig. 1.57), which provides *mechanical negative-pressure respiration*. The patient is enclosed to the neck in an airtight chamber. Air is pumped out of the chamber to lower the pressure and to permit inspiration. When air is allowed to flow into the chamber again, expiration takes place.

One deficiency of these systems is that they hinder *venous return* to the heart, but this can be partly avoided if expiration as well as inspiration is assisted.

Pneumothorax

Pneumothorax occurs when air enters the pleural space. In *open pneumothorax,* when the chest wall is penetrated, the lung on the open side collapses by elastic recoil and does not contribute to ventilation (Fig. 1.58). Air moves in and out of the pleural space when the subject breathes. Gas exchange in the healthy lung is also compromised because (1) air is exchanged in part with that in the collapsed lung instead of with the external atmosphere, (2) the weight of the collapsed lung prevents full

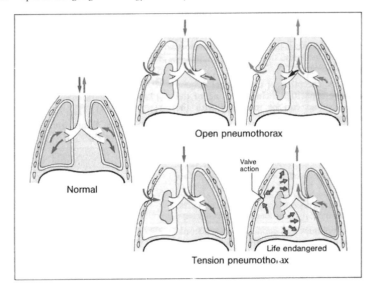

FIGURE 1.58. Pneumothorax.
SOURCE: Despopoulos A, Silbernagl S: *Color Atlas of Physiology,* 4th ed., p. 83. Thieme, New York, 1991.

ventilation, and (3) atmospheric pressure in the pleural space presses the mediastinum into the healthy side. Respiration is stimulated, but distress can be severe. In *tension pneumothorax,* the air entering the pleural space with each respiratory movement is unable to escape (e.g., a flap of tissue on the wound may act as a valve). Pressure in the pleural space on the damaged side becomes positive; the resulting hypoxia elicits a progressive increase in the total ventilatory rate, with the result that pressure may rise to as much as 30 mmHg in the pleural space on the damaged side. The mediastinum shifts to the unaffected side. Cardiac filling is reduced, and peripheral veins distend. Cyanosis develops, and the condition may become fatal if pressure is not relieved by withdrawing air. However, if the hole becomes sealed, Ppl stabilizes, the healthy lung retains its function, and anoxia does not develop. After 1 to 2 weeks, the air pocket is completely absorbed. *Closed pneumothorax* (the most common type of pneumothorax) may develop spontaneously, especially in emphysema, when the lung ruptures through the visceral pleura, so that there is a direct connection between the bronchial system and pleural space. Forced (mechanical) positive-pressure respiration or too rapid surfacing from a dive can also result in closed pneumothorax.

Respiratory Volumes and the Spirometer

In quiet (passive) expiration, the thorax comes to rest at the *resting expiratory level.* Quiet breathing at rest allows a ventilatory exchange of about 0.5 l, the *tidal volume* (VT). An active maximal inspiratory effort allows intake of about 2.5 l of air in excess of the resting VT, the *inspiratory reserve volume.* Beyond the resting expiratory level, however, still more air can be expired; maximum roughly 1.5 l (*expiratory reserve volume*). These two reserve volumes are called upon when, during exertion, the resting tidal volume is inadequate for gas exchange. Even after maximal expiration, some air remains in the lungs; this is the *residual volume*. Sums of these volumes in various combinations are called *capacities*.

The *vital capacity* is the air expired up to maximal expiration following maximal inspiration, and is the sum of the tidal volume + inspiratory reserve volume +expiratory reserve volume (about 4.5 to 5.7 l in a young man 1.8 m in height). The *total lung capacity* includes, in addition to the above three volumes, the residual volume; the *functional residual capacity* is the sum of the expiratory reserve volume and the residual volume.

With the exception of the residual volume and the capacities including it, all of the above values can be measured with the *spirometer* (Fig. 1.59).

It consists of an inverted chamber in a water seal. A subject breathes into and out of the chamber, thus moving an indicator that depicts the magnitude of the corresponding volume change. These movements are recorded as the *spirogram* on a drum moving at a fixed rate, allowing calculations of ventilatory rates as well as volumes, and of values incorporating these data (e.g., compliance, O_2 utilization, dynamic function tests).

These volumes and capacities vary according to height, age, sex, and physical training. The normal value for vital capacity ranges between 2.5 and 7 l in the absence of pulmonary disease.

In order to take into account at least some of the factors that affect the above values, empirical formulae have been introduced for the purpose of standardization. The normal values for VC of Europeans, for instance are:

$$\text{Male: VC (1)} = 5.2\,h - 0.022a - 3.6\,[+ 0.58]$$

$$\text{Female: VC(1)} = 5.2h - 0.018a - 4.6\,[+ 0.42],$$

where h is the height in meters, a the age in years, and the values in brackets represent the standard deviations.

Even with the help of these formulae, only relatively large deviations from the norm are detectable. More informative are the measurements of lung volumes, which, if measured repeatedly in the same subject, reflect for instance the changes accompanying the course of a pulmonary disease.

Conversion of gas volumes. The volume [l] of a quantity of gas n[mol] depends on the absolute temperature $T[K]$ and the total pressure P[kPa], that is, the barometric pressure PB minus water vapor pressure PH_2O:

$$V = n \cdot R \cdot T/P,$$

where R = general gas constant = 8.31 J. $K - 1$. mol $- 1$.

A distinction is made between the following conditions:

STPD: Standard Temperature Pressure Dry (273 K; 101 kPa; $PH_2O = 0$)
ATPS: Ambient Temperature Pressure H_2O-Saturated (Tamb; PB; PH_2O)
BTPS: Body Temperature Pressure H_2O-Saturated (310K; Pb; $PH_2O = 6.25$ kPa)

and hence:

VSTPD = $n \cdot R \cdot 273/101$
VATPS = $n \cdot R \cdot$ Tamb/(PB − PH_2O)
VBTS = $n \cdot r \cdot 310/($PB − 6.25$)$
VSTPD/VBTPS, for example, therefore amounts to 273/310 · PB − 6.25/101.

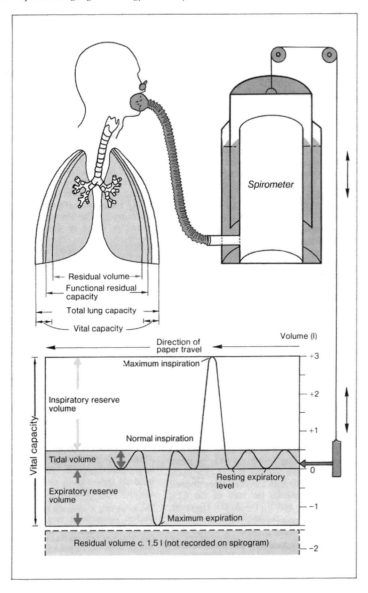

FIGURE 1.59. Measurement of lung volumes.

SOURCE: Despopoulos A, Silbernagl S: *Color Atlas of Physiology,* 4th ed., p. 85. Thieme, New York, 1991.

Anatomy of the Respiratory System

Figure 1.60 ABC

1 **NASAL CAVITY,** "cavitas nasi." **A B C**

2 **Nostrils,** "nares." Framed by nasal wings. **B C**

3 **Posterior nares,** "choanae." **C**

4 **Nasal septum,** "septum nasi." The osseous, cartilaginous, and fibrous nasal septum. **C**

5 **Membranous part,** "pars membranacea." Fibrous portion of nasal septum at tip of nose. **C**

6 **Osseous part,** "pars ossea." Bony section of nasal septum, perpendicular plate of ethmoid bone and vomer. **C**

7 **Vomeronasal** or **Jacobson's organ,** "organum vomeronasale [Jacobsoni]." Occasionally occurring blind sack above incisive canal, a remnant of a phylogenetically earlier accessory olfactory organ. **A C**

8 **Vestibule,** "vestibulum nasi." Anterior section of nasal cavity extending to limen nasi, lined with squamous epithelium that changes into ciliated epithelium at limen nasi. **A B**

9 **"Limen nasi."** Ridge at the end of vestibule formed by margin of greater alar cartilage. **A B**

10 **Olfactory sulcus,** "sulcus olfactorius." Groove between root of middle concha and bridge of nose, extending to olfactory area. **A B**

11 **Superior nasal concha,** "concha nasalis superior." Small, upper concha located in front os sphenoidal sinus. **A B**

12 **Middle nasal concha,** "concha nasalis media." Most of openings of paranasal sinuses lie beneath it. **A B**

13 **Inferior nasal concha,** "concha nasalis inferior." Longest concha; masks opening of nasolacrimal duct. **A B**

14 **Nasal mucosa,** "tunica mucosa nasi." Consists primarily of pseudostratified columnar, ciliated epithelium.

15 **Respiratory region,** "regio respiratoria." Portion of mucosa with ciliated epithelium. Commences in vestibule, and exception for olfactory region, covers entire nasal cavity.

16 **Olfactory region,** "regio olfactoria." Area about the size of a nickel; lies superiorly beneath cribriform plate on nasal septum and lateral nasal wall; equipped with olfactory cells. **A**

17 **Cavernous conchal plexus,** "plexus cavernosi choncharum." Venous plexus, particularly in area of inferior concha and posterior portion of nasal cavity.

18 **Ridge of nose,** "agger nasi." Slightly elevated, rounded remains of an earlier accessory concha located directly in front of middle concha. **A**

19 **Sphenoethmoidal recess,** "recessus sphenoethmoidalis." Recess above superior nasal concha between anterior wall of sphenoidal sinus and roof of nose. **A**

20 **Superior nasal meatus,** "meatus nasi superior." Between superior and middle nasal concha. **A**

21 **Middle nasal meatus,** "meatus nasi medius." Between middle and inferior nasal conchae. **A**

22 **Atrium of middle meatus,** "atrium meatus medii." Area in front of middle and above inferior concha. **A**

23 **Inferior nasal meatus,** "meatus nasi inferior." Between inferior nasal concha and floor of nose. **A**

24 **Nasopharyngeal meatus,** "meatus nasopharyngeus." Junction of three nasal meatus behind conchae. **A**

25 **Incisor duct,** "ductus incisivus." Occasionally occurring blind sack on floor of nasal cavity beside septum, about 2 cm behind external nasal opening. **A**

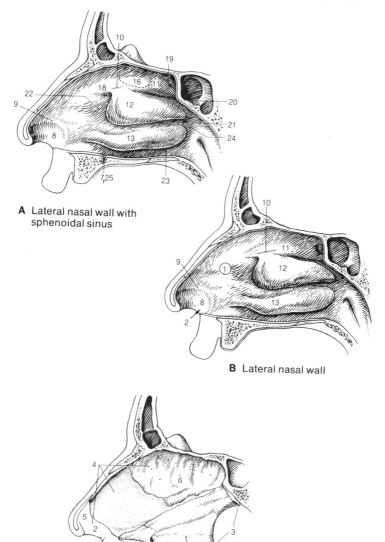

A Lateral nasal wall with sphenoidal sinus

B Lateral nasal wall

C Nasal septum

FIGURE 1.60.
SOURCE: Feneis H: *Pocket Atlas of Human Anatomy,* 2nd ed., p. 137. Thieme, New York, 1985.

Figure 1.61 ABCD

1 **PARANASAL SINUSES**, "nasi paranasales." **A B**

2 **Maxillary sinus**, "sinus maxillaris." Located below orbit and lateral to nose. Opens into middle meatus.

3 **Sphenoidal sinus**, "sinus sphenoidalis." Paired air cells located in body of sphenoid bone behind sphenoethmoidal recess and above nasopharynx; opens into sphenoethmoid recess. **B**

4 **Frontal sinus**, "sinus frontalis." Located in squama of frontal bone, but often also in orbital portion of frontal bone; opens into middle meatus. **A B**

5 **Ethmoid sinus**, "sinus ethmoidales." A system of pea-sized air cells between nasal and orbital cavities comprised of three groups (6–8). **A**

6 **Anterior cells**, "cellulae anteriores." Ethmoidal cells that open under middle concha. **A**

7 **Middle cells**, "cellulae mediae." Ethmoidal cells that open under superior concha. **A**

8 **Posterior cells**, "cellulae posteriores." Ethmoidal cells that open under superior concha. **A**

9 **Ethmoidal bulla**, "bulla ethmoidalis." Rudimentary nasal concha shaped like an ethmoidal air cell that bulges into midline nasal meatus. **B**

10 **Ethmoidal infundibulum**, "infundibulum ethmoidale." Recess in front of ethmoidal bulla beneath middle nasal concha. The maxillary and frontal sinuses open here. **B**

11 **Semilunar hiatus**, "hiatus semilunaris." Sickle-shaped cleft between ethmoidal bulla and uncinate process. **B**

12 **"LARYNX."** Located between pharynx and trachea. **C**

13 **Laryngeal cartilages**, "cartilagines laryngis." Cartilages forming laryngeal skeleton.

14 **Thyroid cartilage**, "cartilago thyroidea." Largest cartilage of larynx, partially surrounding the others. **C D**

15 **Laryngeal prominence**, "prominentia laryngea." Elevation in midline of neck formed by thyroid cartilage. More pronounced in the male (Adam's apple). **C D**

16 **Right and left lamina**, "lamina (dextra et sinistra)." Lateral plates of thyroid cartilage uniting in midline like bow of a ship. **C D**

17 **Superior thyroid notch**, "incisura thyroidea superior." Deep notch in midline; located superiorly between right and left plates of thyroid cartilage. **C D**

18 **Inferior thyroid notch**, "incisura thyroidea inferior." Shallow notch in midline on lower margin of thyroid cartilage. **D**

19 **Superior thyroid tubercle**, "tuberculum thyroideum superius." Small, lateral elevation on upper end of oblique line on outer surface of lamina of thyroid cartilage. **C D**

20 **Inferior thyroid tubercle**, "tuberculum thyroideum inferius." Small, lateral elevant on lower end of oblique line. **C D**

21 **Oblique line**, "linea obliqua." Diagonal ridge on outer surface of thyroid cartilage for attachment of sternothyroid, thyrohyoid m.'s and inferior constrictor m. of pharynx. **C D**

22 **Superior horn**, "cornu superius." Superior process of thyroid cartilage for attachment of thyrohyoid lig. **C D**

23 **Inferior horn,** "cornu inferius." Inferior process on osterior margin of thyroid cartilage for articulation with cricoid cartilage. **C D**

24 **Thyroid foramen,** "formen thyroideum." Occasionally occurring hole located laterally beneath superior tubercle, sometimes providing passage for superior laryngeal a. and vein. **C**

25 **Thyrohyoid membrane,** "membrana thyrohoidea." Elastic membrane between upper posterior margin of hyoid bone and thyroid cartilage. **C**

26 **Medium thyrohyoid ligament,** "ligament thyrohyoideum medianum." Reinforcement of thyrohyoid membrane in midline, with numerous elastic fibers. **C**

27 **Lateral thyrohyoid ligament,** "ligament thyrohyoideum laterale." Connects superior thyrohyoid process to posterior end of greater horn of hyoid bone. Reinforces thyrohyoid membrane laterally. **C**

28 **Triticeal cartilage,** "cartilago triticea." Wheat-kernel-sized elastic cartilage in thyrohyoid ligament. **C**

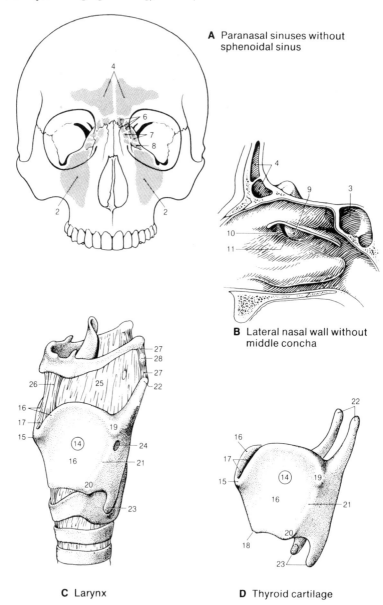

A Paranasal sinuses without sphenoidal sinus

B Lateral nasal wall without middle concha

C Larynx

D Thyroid cartilage

FIGURE 1.61.
SOURCE: Feneis H: *Pocket Atlas of Human Anatomy,* 2nd ed., p. 139. Thieme, New York, 1985.

Figure 1.62 ABCD

1 **Cricoid cartilage,** "cartilago cricoidea." Located at upper end of trachea; articulates with thyroid cartilage. **A B D**

2 **Arch of cricoid cartilage,** "arcus cartilaginous cricoideae." Constitutes anterior and lateral portions of this cartilage. **A B**

3 **Lamina of cricoid cartilage,** "lamina cartilaginis cricoideae." Posteriorly located wide plate or cricoid cartilage. **A B**

4 **Articular surface for arytenoid cartilage,** "facies articularis arytenoidea." Obliquely placed, oval surface located laterally on upper margin of lamina of cricoid cartilage. **A**

5 **Articular surface for thyroid cartilage,** "facies articularis thyroidea." Prominent surface located laterally on lamina. **A**

6 **Cricothyroid articulation,** "articulatio cricothyroidea." Joint between thyroid and cricoid cartilages permitting tilting as well as horizontal and vertical gliding movements. **B**

7 **Articular capsule of cricothyroid articulation,** "capsula articularis cricothyroidea." **B**

8 **Cricothyroid ligament,** "ligament cricothyroideum." Strong vertical band in midline between thyroid and cricoid cartilages. **B D**

9 **Cricotracheal ligament,** "ligament cricotracheale." Elastic membrane between cricoid cartilage and first tracheal cartilage. **B D**

10 **Arytenoid cartilage,** "cartilago arytenoidea." Pyramidal cartilage resting upon the cricoid cartilage. **C D**

11 **Articular surface,** "facies articularis." Concave surface beneath muscular process that guides movement on cricoid cartilage. **C**

12 **Base of arytenoid cartilage,** "basis cartilaginis arytenoideae." **C**

13 **Anterolaterial surface,** "facies anteriolaterlis." Serves as area of m. attachment. **C**

14 **Arcuate crest,** "crista arcuata." Cartilaginous ridge, which starts between oblong and triangular foveae, arches around latter and terminates at colliculus. **C**

15 **"Colliculus."** Small elevation at end of acrucate crest. **C D**

16 **Oblong fovea,** "fovea oblonga." Depression located anteroinferiorly for insertion of thyroarytenoid m. **C**

17 **Triangular fovea,** "fovea triangularis." Depression above oblong fovea filled with glands. **C**

18 **Medial surface,** "facies medialis." Medial surface of arytenoid cartilage. **C**

19 **Dorsal surface,** "facies posterior." Posterior surface of arytenoid cartilage. **C**

20 **Apex of arytenoid cartilage,** "apex cartilaginis arytenoideae." Directed posteriorly. **C D**

21 **Vocal process,** "processus vocalis." Anteriorly directed process for vocal cord attachment. **C**

22 **Muscular process,** "processus muscularis." Short, posterolaterial process for insertion of posterior and lateral cricoarytenoid muscles. **C**

23 **Cricoarytenoid articulation,** "articulatio cricoarytenoidea." Roller-like joint between arytenoid and cricoid cartilages, permitting oscillatory movement around obliquely placed axis and gliding movement parallel to axis. **D**

24 **Cricoarytenoid articular capsule,** "capsula articularis cricoarytenoidea."
   Thin-walled, flaccid capsule between arytenoid and cricoid cartilages. **D**

25 **Posterior cricoarytenoid ligament,** "ligament cricoarytenoideum pos-
   terius." Elastic ligament important for closure of fissure of glottis; runs
   from lamina of cricoid cartilage posteriorly to medial portion of arytenoid
   cartilage. **D**

26 **Cricopharyngeal ligament,** "ligament cricopharyngeum." Fibrous band
   beginning at corniculate cartilage; attaches to posterior surface of cricoid
   cartilage and continues into pharyngeal mucosa covering this surface. **D**

27 **Sesamoid cartilage,** "cartilago sesamoidea." Occasionally occurring
   small elastic cartilages in anterior ends of vocal cords, adjacent to arytenoid cartilage. **D**

28 **Corniculate or Santorini's cartilage,** "cartilago corniculate [Santorini]."
   Small, elastic cartilage on apex of arytenoid cartilage, forming corniculate
   tubercle. **C D**

29 **Corniculate tubercle,** "tuberculum corniculatum." Tubercle, covered by
   mucosa, above the cartilage of same name directly above the typ of the
   arytenoid cartilage.

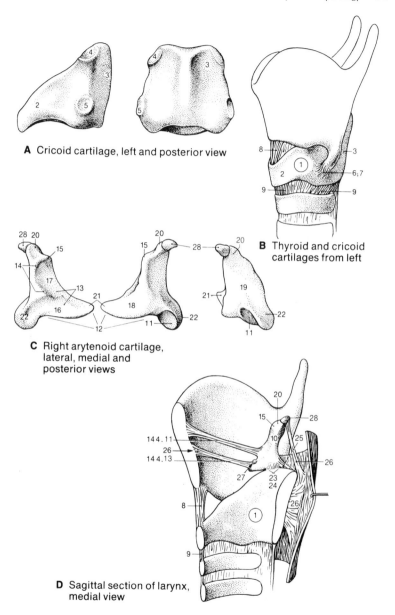

A Cricoid cartilage, left and posterior view

B Thyroid and cricoid cartilages from left

C Right arytenoid cartilage, lateral, medial and posterior views

D Sagittal section of larynx, medial view

FIGURE 1.62.

SOURCE: Feneis H: *Pocket Atlas of Human Anatomy,* 2nd ed., p. 141. Thieme, New York, 1985.

Figure 1.63 ABCDE

1 **Cuneiform or Wrisberg's cartilage,** "cartilago cuneifromis." Small cartilage occasionally present beneath a group of glands in aryepiglottic fold. **D**

2 **Cuneiform tubercle,** "tuberculum cuneiforme." Small elevation in aryepiglottic fold above cuneiform cartilage. In the absence of cartilage it can be formed by glands alone. **B D**

3 **"Epiglottis."** Consists of elastic cartilage shaped like a shoehorn. **B C D E**

4 **Stem of epiglottis,** "petiolus epiglottidis." Directed inferiorly; attaches to thyroid cartilage by connective tissue. **A D**

5 **Epiglottic tubercle,** "tuberculum epiglotticum." Small elevation on posterior mucosal surface over epiglottic stem. **B**

6 **Epiglottic cartilage,** "cartilago epiglottica." Skeleton of epiglottis made up of elastic cartilage. **A C D**

7 **Thyroepiglottic ligament,** "ligament thyroepiglotticum." Serves to fix stem of epiglottis on posterior surface of thyroid cartilage. **A D**

8 **Hyoepiglottic ligament,** "ligament hyoepiglotticum." Between hyoid bone and epiglottis. **C**

9 **Corniculate tubercle,** "tuberculum corniculatum." Mucosal elevation over corniculate cartilage immediately above apex of arytenoid cartilage. **B D**

10 **Muscles of larynx,** "mm. laryngis." **B C D E**

11 **Aryepiglottic muscle,** "m. aryepiglotticus." O: apex of arytenoid cartilage. I: lateral margin of epiglottis. Forms base of aryepiglottic fold. A: lowers epiglottis. **B D**

12 **Cricothyroid muscle,** "m. cricothyroideus." O: anteriorly on outer side of cricoid cartilage. I: inferiorly on outer and inner surfaces of lamina of thyroid cartilage. A: tenses the vocal cords by lowering and drawing thyroid cartilage forward. **C E**

13 **Straight part,** "pars recta." Anterior, more vertically oriented fibers. **C**

14 **Oblique part,** "pars obliqua." Posterior, more horizontally oriented fibers. **C**

15 **Posterior cricoarytenoid muscle,** "m. cricoarytenoideus posterior." O: posterior surface of cricoid cartilage. I: muscular process of arytenoid cartilage. A: opens glottis by swinging vocal process upward and outward. **B D**

16 **Ceratocricoid muscle,** "m. ceratocricoideus." Variation. O: inferior horn of thyroid cartilage. I: lower margin of cricoid cartilage. **B**

17 **Lateral cricoarytenoid muscle,** "m. cricoarytenoideus lateralis." O: upper portion of lateral margin of cricoid cartilage. I: anteriorly, on muscular process of arytenoid cartilage and adjacent area. A: aids in closing of glottis. **D**

18 **Vocal muscle,** "m. vocalis." O: inner surface of thyroid cartilage near midline. I: vocal process and oblong fovea of arytenoid cartilage. A: varying degrees of tension alter the quality of vibration of vocal cord. **E**

19 **Thyroepiglottic muscle,** "m. thyroepiglotticus." O: inner surface of anterior part of thyroid cartilage. I: epiglottis and quadrangular membrane. **D**

20 **Thyroarytenoid muscle,** "m. thyroarytenoideus." O: anterior, inner surface of thyroid cartilage. I: muscular process and lateral surface of arytenoid cartilage. A: aids in closure of glottis. **D E**

21 **Oblique arytenoid muscle,** "m. arytenoideus obliquues." O: posterior surface of muscular process. I: apex of opposite arytenoid cartilage. A: brings the arytenoid cartilages together and aids in closure of glottis. **B**

22 **Transverse arytenoid muscle,** "m. arytenoideus transversus." O: posterior surface of arytenoid cartilage. I: same as origin. A: brings the arytenoid cartilages together and aids in closure of glottis. **B**

23 **Laryngeal cavity,** "cavitas laryngis." Internal space of larynx. **E**

24 **Entrance to larynx,** "aditus laryngis." Between epiglottis, the aryepiglottic folds and interarytenoid inncisure. **B E**

25 **Aryepiglottic fold,** "plica aryepiglottica." Mucosal fold over homonymous m., of running from apex of arytenoid cartilage to lateral margin of epiglottis. **B D**

26 **Interoarytenoid incisure,** "incisura interarytenoidea." Mucosal slit between both tips of the arytenoid cartilage. **B**

27 **Laryngeal vestibule,** "vestibulum laryngis." Upper part of laryngeal cavity down to vestibular [ventricular] fold. **E**

28 **"Rima vestibuli."** Cleft between the two vestibular folds [plicae vestibulares]. **E**

29 **Vestibular or ventricular fold,** "plica vestibularis [ventricularis]." False vocal cord. Fold caused by vestibular ligament located between laryngeal ventricle and vestibule. **E**

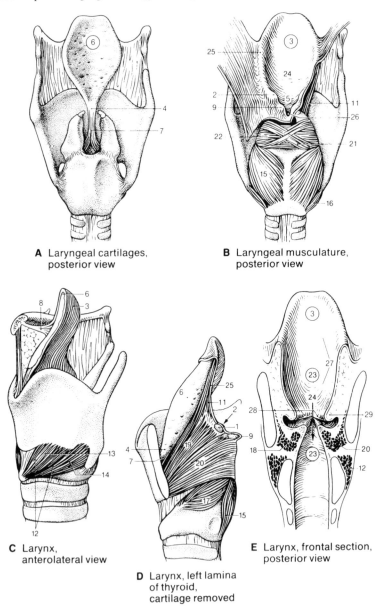

A Laryngeal cartilages, posterior view

B Laryngeal musculature, posterior view

C Larynx, anterolateral view

D Larynx, left lamina of thyroid, cartilage removed

E Larynx, frontal section, posterior view

FIGURE 1.63.

SOURCE: Feneis H: *Pocket Atlas of Human Anatomy,* 2nd ed., p. 143. Thieme, New York, 1985.

Figure 1.64 ABCDEFGH

1 **Laryngeal ventricle,** "ventriculus laryngis." Lateral recess between the vocal and ventricular folds. **B D C**

2 **Laryngeal sacuule,** "sacculus laryngis [appendix ventriculi laryngi]." Small, blind sack of laryngeal ventricle directed upward. **B**

3 **"Glottis." Voice-producing part of larynx, including the two vocal folds.** A

4 **Fissure of glottis,** "rima glottidis." Cleft between the two arytenoid cartilages and the vocal cords. **A**

5 **Vocal fold,** "plica vocalis." Mucosal fold supported below by vocal ligament and laterally by vocal m. **A**

6 **Intermembranous part,** "pars intermembranacea." Part of fissure of glottis running from thyroid cartilage to apex of vocal process. **A**

7 **Intercartilaginous part,** "pars intercartilaginea." Part of fissure of glottis lying between arytenoid cartilages. **A**

8 **Infraglottic space,** "cavitas infraglottica." Space below fissure of glottis surrounded by elastic cone. **C**

9 **Fibroelastic membrane of larynx,** "membrana fibroelastica laryngis [membrana elastica laryngis]." Tela submucosa of larynx, richly supplied with elastic fibers; starts at quadrangular membrane and terminates at lower edge of elastic cone. **B**

10 **Quadrangular membrane,** "membrana quandrangularis." Membrane between epiglottis and aryepiglottic and ventricular folds. **D**

11 **Vestibular ligament,** "ligament vestibulare." Reinforces inferior margin of quadrangular membrane. **C**

12 **Elastic cone,** "conus elasticus." Reinforced fibroelastic membrane between vocal lig. and cricoid cartilage. **D**

13 **Vocal ligament,** "ligament vocale." Vocal cord stretched between vocal process of arytenoid and thyroid cartilage. Forms upper limit of elastic cone. **C**

14 **Mucosa,** "tunica mucosa." Only posterosuperior surface of epiglottis and the vocal folds are covered with noncornified, stratified squamous epithelium; rest of larynx is lined with pseudostratified ciliated columnar epithelium. **B**

15 **[Laryngeal glands,** "glandulae laryngeae."] Submucosal mixed glands of laryngeal tunica mucosa. **B**

16 **Laryngeal lymphatic follicles,** "noduli (folliculi) lymphatici laryngis." Located principally in submucosa of ventricle. **B**

17 **"TRACHEA." Trachea and its branches, the bronchial tubes.** E

18 **Cervical part,** "pars cervicalis." Portion of trachea located between 6th and 7th cervical vertebrae.

19 **Thoracic part,** "pars thoracica." Chest section of trachea, reaching from 1st to 4th thoracic vertebrae inclusive.

20 **Tracheal cartilages,** "cartilagines tracheales." Horseshoe-shaped cartilages supporting tracheal wall. **E F H**

21 **Tracheal muscle,** "m. trachealis." Smooth m. fibers between free ends of tracheal cartilages. **H**

22 **Annular ligaments,** "ligamenta annularia (trachealia)." Connective tissue bridges between tracheal cartilages. **E F**

23 **Membranous wall,** "paries membranaceus." Posterior wall of trachea. **F**

24 **Bifurcation of trachea,** "bifurcatio tracheae." At level of T 4. **E G**

25 **Carina of trachea,** "carcina tracheae." Crest projecting into tracheal lumen at point of bifurcation, exerting an aerodynamic effect. **G**

26 **Mucosa,** "tunica mucosa." Ciliated columnar epithelium lining air passages. **H**

27 **Tracheal glands,** "glandulae tracheales." Mixed submucosal glands. **H**

28 **"BRONCHI."** Branches of trachea.

29 **Bronchial system,** "arbor bronchialis." Complete branching system of bronchi.

30 **Right and left primary bronchus,** "bronchus principalis (dexter et sinister)." Stem bronchus arising directly from trachea. **E**

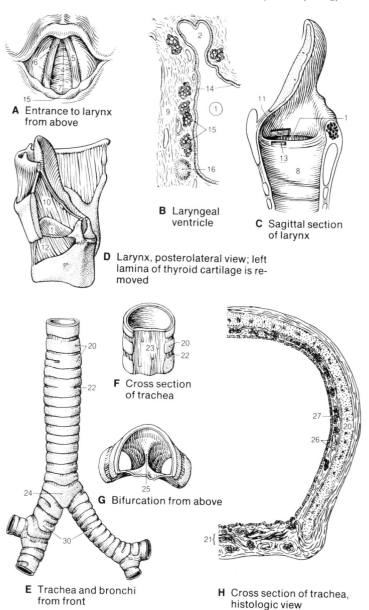

A Entrance to larynx from above

B Laryngeal ventricle

C Sagittal section of larynx

D Larynx, posterolateral view; left lamina of thyroid cartilage is removed

F Cross section of trachea

G Bifurcation from above

E Trachea and bronchi from front

H Cross section of trachea, histologic view

FIGURE 1.64.

SOURCE: Feneis H: *Pocket Atlas of Human Anatomy,* 2nd ed., p. 145. Thieme, New York, 1985.

The Nervous System

Brain Function (*Figure 1.65A–C*)

The central nervous system helps the organism to adapt to its environment and survive. It receives stimuli from outside and inside the body through the sense organs, filters them, and processes them into information. In accordance with the information received, it sends back impulses to the periphery of the body, so that the organism can react appropriately to constantly changing situation. The functional systems described below are in no sense independent, isolated apparatuses. The highly simplified, schematic information presented here can only serve as an approximation of the extraordinarily complex interrelationships between billions of nerve cells.

The simple, mechanistic idea that sensory impressions reach the brain, which then produces motor reactions in response, has existed for centuries. According to *Descartes*, optical stimuli are transmitted from the eye to the pineal body (epiphysis), from which impulses are sent to the musculature (**A**). He considered the pineal body to be the seat of the soul. *Franz Gall* was the first to postulate that the convolutions of the brain and the cortex were significant for brain function. He localized the "organs of the soul" as being on the surface of the hemispheres and believed he could demonstrate their varying degrees of development by examining the external surface of the skull (phrenology) (**B**). His localizations, in Roman numerals, included I, reproductive instinct; II, love for offspring; III, friendship; IV, bravery; V, the instinct to eat meat; VI, intelligence; VII, greed; kleptomania; VIII, pride, arrogance; IX, vanity, ambitiousness, and so on.

On the basis of injuries to the brain, *Kleist* produced a localization of the higher cerebral functions (**C**). He assumed that, corresponding to the negative findings in pathological deficits of cognition, thinking, motivation, action, and so on, there must be positive capacities, termed "functions." This is not the case. Symptoms of deficits can be localized, but not functions (*von Monakow*). Critics of the theory of localization and brain centers spoke of a "brain mythology." Ultimately, specific functions are not attributable to specific areas of the brain because innumerable other groups of neurons constantly influence a particular capacity by stimulating it, inhibiting it, or modulating it. The various so-called "centers" can at best only be seen as important relay stations for a specific capacity. Nor is the central nervous system a rigid apparatus; it shows considerable *plasticity*. Especially in infant brains, other centers can take over functions vicariously when injuries occur. A degree of plasticity in the central organ is also a prerequisite for the ability to learn (language, writing, physical abilities).

Information processing in the telencephalon is termed *integration*. This is a combination and interconnection of all the sense impressions that incorporate stored experience to form a higher, complex functional unit. In this way, the organism's various abilities are controlled through meticulous mutual coordination between groups of neurons. During the course of evolution, these integrative processes in man have developed from regulating and coordinating elementary biological tasks into conscious knowledge, thinking, and action. Cybernetics and computer technology have provided us with models of brain function (cognitive science). These suggest that the various "functions" are based on constantly alternating stimulation in interconnected neuronic control circuits.

In spite of highly developed instrument technology, only one instrument is ultimately available to us for research on the brain: the brain itself. Thus, one of the organs of the human body is involved in an attempt to discover its own structure and functioning.

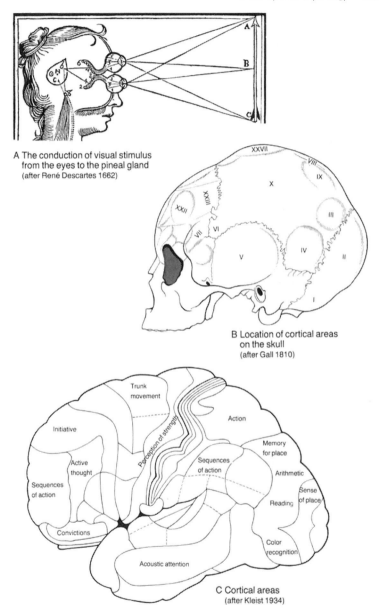

A The conduction of visual stimulus
from the eyes to the pineal gland
(after René Descartes 1662)

B Location of cortical areas
on the skull
(after Gall 1810)

C Cortical areas
(after Kleist 1934)

FIGURE 1.65.
SOURCE: Kahle W, Leonhardt H, Platzer W: *Color Atlas/Text of Human Anatomy, Vol. 3: Nervous System and Sensory Organs,* 4th rev. ed., p. 285. Thieme, New York, 1993.

Motor Systems

Pyramidal Tract (Figure 1.66 A and B)

The *corticospinal tract* and the *corticoconuclear fibers* are regarded as the pathways for control of voluntary movement. Through them the cortex regulates the subcortical motor centers. It may have a retarding or inhibitory effect, but also produces a constant tonic excitation through which sudden, rapid movements are promoted. Automatic and stereotyped movements, which are under the control of subcortical motor centers, are thought to be modified by the influence of pyramidal tract impulses, so that purposeful and directly controlled movements are achieved.

The pyramidal tract fibers arise in the precentral fields 4 and 6 (**A1**), in parietal lobe fields of areas 3, 1, and 2, and in the secondary sensorimotor region (area 40). About two-thirds stem from the precentral region and one-third from the parietal lobe. Only 60% of the fibers are myelinated, and the remaining 40% are unmyelinated. The thick fibers of the giant pyramidal cells in area 4 comprise only 2–3% of all myelinated fibers. All the other fibers arise from smaller pyramidal cells.

Fibers of the pyramidal tract traverse the internal capsule. At the transition to the midbrain, they occupy the base of the brain where, together with the corticopontine tracts, they form the cerebral peduncles. The pyramidal tract fibers occupy the middle of the peduncles and most laterally lie the fibers from the parietal cortex (**B2**). Next to them in sequence, are the corticospinal tracts for the lower limb (**LS**), trunk (T), upper limb (C), and corticobullar fibers for the face region (**B3**). During their passage through the pons, they rotate so that the corticobulbar fibers now lie dorsally, followed by the bundles that run to the cervical, thoracic, lumbar, and sacral regions. In the medulla, the corticonuclear fibers terminate on cranial nerve nuclei. Seventy to 90% of fibers cross to the opposite side in the pyramidal decussation (**AB4**) and form the *lateral corticospinal tract* (**AB5**). The fibers for the upper limb cross dorsal to the fibers to the lower limb. In the lateral pyramidal tract, fibers for the upper limb lie medially, and the long fibers for the lower limb lie laterally. The uncrossed fibers run on in the *ventral corticospinal tract* (**AB6**) and cross in the white commissure to the other side only at the level at which they terminate. The ventral tract is variable in size and may be asymmetrical, or may be completely absent. It only extends in the spinal cord as far as the cervical or thoracic region.

The majority of pyramidal tract fibers end on interneurons in the intermediate zone between the anterior and posterior horns. Only a small number reach the motor anterior horn cells, principally those which supply the distal parts of the extremities. They are particularly under the discrete influence of the pyramidal tract. Pyramidal tract impulses activate neurons that supply flexor muscles and inhibit those neurons that supply extensors. Fibers that arise in the parietal lobe end in posterior funicular nuclei (*nucleus gracilis* and *nucleus cuneatus*) and the *substantia gelatinosa* of those posterior horn. They regulate the input of sensory impulses. The pyramidal tract is therefore not a single motor tract but contains a number of functionally different descending systems.

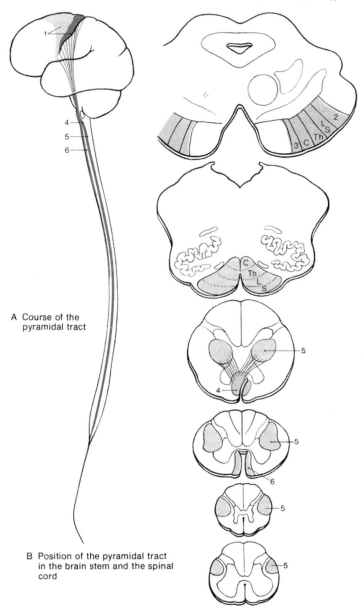

A Course of the pyramidal tract

B Position of the pyramidal tract in the brain stem and the spinal cord

Figure 1.66.
Source: Kahle W, Leonhardt H, Platzer W: *Color Atlas/Text of Human Anatomy, Vol. 3: Nervous System and Sensory Organs,* 4th rev. ed., p. 287. Thieme, New York, 1993.

Extrapyramidal Motor System (Figure 1.67)

Definition. In addition to the precentral region and the pyramidal tract, many other regions and tracts influence the motor activity. They are known collectively as the *extrapyramidal motor system.* Phylogenetically, this is older than the pyramidal tract and, unlike it, consists of multisynaptic neurons. Originally, a group of nuclei that had characteristically high iron content was regarded as the extrapyramidal system: the striatum (putamen **1** and caudatum **2**), pallidum **3**, subthalamic nucleus **4**, red nucleus **5**, and substantia nigra **6** (*striatal system or extrapyramidal system in the narrow sense*).

Other centers of importance for the motor system are connected with this group of nuclei, but they are integration centers and not motor nuclei: the cerebellum **7**, thalamic nuclei **8**, reticular formation, vestibular nuclei **9**, and certain cortical regions. Together, these structures are regarded as the *extrapyramidal system in the broad sense.*

Function. During voluntary movements of one limb, there is simultaneous stimulation of muscle groups in other limbs and in the trunk, in order to maintain balance and the upright posture under the changed static conditions, and to permit the movement to occur smoothly. These concomitant muscular actions, which are often only an increase or decrease of tone in the muscle groups, are not under voluntary control and are not performed consciously, but without them no coordinated movement would be possible. Other movements performed unconsciously are the associated movements (movement of the arms during walking). They are all controlled by the extrapyramidal system, which is comparable to a servomechanism acting independently and involuntarily to support voluntary movements.

Tracts. Afferent tracts reach the system through the cerebellum. Cerebellar tracts end in the red nucleus (dentatorubral tract **10**) and in the centramedian nucleus of the thalamus **11**, whose fibers extend into the striatum. From the cortex fibers project to the striatum **12**, red nucleus **13,** and substantia nigra **14**. Vestibular fibers terminate in the interstitial nucleus of Cajal **15**.

The central tegmental tract **16** is regarded as the efferent tract of the system. Other descending tracts are the reticulospinal tract **17**, the rubroreticulospinal tract **17**, the rebrureticulospinal tract, the vestibulospinal tract **18** and the interstitiospinal fasciculus **19**.

The extrapyramidal centers are connected to each other by numerous neuronal circuits, which permit reciprocal control and adjustment of activity. There are two-way connections between the pallidum and the subthalamic nucleus, and between the striatum and the substantia nigra **20**. A large neuronal circuit extends from the cerebellum through the centromedian nucleus of the thalamus to the striatum, and from there back to the cerebellum via the pallidum, red nucleus and olive **21**. Other functional circuits are formed by cortical fibers to the striatum, which produce a recurrent circuit to the cortex through the pallidum and the anterior and lateral ventral thalamic nuclei.

The frontal and occipital visual fields, together with certain regions of the parietal and temporal lobes, from which complex mass movements can be elicited by strong electrical currents, are known as the "extrapyramidal cortical fields." There is still disagreement about the inclusion of cortical regions in the extrapyramidal system.

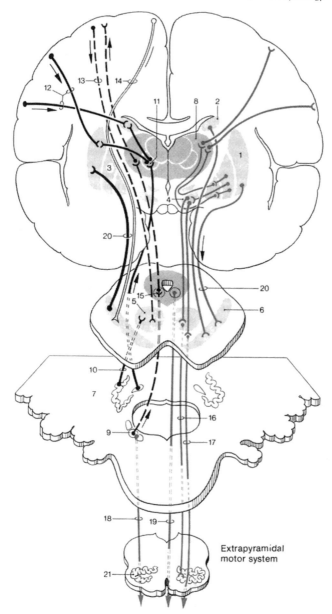

FIGURE 1.67.

SOURCE: Kahle W, Leonhardt H, Platzer W: *Color Atlas/Text of Human Anatomy, Vol. 3: Nervous System and Sensory Organs,* 4th rev. ed., p. 289. Thieme, New York, 1993.

Motor End Plates (Figure 1.68 A–G)

Motor nerve fibers **A1** branch in the muscles so that every muscle fiber **ABC2** is supplied by an axonal branch **A3**. The number of muscle fibers supplied by a single axon is very variable. In the eye and the finger muscles, one axon innervates two or three muscle fibers and in other muscles, 50 to 60 muscle fibers. The group of muscle fibers innervated by the axon from one anterior horn cell together with the cell itself form a *motor unit*. The muscle fibers contract in unison when the neuron is stimulated. The terminal branches of each axon lose their myelin sheath before ending by splitting into terminal ramifications. In the terminal zone there is an aggregation of cell nuclei, and the surface of the muscle fibers form a flat elevation (hence the term *end plate* **A4**).

A number of cell nuclei lie in the region of the axonal ramifications **B5**. The nuclei that lie on the axonal ramifications belong to Schwann cells surrounding the axonal endings (*telogia* **CB6**), and the nuclei which lie beneath **B7** are the muscle fiber nuclei in the region of the end plate. At the border zone between the axoplasm and the sarcoplasm, the axon branches are enfolded by a palisaded layer **B8**, which electron microscopy shows to be composed of sarcolemmal folds.

The axons end with nodular swellings **C9**, which bury themselves in the end plate. The cavities in which they lie are covered by a sarcoplasmic membrane and a basement membrane, so that the axon endings are always extralemmal. In the cavities there is much folding of the sarcolemma (subneural junction folds **CD10**), which serves to greatly enlarge the surface area of the membrane of the muscle fiber.

The motor end plate is a specialized form of synapse; the presynaptic membrane is the axoplasmic membrane **D11**, and the postsynaptic membrane is the folded sarcoplasmic membrane **D12**. The basement membranes of the axon ending **C13** and the muscle fiber **C14** join in the synaptic fissure to form a dense zone **D15**. The neurotransmitter substance that conveys the nerve stimulus to the muscle fiber is *acetylcholine*. It is contained in clear vesicles **C16**, which empty into the synaptic fissure during stimulation of the axon and cause depolarization of the muscle fiber membrane.

Tendon Organs

The Golgi organ in tendons lies at the transition between the tendon and muscle. It consists of a group of collagen fibers **E17** surrounded by a thin connective tissue tunic and supplied by a myelinated nerve fiber **E18**. The latter loses its myelin sheath after passing through the capsule and divides into a number of branches, which coil among the collagen fibers. It is thought that the loosely arranged collagen fibers **F** are compacted when stretched **G** and so cause pressure on the nerve fibers. The nerve impulse that results is passed from the nerve fiber through the posterior root to the spinal cord, where it has an inhibitory effect on the motor neuron. In this way it prevents excessive stretching or contraction of the muscle.

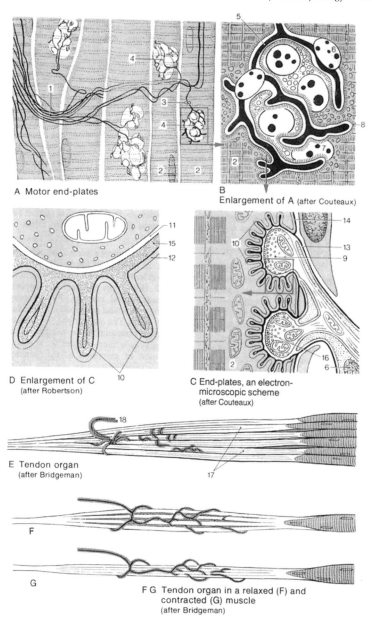

A Motor end-plates

B
Enlargement of A (after Couteaux)

D Enlargement of C
(after Robertson)

C End-plates, an electron-
microscopic scheme
(after Couteaux)

E Tendon organ
(after Bridgeman)

F

G

F G Tendon organ in a relaxed (F) and
contracted (G) muscle
(after Bridgeman)

FIGURE 1.68.

SOURCE: Kahle W, Leonhardt H, Platzer W: *Color Atlas/Text of Human Anatomy, Vol. 3: Nervous System and Sensory Organs,* 4th rev. ed., p. 291. Thieme, New York, 1993.

Muscle Spindle *(Figure 1.69 A–F)*

A muscle spindle consists of 5–10 fine, transversely striated muscle fibers (*intrafusal fibers* **A1**), surrounded by a fluid-filled connective tissue capsule **A2**. The fibers of the spindles, which are up to 10 mm long, lie parallel to the other fibers of the muscle (*extrafusal fibers*). They are attached either to the muscle tendon or to the connective tissue poles of the muscle capsule. Since the intrafusal fibers lie in the same longitudinal direction as the extrafusal fibers, they are affected in the same way by elongation and shortening of the muscle. The number of spindles in each individual muscle is quite variable. Those muscles that are concerned with fine, highly differentiated movements (finger muscles) have a large number of spindles, whereas muscles that perform only simple movements (trunk muscles) contain far fewer spindles.

In the middle or equatorial zone **A3** of the intrafusal fiber, which contains a number of cell nuclei, myofibrils are lacking; this part is not contractile. Only the two distal parts **A4**, which contain cross-striated myofibrils, are able to contract. A large sensory nerve fiber **A5** ends in the middle part of the muscle fiber and is wound spirally around, forming the *anulospiral ending* **AC6B**. On one or both sides of the annulospiral ending a finer sensory nerve fiber **A7** may form a type of umbelliform attachment (*flower-spray ending* **A8D**).

Both distal contractile regions are supplied by fine motor fibers (Y-fibers **A9**). Their small motor end plates are marked by poorly developed junctional folds, but as in the extrafusal muscle fibers, their end plates are still epilemmal. The sensory annulospiral endings, on the other hand, lie beneath the basement membrane of the muscle fiber **C10** and are thus hypolemmal. The Y-fibers for these specialized motor endings stem from small motor cells in the anterior horn, the Y-neurons, whose impulses produce contraction of the distal parts of the muscle fibers. The resultant stretch of the sensory equatorial part not only stimulates the annulospiral ending, but also alters the sensitivity of the spindle.

The muscle spindle is a stretch receptor that is stimulated by elongation of the muscle and ceases to be active when the muscle contracts. During stretching of a muscle, the frequency of the impulses increases with the change in length. In this way the spindle transmits information about the current length of the muscle. The stimuli are not only transmitted via the spinocerebellar tracts to the cerebellum but are also transmitted directly via reflex collaterals to the large anterior horn cells. Their stimulation by sudden stretching of the muscle produces an immediate contraction response of the muscle.

The muscle spindle contains two different types of intrafusal fibers: the *nuclear chain fiber* **EF11** and the *nuclear bag fiber* **EF12**. Both types of fibers are supplied by annulospiral endings. Flower-spray endings are found principally on nuclear chain fibers. The nuclear bag fibers react to active extension of the muscle, while nuclear chain fibers register the continuing state of extension of the muscle. Muscle spindles transmit not only information about the length of the muscle but also convey to the cerebellum information about the velocity of contraction.

In addition to the tendon organs and muscle spindles, sensory terminal organs in articular capsules and ligaments (tension receptors) constantly send messages about the movement and posture of the trunk and extremities to the cerebellum (dorsal and ventral spinocerebellar tracts).

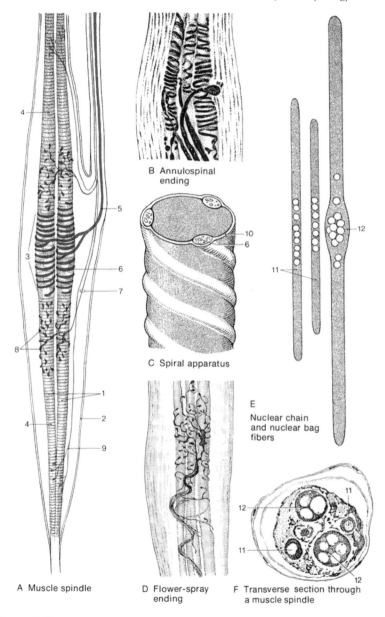

A Muscle spindle

B Annulospinal ending

C Spiral apparatus

D Flower-spray ending

E Nuclear chain and nuclear bag fibers

F Transverse section through a muscle spindle

FIGURE 1.69.

SOURCE: Kahle W, Leonhardt H, Platzer W: *Color Atlas/Text of Human Anatomy, Vol. 3: Nervous System and Sensory Organs,* 4th rev. ed., p. 293. Thieme, New York, 1993.

Final Common Motor Pathway *(Figure 1.70)*

The final common motor pathway for all the centers involved in motor activity is the large anterior horn cell **1** and its axon (a-neuron), which innervates the voluntary skeletal musculature. The majority of all tracts that run to the anterior horn do not terminate directly on anterior horn cells but on interneurons. These influence the neuron either directly, or may act by inhibiting or activating reflexers between the muscle receptors and the motor neurons. Thus, the anterior horn is not a simple synaptic center but a complex integration apparatus for regulation of motor activity.

The central regions that influence the motor system through descending tracts are associated with each other in many ways. The most important afferent tracts stem from the cerebellum. These receive impulses from muscle receptors via the spinocerebellar tracts **2** and stimuli from the cerebral cortex via the corticopontine tracts **3**. Cerebellar impulses are transmitted via the small-celled part of the dentate nucleus **4**, and the ventrolateral thalamic nucleus **5**. The pyramidal tract **7**, descending from area 4 to the anterior horn, sends off collaterals in the pons **8** back into the cerebellum. Other cerebellar impulses run through the emboliform nucleus **9** and the centromedian nucleus of the thalamus **10** to the striatum **11**, and through the large-celled part of the dentate nucleus **12** to the red nucleus **13**. From there fibers pass in the central tegmental tract **14**, through the olive **15** and back to the cerebellum, and in the rubroreticulospinal tract **16** to the anterior horn. Fibers pass from the nucleus globosus **17** to the interstitial nucleus of Cajal **18** and from it via the interstitiospinal fasciculus **19** to the anterior horn. Finally, cerebellofugal fibers make contact in the vestibular nuclei **20** and the reticular formation **21** with, respectively, the vestibulospinal tract **22** and the reticulospinal tract **23**.

The descending tracts may be divided into two groups according to their effects on the muscles: one group, which stimulates flexor muscles, and the other, which stimulates extensors. The pyramidal tract and rubroreticulospinal tract principally activate neurons of flexor muscles and inhibit neurons of the extensors. This corresponds to the functional importance of the pyramidal tract for fine, precise movements, particularly of the hand and finger muscles, in which the flexors play a decisive role. On the other hand, the fibers of the vestibulospinal tract and of the reticular formation of the pons inhibit flexors and activate extensors. They belong to a phylogenetically older part of the motor system, which is concerned with opposing the effects of gravity, and thus is of particular importance for body posture and balance.

Peripheral fibers that run through the posterior root to the anterior horn system form muscle receptors. Collateral branches of the afferent fibers from the annulospiral endings **24** terminate directly on the A-neurons; the fibers of the tendon organs **25** end on intermediate neurons. Many descending tracts influence the A-neurons via the spinal reflex apparatus. They end of the large A-cells and the small Y-cells **26**. As the Y-neurons have a low threshold, they begin to fire first, thus activating the muscle spindles. These send impulses directly to the A-neurons. Y-neurons and muscle spindles thus have a type of "starter" function for voluntary movement.

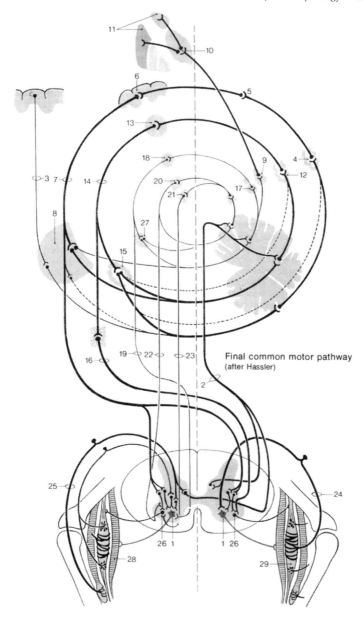

Final common motor pathway
(after Hassler)

FIGURE 1.70.

SOURCE: Kahle W, Leonhardt H, Platzer W: *Color Atlas/Text of Human Anatomy, Vol. 3: Nervous System and Sensory Organs,* 4th rev. ed., p. 295. Thieme, New York, 1993.

Neurology
Special Cerebral Symptoms and Signs
Dementia and Dementing Neurological Diseases

Dementia may be defined as the secondary loss of intellectual faculties, as opposed to mental retardation (oligophrenia) which is the primary defect. There is a gradual transition from the normal to various (e.g., age-related) states of reduced functional capacity, which end in dementia.

Psychopathological signs of dementia. The following signs, which are characteristic features of an *organic mental syndrome* of greater or lesser degree, belong to this group, largely irrespective of the cause:

- Rapid exhaustion
- Loss of interest in recent events
- Lack of persistence in carrying out personal tasks
- Disinterest in people and environment, and in extreme cases
- Sloppiness in dress, unrestrained and aggressive behavior, loss of insight, and a presumptuous and intrusive manner
- Loss of refinement in behavior with improper, crude, and tactless attitudes
- Emotional lability, irritability, and anxiety, and
- Hypochondriacal, depressive, or paranoid features.

Subcortical dementia. This condition is characterized by prolongation of the thought process ("mental akinesia"), indifference, memory disturbances, and sometimes obsessive behavior. The syndrome accompanies bilateral lesions of the basal ganglia, irrespective of their etiology.

Neurological signs of dementia. These signs, none of which is necessarily present, may accompany dementia and depend upon the underlying cause of the disease. Focal neurological findings (often accompanying posttraumatic dementia) need not be present. Neuropsychological deficits are practically always present. A variety of abnormal reflexes are found in cases of diffuse damage, including an accentuated facial reflex (snout reflex), sucking reflex, abnormal nuchocephalic reflex, positive grasp reflex, and increased palomental reflex.

Examination in organic mental syndrome. The following simple procedure and questions will reveal dementia or an organic mental syndrome.

- It should be noted if the patient is oriented in time, place, situation, and person.
- Disturbances in the attention span and memory capacity occasionally become obvious while taking the patient's history. The attention span may be evaluated further by the following: repeating a six-digit number; recalling a four-digit number after an interval of 5–10 minutes; naming eight diagrams shown to the patient; recalling a four-word phrase after an interval of 10 minutes; solving a complex mental arithmetic problem.
- Evaluation of recent memory: menu of the previous evening, names of the doctors, time patient arrived, recent news items.
- Evaluation of concentration ability: months of the year in reverse order; subtracting serial 7's from 100; checking off a particular letter of the alphabet in a long text (Bourdon's test).

• Evaluation of higher intellectual functions including abstract thinking: combining several words into a meaningful phrase; simple questions to verify power of discrimination (e.g., child/dwarf, tree/bush, river/lake, greed/thrift); interpreting a complicated picture; repeating and explaining the meaning of a story.

• Arranging objects according to their size, shape, or mutual affinity.

• In patients with organic mental syndromes, it is always important to obtain information about their behavior from relatives or friends.

The most important etiological causes of dementia. The most important etiological groups for the neurologist are shown in Table 1.15, which will serve as a guideline in the assessment of dementia. While most of the clinical syndromes are dealt with in other chapters of this book, only some will be discussed here which belong to the category of *senile or presenile dementia.* Their etiology is not clear. Basically, a genetic defect in the cell structure, a disturbance of the cell metabolism, a slow viral infection, or an autoimmune process have been postulated.

Arteriosclerotic Dementia. In this condition, the onset of the mental symptoms mentioned above is often fluctuating and not infrequently accompanied by physical signs of the underlying disease. The patients are over 60 years of age. The case history and physical examination often reveal evidence of previous vascular accidents. Hydrocephalus is not marked, and it may be absent. Histopathological study shows the smaller blood vessels to be more severely affected than the larger ones, and small parenchymal lesions are present, usually foci of softening in the cortical gray matter.

Multi-Infarct Dementia. This concept in the modern literature serves either as a substitute for arteriosclerotic dementia or is used in those patients in whom evidence can be demonstrated of previous multiple insults. In a series of 77 patients with multiple infarcts examined by CT scanning, 37 showed dementia. Dementia was significantly commoner in lesions of the dominant hemisphere. In 10 patients, with a clear history of previous insult, the CT revealed evidence only of diffuse atrophy.

Subcortical Encephalopathy. (Binswanger)

Thromboangiitis Obliterans. (von Winiwarter–Buergener)

Alzheimer's Disease. This is a presenile dementia, usually starting after the 50th year of life, but also affecting younger subjects. This pattern of incidence previously served to differentiate it from *senile dementia,* which presents after the age of 65 years. On the basis of transitional patterns and histological criteria, both forms nowadays are grouped together and called senile dementia of the Alzheimer type (SDAT). It is the *commonest cause* of a dementia. The disease is present in about 20% of all patients attending psychiatric clinics and is encountered in about 5% of subjects up to the 80th year. Familial cases are not unusual and probably account for 5–10% of Alzheimer's disease. Women appear to be more commonly affected than men. Clinically, the patient initially is often restless and agitated, and then within a year exhibits severe progressive memory disturbances, confusion, disorientation, and the other above-mentioned signs and symptoms of a dementia. Neurological signs are by no means invariably present and may at most be slight: pyramidal signs, extrapyramidal features, anomalies of muscular tone, oral automatisms, and so on. The average duration of the disease is 2–5 years. *Autopsy*

TABLE 1.15. Etiologic causes and differential diagnosis of dementing lesions.

Disease	Age	Main Clinical Features	Remarks
Arteriosclerotic dementia	Over 60	Fluctuating	Signs of generalized arteriosclerosis. Often brain CT reveals infarcts. Primitive reflexes
Multi-infarct dementia	Over 60	Cerebral infarcts in case history or CT	Similar to arteriosclerotic dementia but infarcts always present
Binswanger's disease (subcortical encephalopathy)	Middle age and the elderly	Mood fluctuation, small insults, pseudobulbar signs	Hypertension especially important. Survive up to 10 years. Brain CT shows attenuated density of white matter
Thromboangiitis obliterans	60 or younger	Vascular symptoms of other organs	Similar to cerebral arteriosclerosis. Also called Buerger's disease
Alzheimer's disease (and senile dementia)	50 or younger	Increasing dementia	Commonest cause of dementia! Over 2–5 years of increasingly severe memory disturbance, periodic confusion, and disorientation
Pick's disease	40 or younger	Dementia and focal neurologic deficits	Particularly clear-cut personality change. Apart from diffuse involvement, the brain CT reveals area of focal atrophy
Progressive paralysis	30 or younger	Expansive, grandiose ideas	Neurologic deficits, pupillary abnormalities, abnormal CSF
Creutzfeld-Jakob disease	Young and middle-aged adults	Pyramidal and extrapyramidal signs, fasciculation, myoclonic features	In about 70% typical EEG. Rapidly progressive coma. Transmissible
Normal pressure hydrocephalus (nonresorptive hydrocephalus)	Any age	Dementia, apractic gait, disturbances of urination	Seek causes of nonresorptive hydrocephalus. Transient improvement follows LP. Internal hydrocephalus while extraventricular CSF spaces are reduced.

	Age	Clinical features	Remarks
Normal pressure hydrocephalus (nonresorptive hydrocephalus)	Any age	Dementia, apractic gait, disturbances of urination	Seek causes of nonresorptive hydrocephalus. Transient improvement follows LP. Internal hydrocephalus while extraventricular CSF spaces are reduced.
Brain tumor	Any age	Focal neurologic deficits, epileptic attacks	Especially in slowly growing benign tumors, e.g., meningioma
Craniocerebral trauma	Any age	History of injury	Neurologic deficits or abnormal findings in brain CT not essential for the diagnosis. Watch for epileptic attacks!
Chronic exogenous poisons	Any age	Contact with toxic substances	e.g., bromide, cannabis, alcohol, barbiturates
Endocrinopathies	Any age	Other clinical signs	e.g., Cushing's disease, hypercalcemia, hypothyroidism
Metabolic disorders	Any age		e.g., Kinnier-Wilson disease
Malnutrition	Any age		e.g., pellagra, vitamin B_{12} deficiency
As part of another neurologic disease	Preceding illness		e.g., parkinsonian syndrome, Huntington's chorea, myoclonic epilepsy, sphingolipidoses, leukodystrophies, hereditary system degenerations, various vascular lesions, chronic meningoencephaliitides

SOURCE: Mumenthaler M: *Neurology*, pp. 166–167. Thieme, New York, 1990.

reveals a diffuse cerebral atrophy involving the frontal and occipital lobes most severely. Histological study shows the presence of placques and a great number of neurofibrillary (Alzheimer's) tangles, as well as diffuse cell necrosis, granulovacuolar degeneration, and occasionally a congophili amyloid angiography.

Pick's Disease. This disease belongs to the systematic degenerative processes such as Huntington's chorea. It occurs twice as commonly in women as in men, usually in younger individuals than Alzheimer's disease; also, it is far less common. The *personality changes* in Pick's disease are more severe than those in Alzheimer's disease, and the grossly disturbed behavior may occasionally in individual cases give rise to severe ethical problems (differential diagnosis of tertiary neurosyphilis). Apart from these mental changes, *focal neurological signs* are often present, notably aphasia and parietal lobe involvement. The disease lasts 2–10 years. Neuroradiological examination reveals an internal hydrocephalus combined with wide subarachnoid spaces over the surface of the frontal and parietal lobes, with the posterior two-thirds of the first temporal convolution being spared. The caudate nucleus may be atrophic. Apart from loss of ganglion cells and gliosis, the diseased areas of the brain contain Alzheimer's fibrils and senile placques.

Creutzfeldt–Jakob Disease. This is a rare, rapidly progressive disease that involves men and women with equal frequency. It commences in early adulthood or middle life. The onset is heralded by nonspecific or *uncharacteristic symptoms* such as mood fluctuations, depression, tiredness, sleep disturbances, and increasing forgetfulness. Soon these features are combined with objectively demonstrable *neurological signs:* anomalies of muscular tone, pyramidal signs, extrapyramidal features, neuropsychological deficits, muscular fasciculation, and later myoclonic contractions. In parallel, the patient's signs of dementia increase and mental activity progressively ceases, leading to decorticate status and terminal coma. Diagnostically important is a characteristic *EEG pattern;* however, this may only appear in the later stages. About three-fourths of cases show bilaterally synchronous, diffuse frontal periodic activity comprising sharp, polyphasic potentials repeated with a frequency of 1/s (Fig. 1.71). In the later stages, these periodic complexes are replaced by diffuse slowing. The disease lasts no longer than 6–30 months.

Pathological anatomy. Naked-eye examination of the brain reveals spongiform changes of the neurophil with loss of ganglion cells and compensatory astrocytosis. The degree of severity of these changes corresponds to the clinical details and varies from case to case. It has been possible in more than 100 cases to *transmit* the disease to primates and other laboratory animals; human-to-human transfer occurring accidentally during surgical operation has also been observed. The etiological role of virus particles in the disease is nowadays widely accepted. These particles have been identified as "prions," which are found in laboratory animals infected with scrapie. For those in contact with patients, it is recommended that excreta and body fluids should be handled with the same precautions applied to viral hepatitis.

Presenile Spongiform Cerebral Atrophy. This is a fatal, progressive type of dementia in which choreiform and myoclonic or epileptic features are present. The characteristic pathological picture, in the presence of intact nerve cells and the absence of signs of Alzheimer's disease, is multiple cystic cavitation of the cerebral cortex. The condition has a complex relationship to Creutzfeldt–Jakob disease.

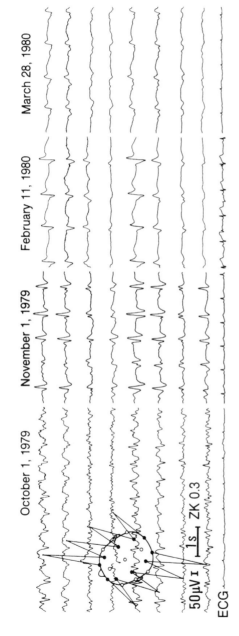

FIGURE 1.71. Serial EEG examinations in a 57-year-old with autopsy-proven Creutzfeld-Jakob disease.

The examination 6 weeks from the onset of the prodromal stage (October 1, 1979) revealed only periodic activity. One month later (November 1, 1979) this activity was most marked, and in the succeeding months it showed a tendency toward gradual attenuation.

SOURCE: Mumenthaler M: *Neurology*, pp. 170. Thieme, New York, 1990.

Prolonged Steroid Medication. Steroid preparations administered over a long period cause diffuse shrinkage of the brain, which is visible on CT scanning as surface atrophy and hydrocephalus. This abnormal picture disappears completely upon withdrawal of medication.

Neuropsychological Syndromes

General. Disturbances of complex psychical functions, possessing an organic background, are included in this concept. None of these syndromes presents primarily as disturbances of consciousness, mood, or thought processes—instead, they usually manifest as disturbances of recognition and processing of information and secondary effects on the behavior of the individual. These neuropsychological syndromes are identified by the technique of neuropsychological testing. The scientific substrate of this field is experiences gained from experimental psychology. It is only partly possible to relate topographically specific syndromes to specific regions of the brain. Experience has confirmed that neuropsychological testing permits only organic brain damage as such to be demonstrated and evaluated quantitatively, as well as sometimes to be lateralized with a certain degree of accuracy. Abnormalities previously accepted as isolated syndromes (finger agnosia, autopagnosia, right–left confusion, Gerstmann's syndrome) are so closely linked to other basic neuropsychological disturbances that they cannot be interpreted as independent entities.

One of the complex integrating functions of the brain, of which the abnormalities are particularly striking, is the ability of humankind to communicate by means of speech and other forms of information transfer with his others and the environment. *Speech disturbances* not caused by cortical lesions must be briefly mentioned in this section, in view of their differential diagnostic importance.

• *Nonorganic speech disturbances* (speech disorders in schizophrenic psychoses, monotonous scant speech depression, mutism in catatonia, aphonia in hysteria).

• *Developmental speech disorders* are disturbances of speech development, one of which is stammering.

• Lesions of the *speech-forming structures:* The choice of words is correct but there are changes in the tone and clarity of utterance (hoarseness in laryngeal lesions; blocked nasal passages with enlarged adenoids; epiphyarngeal tumors or patent nasal passages in cleft palate; spastic dysphonia with irregular phonation accompanied by contractions of the facial and neck muscles—presumably a functional anomaly of phonation).

• Lesions of the *muscles of phonation,* provoking similar symptoms (involvement of muscles of the soft palate in myasthenia gravis with patent nasal passages, progressively increasing exhaustion of the patient, and other myasthenic manifestations).

• Lesions of the *lower cranial nerves,* with paralysis of the muscles of phonation, which they supply, causing dyarthria (unilateral hypoglossal palsy affects speech only slightly; paralysis of one vocal cord due to unilateral recurrent laryngeal nerve palsy causes hoarseness but is rapidly compensated; bilateral paralysis of the soft palate, e.g., in diphtheria).

• Lesions of the *nuclei in the medulla oblongata:* "bulbar speech" (i.e., nasal, slurred, poorly articulated, and often babbling speech, as if the patient has an egg in his or her mouth). The consonants *R* and *L* are most likely to be slurred (this type of speech is a typical feature of the bulbar type of amyotrophic lateral sclerosis). A unilateral lesion of the bulbar nuclei (e.g., a vascular accident in the vertebrobasilar territory) produced only transient hoarseness.

• *Upper motor neuron palsy* of muscles of phonation ("pseudobulbar palsy"): Articulatory disturbances that cannot be distinguished from those in bulbar palsy (anarthria, dysarthria) accompany this type of lesion, which usually results from vascular damage to the corticobulbar tracts. The onset is usually sudden, unlike that of true bulbar palsy. The picture of (childhood) brain-stem encephalitis is similar

• *Cerebellar lesions:* The coordinating and regulating function exerted by the cerebellum is abolished. Syllables and words are uttered too loudly and too rapidly in an irregular way (i.e., they are articulated explosively). In advanced cases of *multiple sclerosis,* involvement of the cerebellum sometimes leads to scanning speech.

• The parkinsonian syndrome and other *lesions of the basal ganglia* hamper the harmonious and coordinated utterance of speech. The poverty of movement of the parkinsonian patient is expressed as soft and monotonous, slow and scarcely modulated speech (bradylalia; in extreme cases, mutism). Rarely, logoclonia (compulsive repetition of end syllables) and palilalia (repetition of individual words or phrases) may occur. Such repetitive speech may also accompany diffuse cerebrovascular disturbances and senile dementia. The slow, slurred speech of general paresis is similar. However, it must be stressed that this early symptom is a nonspecific feature of general paresis.

• Damage in the vicinity of the *periaqueductal gray matter:* failure of the speech impulse with preservation of movement of the organs of speech and no obvious disturbance of consciousness; in extreme cases, akinetic mutism after encephalitis involving the basal ganglia, especially encephalitis lethargica, vertebrobasilar insufficiency, and subarachnoid hemorrhage. A similar clinical picture is produced by lesions of the limbic system.

• The term *aphemia* is used to describe dysarthria without aphasia. It is observed in left-hemisphere lesions of the pars opercularis, the inferior precentral gyrus, and the white matter immediately below it.

• *Bilateral cortical damage in the anterior operculum* leads to a central diplegia of the mouth and throat muscles, the Foix–Chavany–Marie syndrome.

Disturbances of Language, Speech, and Other Allied Forms of Communication

General. Aphasia, in the context of expressing a disturbance of higher integrative cortical function, should be discussed together with the other complex deficiencies of communication between the individual and the environment that do not directly affect speech. Speech is only possible if the information that is hidden in various parts of the brain is integrated. The integrity of various cortical areas and the tracts connecting them is essential for this function. Even if no precise localizing significance can be attributed to speech disorders, it is justifiable and clinically relevant to attribute certain forms of aphasia and other communication defects to specific areas of the brain (Fig. 1.72). In right-handed individuals, the cortical centers responsible for language are nearly always localized in the left hemisphere, and only in 1% are they on the right side. In contrast, only about 25% of left-handed persons have their language center in the right cerebral hemisphere.

Examination of Communication Disorders. The practical method of testing must be adequate to ensure that any defect encountered can be diagnosed and localized. The following is a simplified scheme suitable for quick bedside orientation.

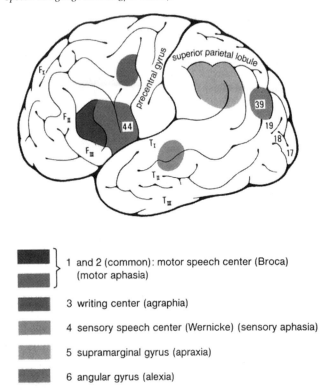

■■ } 1 and 2 (common): motor speech center (Broca)
(motor aphasia)

■ 3 writing center (agraphia)

■ 4 sensory speech center (Wernicke) (sensory aphasia)

■ 5 supramarginal gyrus (apraxia)

■ 6 angular gyrus (alexia)

FIGURE 1.72. **Several areas of the cerebrum significant in speech function.**
SOURCE: Mumenthaler M: *Neurology,* pp. 174. Thieme, New York, 1990.

1. *Preliminary examination:* Verify that

- The *sensorium* is intact, that no obtundation or stupor is present
- No *severe defect of intelligence* is present (retardation, dementia)
- *Hearing and vision* are adequate
- *Function of the speech organs* is intact (no severe dysarthria), and
- No (other) *neurological defects* are present (e.g., hemianopsia or hemiplegia).

2. *Aphasia testing:* First, *spontaneous speech* should be tested by drawing the patient into conversation.

2.1. Verify that conversation is *fluent* that is, consists of a normal speech production (more than 90 words a minute), possesses a normal prosody (melody and intonation), and that the sentences have a normal length (more than five words) and no excess of nouns.

2.1.1. If, in addition, there are no anomalies in the choice or construction of words, then no aphasia is present.

2.1.2. If spontaneous speech is fluent but paraphasias (sense approximately correct but words altered or incorrect) and *neologisms* are present, the picture points to a left-sided postcentral lesion. Greater precision is possible by *testing speech comprehension,* which may be carried out by asking the patient to point out specific objects, arrange objects in order, answer complex questions, and so on.

    2.1.2.1. Confirm that *speech reception* is intact, as well as speech repetition (of sounds, words, and sentences).

- If *undisturbed,* an anomic aphasia is present that possesses only slight localizing value (second temporal convolution or angular gyrus?).
- If *speech repetition* is severely *disturbed,* conduction of aphasia may be presumed to be present due to damage to the arcuate fasciculus, which connects the posterior part of the temporal lobe to the operculum.

    2.1.2.2. If *speech comprehension* is *disturbed,*

- but *speech repetition* is undisturbed, then a transcortical sensory aphasia is present, localizing the lesion to the angular gyrus.
- and *expression is equally disturbed,* then Wernicke's aphasia is present, and it may be assumed that the lesion lies in the sensory speech center in the first temporal convolution.

    2.2. Spontaneous speech may not be fluent: Speech production may be reduced to less than 50 words per minute, with dysprosody (disturbances of speech melody and intonation of sentences), visible (mimicry) and audible (dysarthria) strained speech, short sentences (fewer than five words), and impaired construction (agrammatism). These features point primarily to a precentral lesion.

    2.2.1. If in this situation *speech repetition is intact* (see above), then in the presence of

- *Disturbed expression, Broca's aphasia* is indicated, caused by a cortical lesion in the upper perisylvian region; or in the presence of
- *Normal expression, transcortical motor aphasia* is present, caused by a lesion situated rostrally and more superficially to Broca's area.

    2.2.2. If, in addition to defective spontaneous speech, *speech comprehension is disturbed,* then either

- *A transcortical sensorimotor aphasia* is present (which marked difficulty) in finding names and echolalia), indicating an extensive lesion interrupting the connection of the cortical speech center with the rest of the brain, and particularly cutting off the associated sensory centers (isolation aphasia) or
- *A global (total) aphasia* is present, which is always the result of an extensive lesion in the territory of supply of the middle cerebral artery. The procedure for testing an aphasia speech disturbance is shown in Figure 1.73. The treatment of aphasia continues to undergo intensive development, while its efficacy continues to be challenged, especially in cases of aphasia following vascular accidents.

    3. *Apraxia examination:* Apraxia is defined as the inability of the patient to execute appropriate movements upon command.

- *Ideomotor apraxia* indicates inability of the face (facial apraxia, in 80% of aphasics) or the extremities to carry out a command or to imitate it by a specific motor response. This inability indicates a lesion of the dominant hemisphere (e.g., Wernicke's region, subcortical beneath the operculum, beneath the motor association center, the commissural tracts to the opposite hemisphere).

- *Ideational apraxia,* far more infrequent, describes the situation in which more complex sequences of movements cannot be successfully executed (e.g., preparing a cup of coffee, opening a letter and filing it, keeping a file in order, etc.)

4. *Agnosia examination:* Agnostic disturbances (i.e., disturbances of recognition) affect the various modalities of sensation. Thus,

- *Visual object agnosias* indicate that although vision is intact, the patient fails to recognize objects that can be identified by touch or hearing (rattling a bunch of keys). The cause is usually a right-sided or bilateral parieto-occipital lesion.
- *Spatial agnosia* implies a disturbance of spatial orientation. It may be manifest as follows: Patients lose their way, are less observant, are unable to copy simple or more complicated drawings, are disoriented concerning their own body, exhibiting finger agnosia or dressing apraxia. This feature points to a lesion in the posterior part of the right parietal lobe.
- *Prosopagnosia* is the term used to identify an isolated disturbance, namely, failure to recognize familiar faces. It points to a lesion of the occipitotemporal region of the right hemisphere, extending into the cerebral cortex.
- *Anosognosia* is the inability of the patient to recognize an abnormal function of his body (e.g., the patient explains failure to move a paralyzed left arm as "not wanting to move it"). Although mostly seen with lesions of the right hemisphere, in 20% of cases, this symptom also occurs with damage to the left hemisphere. It is not exclusively an expression of a parietal lesion. Rather, it can be the result of diffuse brain damage, combined with a focal lesion.
- *Auditory, tactile, and color agnosias* as isolated disturbances are debatable entities.

5. *Disconnection syndrome:* This syndrome is not caused by a lesion of the cortical associated centers but by an interruption of the connections linking these centers. In particular, the connections linking the sensory and motor centers of the right hemisphere with the cortical speech center in the left hemisphere are severed. Some of these disturbances include the following:

- *True alexia* (alexia without agraphia, i.e., no disturbance of writing, but an inability to read the written word). The lesion may be situated in the splenium of the corpus callosum and left striate cortex.
- Also, *alexia* combined with an *inability to name colors* and *hemianopsia* to the right side may accompany a lesion of the left visual center and the splenium of the corpus callosum (territory of supply of the left posterior cerebral artery).
- *Alexia with agraphia* is not a disconnection syndrome; this combination points to a lesion of the angular gyrus.
- *Pure word blindness* in the presence of intact recognition of nonverbal auditory stimuli and in the presence of an intact cortical Wernicke's area points to a lesion in the left auditory radiation and the commissural fibers of the corpus callosum.

Syndromes of Individual Areas of the Cerebral Cortex

Lesions of specific areas of the cerebral cortex produce focal neurological signs as well as a focal and sometimes generalized mental syndrome. However, additional specific features point to involvement of specific cortical areas.

Precentral Region of the Frontal Lobe. Lesions of this region may implicate parts of the pyramidal cell layers and therefore involve motor function of the

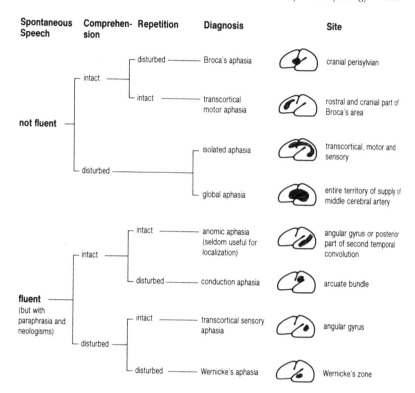

Spontaneous Speech	Comprehension	Repetition	Diagnosis	Site
	intact	disturbed	Broca's aphasia	cranial perisylvian
		intact	transcortical motor aphasia	rostral and cranial part of Broca's area
not fluent	disturbed		isolated aphasia	transcortical, motor and sensory
			global aphasia	entire territory of supply of middle cerebral artery
	intact	intact	anomic aphasia (seldom useful for localization)	angular gyrus or posterior part of second temporal convolution
		disturbed	conduction aphasia	arcuate bundle
fluent (but with paraphrasia and neologisms)	disturbed	intact	transcortical sensory aphasia	angular gyrus
		disturbed	Wernicke's aphasia	Wernicke's zone

FIGURE 1.73. Procedure for examining a patient with an aphasic speech disturbance.
SOURCE: Mumenthaler M: *Neurology*, pp. 176. Thieme, New York, 1990.

trunk. Such lesions give rise to focal *paralyses*. The more localized the paralysis, the more superficial is the site of the lesion likely to be (e.g., facial monoplegia or crural monoplegia). The situation may arise, for example, in which a distinction must be made between a central paralysis of the foot and a peroneal palsy. This illustrates the fact that isolated damage to area 4 may be unaccompanied by an increase in muscular tone and present simply as a flaccid weakness. *Disturbances of gaze* accompany lesions of the cortical gaze center at the foot of the second frontal convolution. Gaze is directed initially to the affected side. Sometimes *signs of cerebral irritation* may be present in the form of focal motor epilepsy, often referred to as adversive attacks, although the eyes turn away from the discharging focus (aversive movement).

Convexity of the Frontal Lobe. Lesions of the convexity of the frontal lobe give rise to the following disturbances:

Changes in motor behavior: Grasp automatisms of the mouth and hand appear at an early stage. The lips and jaws reflexly close when touched or even when an object is brought to the mouth. An object laid in the hand is touched intentionally in a purposeful manner, the fingers following it like a magnet and grasping the object as if obeying a reflex. These features usually affect both hands but are more marked on the side of the lesion. If the frontopontocerebellar tracts are interrupted, *ataxia* develops, which is most obvious in the lower limbs. Coordination of movements of the opposite side of the body is limited, especially in walking; if the legs are crossed, abduction and adduction are exaggerated, and there may even be abasia. Patients show a type of passive resistance during passive positioning of their limbs, which is called *gegenhalten* (paratonia), and reaction that may resemble catatonia. Once a limb has been placed in a particular position, that position is maintained for an unusually long time (*postural retention*), and passive repetitive movements are actively continued by the patient (Kral phenomenon). Also, movements observed may be imitated (*echopraxia*), and words and sentences heard may be repeated (*echolalia*).

Psychopathological and neuropsychological features: There is a general *loss of interest and drive, spontaneity, and activity*, leading to an indifferent, unobservant, and detached attitude. Contact with the environment diminishes, and personal initiative and the patient's reaction to external stimuli may disappear. Instead, an impulsive behavior pattern emerges. Lesions of the basal part of the frontal lobe, the so-called *orbital brain*, bilaterally influence affect and judgmental instincts, especially those concerned with social conventions. This leads to a progressive mental blunting and a picture of impulsive behavior, humorlessness, and moral decay, and ultimately to affective dementia. If the opercular part of the foot of the third frontal convolution (area 44) is also involved, then a lesion of the Broca's speech center leads to *motor aphasia*.

Parietal Lobe. The parietal lobe is not clearly demarcated in the cerebral hemisphere from either the temporal lobe below or the occipital lobe behind. It contains the postcentral gyrus with sensory cortical representation, the circumflex or supramarginal gyrus and the angular gyrus, the latter being important for gnostic function. In lesions involving the postcentral region and upper part of the lobe, the following symptoms and signs may be found.

Neurological deficits: These include a *sensory* or a *sensorimotor hemisyndrome*, the *avoidance phenomenon* of contralateral hand (abnormal resting position, clumsy movements, absent grasp reflex on tactile simulation), homonymous *quadrantic field defect* inferiorly, inattention hemianopsia to the opposite side, and a reduced response of *optokinetic nystagmus* to stimuli, affecting the motion of the eyes toward the contralateral half of the visual field.

Epileptic attacks: These attacks in parietal lobe lesions commence as sensory jacksonian seizures. They may be followed by motor hemiseizures, with conjugate deviation of the eyes, head, and trunk to the opposite side. A lesion situated on the medial surface, at the paracentral lobule, causes parasthesias in the anogenital region with urinary and fecal urgency.

Neuropsychological disturbances: A disturbance of spatial orientation and right–left discrimination may be present, as well as tactile agnosia, a constructional apraxia, if the lesion affects the dominant hemisphere, and an amnesic aphasia and dyslexia.

Temporal Lobe. The convexity of the temporal lobe contains cortical areas that are associated with speech comprehension (Wernicke's area in the superior temporal gyrus) and are connected with the sensory auditory pathway and the central pathway of olfaction. The floor of the temporal lobe forms part of the limbic system, and fibers from the sensory cortex and enteroceptive autonomic afferent pathways terminate here. The visual pathway passes through the basal white matter, with fibers arising from the lower half of the retina.

Neurological deficits: These include homonymous field defects, especially of the upper quadrant. No impairment of the senses of smell or hearing accompanies unilateral lesions. Lesions extending into the depth of the globus pallidus present with incoordination of movement and involuntary choreoathetoid movements.

Epileptic attacks: These attacks possess the features of psychomotor epilepsy and may become generalized. Attacks of auditory sensation may occur (Heschl's convolution), also attacks of altered sensation of taste and smell (uncinate fits).

Psychopathological and neuropsychological disturbances: Memory disturbances accompany lesions of the mediobasal part of the temporal lobe (hippocampus). Other features are disturbances of mood such as depression and irritability, occasionally disinhibition and aphasic disturbances of the amnestic type. Neglect phenomena are typical. They primarily involve the left side with a right-sided hemisphere lesion, rarely the reverse. This includes not seeing people on the neglected side, not hearing acoustical stimuli, not feeling sensory stimuli, and not paying attention to this side of an object during tactile exploration with the eyes closed. One also finds decreased motor activity on the corresponding half of the body and neglect of it, for instance, while washing and dressing, as well as perhaps on anosognosia.

Occipital Lobe. The major part of the occipital lobe lies on the median surface of the hemisphere, and only a small part faces the cerebral convexity. Within it ends the secondary sensory neuron on the visual pathway, the optic radiations terminate in the striate area in the vicinity of the calcarine fissure. In areas 18 and 19, fields are present that are responsible for processing incoming visual stimuli.

Neurological deficits: Lesions of areas 18 and 19 lead to a transient conjugate deviation to the side of the lesion and a gaze palsy to the opposite site. Tracking or pursuit movements of the eyeballs may remain limited for a long period (while the eyes continue to function normally to command). This leads to disturbances of reading (dyslexia).

Signs of irritation take the form of attacks of abnormal visual sensations. In lesions of area 17, they possess a primitive character (flashes, sparks). In lesions of area 18, they consist of hallucinations of objects. In lesions of area 19, they may give rise to complex science hallucinations. They may also be combined with conjugate eye and head movements to the opposite side, and they may become generalized.

Neuropsychological disturbances: Disturbances of visuospatial orientation, color agnosia or visual agnosia, so-called "psychic blindness," or alexia may occur.

2

Phonology, Respiration, and Articulation-Child

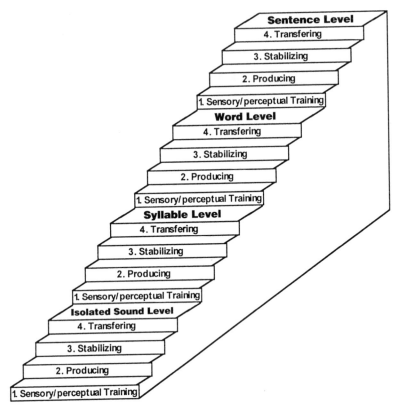

Figure 2.1. Articulation therapy: traditional training levels.

Source: From Van Riper C, Erickson RL: *Speech Correction: An Introduction to Speech Pathology and Audiology,* 9th ed. Copyright © 1996 by Allyn & Bacon. Reprinted/adapted by permission.)

TABLE 2.1. Articulatory errors most often found in preschool children: comparisons with and without cleft palate.

Speech sound element tested	Templin norm	Pool norm	Errors of control subjects (N = 120, 3–6 yr.)	Errors of cleft palate subjects in order of frequency of occurrence (N = 60, 3–6 yr.)
/p/	3	3.5	None	ʔ/p, PF*
/b/	4	3.5	p/b	m/b, ʔ/b
/t/	6	4.5	d/t	ʔ/t, PF, k/t
/d/	4	4.5	t/d	ʔ/d, PF, n/d
/k/	4	4.5	t/k	ʔ/k, PF, t/k
/g/	4	4.5	k/g, d/g	ʔ/g, d/g, PF
/f/	3	5.5	p/f, b/f, s/f	ʔ/f, PF, p/f
/v/	6	6.5	b/v, f/v	b/v, ʔ/v, m/v
/θ/	6	7.5	t/θ, s/θ, fθ	ʔ/θ, PF, t/θ
/ð/	7	6.5	d/ð	d/ð, ʔ/ð, PF
/s/	4.5	7.5	θ/s, t/s	PF, ʔ/s, t/s
/z/	7	7.5	s/z, θ/z, d/z	PF, ʔ/z, s/z
/ʃ/	4.5	6.5	s/ʃ, tʃ/ʃ	PF, ʔ/ʃ
/tʃ/	4.5	-	ʃ/tʃ, s/tʃ, t/tʃ	PF, ʔ/tʃ, ʃ/tʃ
/dʒ/	7	-	tʃ/dʒ, d/dʒ, ʒ/dʒ	PF, ʔ/dʒ, ʒ/dʒ
/l/	6	6.5	w/l	w/l, ʔ/l
/j/	3.5	4.5	ʔ/j	ʔ/j, w/j, l/j
/r/	4	7.5	w/r	w/r, j/r, PF
/w/	3	3.5	j/w	ʔ/w, l/w
/m/	3	3.5	b/m	PF, ʔ/m
/n/	3	4.5	m/n	ʔ/n, j/n
/ŋ/	3	4.5	n/ŋ	n/ŋ

SOURCE: With permission from Aronson AE: *Clinical Voice Disorders*, p. 222. Thieme, New York, 1990.
*PF = either pharyngeal or velar fricative substitution.

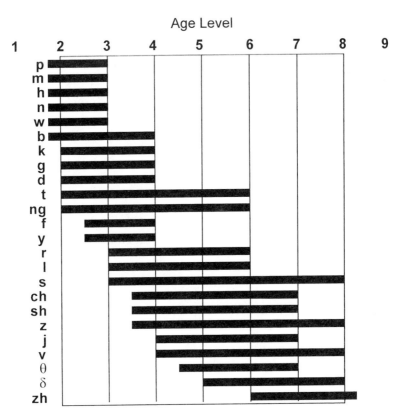

FIGURE 2.2. Consonant acquisition (Sander's study): average age estimates and upper age limits of customary consonant production.*

The solid bar corresponding to each sound starts at the median age of customary articulation; it stops at an age level at which 90% of all children are customarily producing the sound.

*Customary production refers to that point when a child is producing a sound correctly more often than misarticulating or omitting it.

SOURCE: Adapted with permission from Sander E: When Are Speech Sounds Learned? *Journal of Speech and Hearing Disorders* 1972; 37:62.

TABLE 2.2. **Consonant classification: manner, place, and voice.**

Manner	Place	Voiced	Voiceless
Stop	Bilabial	b	p
	Alveolar	d	t
	Velar	g	k
	Glottal	------ʔ----------	-----------
	Labiodental	v	f
	Linguadental	ð	θ
Fricative	Alveolar	z	s
	Palatal	ʒ	ʃ
	Glottal		h
Affricate	Palatal	dʒ	tʃ
	Bilabial	m	
Nasal	Alveolar	n	
	Velar	ŋ	
Lateral	Alveolar	l	
Rhotic	Palatal	r	
	Palatal	j	
Glide	Labial/Velar	w	ʌ

SOURCE: From Kent R: Normal Aspects of Articulation. In Bernthal JE, Bankson NW: *Articulation and Phonological Disorders,* 3rd ed. Copyright © by Allyn & Bacon. Reprinted/adapted by permission.

TABLE 2.3. **Consonants: frequency of occurrence in American English.**

Sound	Percentage of occurrence	Cumulative percentage
n	12.0	12.0
t	11.9	23.9
s	6.9	30.8
r	6.7	37.5
d	6.4	43.9
m	5.9	49.8
z	5.4	55.2
ð	5.3	60.5
l	5.3	65.8
k	5.1	70.9
w	4.9	75.8
h	4.4	80.2
b	3.3	83.5
p	3.1	86.6
g	3.1	89.7
f	2.1	91.8
ŋ	1.6	93.4
j	1.6	95.0
v	1.5	96.5
ʃ	0.9	97.4
θ	0.9	98.3
dʒ	0.6	98.9
tʃ	0.6	99.5
ʒ	< 0.1	99.6

SOURCE: With permission from Shribery LD, Kwiatowski J: Computer-Assisted Natural Process Analysis (NPA): Recent Issues and Data. *Seminars in Speech and Language* 1983; 4(4):389–406.

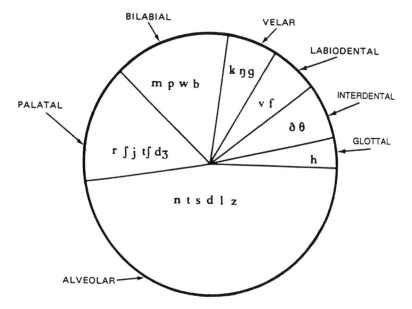

FIGURE 2.3. Consonants: frequency of occurrence made at different places of articulation based on data from Dewey (1923).

SOURCE: From Kent R: Normal Aspects of Articulation. In Bernthal JE, Bankson NW (eds.): *Articulation and Phonological Disorders,* 3rd ed. Copyright © 1993 by Allyn & Bacon. Reprinted/adapted by permission.

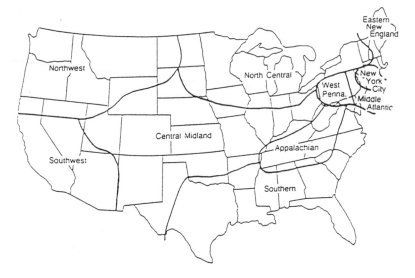

FIGURE 2.4. Dialects: major American geographic divisions.

SOURCE: From Owens RE Jr.: *Language Development: An Introduction,* 4th ed. Copyright © 1996 by Allyn & Bacon. Reprinted/adapted by permission.

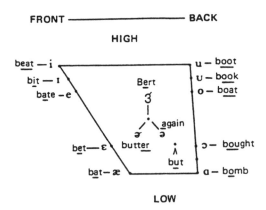

FIGURE 2.5. English vowels: identified by phonetic symbol and key word and plotted within vowel quadrilateral.

SOURCE: From Kent R: Normal Aspects of Articulation. In Bernthal JE, Bankson NW: *Articulation and Phonological Disorders,* 3rd ed. Copyright © 1993 by Allyn & Bacon. Reprinted/adapted by permission.

TABLE 2.4. Development of speech sound variables: early utterances of preterm infants.

Variable	Normal age of establishment	Reference source
Vocal laughter	4 months	Sroufe & Water, 1976; Coplan et al., 1982
Vowels	Prephonological	Burh, 1980; Stark, 1979
Front	2–7 months	
Medium		
Back	Phonological 30+ months	Cruttenden, 1979
Diphthongs	No early data	
	12 months	Byers, Brown, & Lewis, 1984;
	12–18 months	Stark & Bond, 1985
Consonants	Prephonological 4 months	Stark, 1979
	Phonological 18–32 months	Ingram, 1976; Hedrick et al., 1975
Plosives	Prephonological 3–7 months	Glazewski & McCune, 1984; Stark, 1979
	Phonological 18–36 months	Hedrick et al., 1975
Fricatives	Prephonological 4 months	Stark, 1979
	Phonological 24–48 months	Ingram, 1976; Hedrick et al., 1975
Liquids	Prephonological	Irwin, 1947; Locke, 1980
	Phonological 32–36 months	Ingram, 1976; Hedrick et al., 1975
Glides	Prephonological 6 months	Stark, 1979
	Phonological 18 months	Ingram, 1976; Hedrick et al., 1975
Pitch variation	6–12 months	Crystal, 1979; Cruttenden, 1979
Melodic cadences derived from vowels + intonation		Byers, Brown, & Lewis, 1984 Crystal, 1979; Cruttenden, 1979
Vowel sequences (vowel stammer, vocable)	6 months	Elbers, 1982; Carter, 1979; Byers, Brown, & Lewis, 1984; Ferguson, 1978
Babbling	4–10 months	Coplan et al., 1982
Monosyllabic	4–12 months	Stark, 1979; Byers, Brown, &
Polysyllabic-repetitive (reduplicated)		Lewis, 1984; Waterson, 1981

(continued)

TABLE 2.4. (*continued*)

Variable	Normal age of establishment	Reference source
Polysyllabic nonrepetitive (nonreduplicated, variegated)	9–18 months	Stark, 1979; Byers, Brown, & Lewis, 1984
Jargon	9–18 months	Stark, 1979; Menyuk, 1972; Bzoch & League, 1971
1 word utterances	10–18 months	Cruttenden, 1979; Grieve & Hoogenraad, 1979; Coplan et al., 1982
2 word utterances	18–24 months	Rescoria, 1984; Bloom, 1973; Griffiths, 1979

SOURCE: With permission from Brown BB, Bendersky M, Chapman T: The Early Utterances of Preterm Infants. *British Journal of Disorders of Communication* 1986; 21:310.

TABLE 2.5. **Developmental verbal dyspraxia (DVD): basic principles of a speech production treatment program for children.**

1. Main focus of treatment should be syllable structure control and organization within a variety of dynamic linguistic contexts.
2. A successful program is one that will facilitate correct production of varying syllable shapes and the organization of these shapes into longer and increasingly complex phonotatic patterns.
3. A sound-by-sound treatment plan that emphasizes phoneme production in isolation prior to moving to words and phrases does not address the hierarchical dynamic movement problem in DVD.
4. Auditory discrimination training does not address the problem.
5. Frequent, short sessions with breaks are most successful. Because DVD is a dynamic disorder, system fatigue is a problem.
6. Sessions should be divided into short parts:
   a. Warm-ups: Imitation of body and/or oral motor sequences.
   b. Practicing the scales: Syllable sequence drill activities. Establish consistent connected syllable productions from within the child's repertoire. Include sequences that vary articulatory positions, for example, from front to back ([bʌdʌgʌ] or "buttercup") or vice versa ([gʌdʌbʌ] or "go to bed").
   c. Learning the song: Meaningful single-word activities to include a core group of words that would increase overall intelligibility of speech.
   d. Changing the song: Short sentence activities starting with a key carrier phrase and changing one word, gradually increasing in length and complexity.

SOURCE: With permission from Velleman SL, Strand K: Developmental Verbal Dyspraxia. In Bernthal JE, Bankson NW (eds.): *Child Phonology: Characteristics, Assessment, and Intervention with Special Populations*, p. 131. Thieme, New York, 1994.

TABLE 2.6. **Developmental verbal dyspraxia (DVD): characteristics of early history.**

1. Poor coordination of sucking response.
2. *Very* quiet baby.
3. Little or no babbling but vowel-like vocalizations may be heard.
4. Limited differentiation of consonants and vowels in the babbling repertoire.
5. Little spontaneous imitation of syllables.
6. Excessive drooling in spite of adequate feeding skills.
7. Language comprehension within normal limits for age.
8. Early expressive language milestones may or may not be delayed.
9. Pointing accompanied by "vowel-like" vocalization or single syllable to request or comment.
10. Natural gesture or pantomine system.
11. Isolated productions: On rare occasions the child has said a word or phrase clearly that (s)he could not repeat upon request.
12. By 24 months, excessive frustration is noted; problems with behavior management may be present.
13. Often reported to be excessively dependent or shy, especially in unfamiliar social settings.
14. Family member often cited as interpreter.

SOURCE: With permission from Velleman SL, Strand K: Developmental Verbal Dyspraxia. In Bernthal JE, Bankson NW (eds.): *Child Phonology: Characteristics, Assessment, and Intervention with Special Populations,* p. 131. Thieme, New York, 1994.

TABLE 2.7. **Diacritics and international phonetic alphabet cover symbols.**

Diacritics symbol	Meaning	Symbol	Meaning
V\	Labialized	::	Overlong
(+) w	Rounded	-	Short/checked
< >	Spread	--	Very short
pr	Protruded	=	Unreleased
d	Dentalized		
D	Interdentalized	(+) v	Voiced
ap	Apical	−v	Devoiced
lm	Laminal	hv	Breathy (murmured)
dr	Dorsal	?v	Creaky (laryngealized)
j	Palatalized	h (−)	(Post-) aspirated
g	Velarized	h+	Preaspirated
G	Uvularized	−h	De-/unaspirated
H	Pharyngealized	v>	Ingressive
?	Glottalized	v<	Egressive
		?>	Implosive
(+) n	Nasalized	?<	Ejective
−n	Denasalized	!(>)	Velaric (ingressive)
n+	Mprenasalized		
n−	Nasal release	s	Syllabic
ne	Nasal emission	AS	Ambisyllabic
(+) l	Lateralized	gl	Glide (vocalic)
l−	Lateral release	os	On-/offset (consonantal)
r	Retroflexed, rhoticized		
−r	Dewoticized	L	Lenis (weak)
f	Fricated	LL	Very weak
s	Stopped	F	Fortis (strong)
t	Tapped, flapped	FF	Very strong
rr	Trilled		
qr	Quick release		
lk	Leaky (stop)	*Cover Symbols*	
wh	Whistled		
wt	Wet	CN—consonant	
		VL—vowel	
/, up	Raised	AP—approximant	
\, dn	Lowered	RS—resonant	
<, fr	Fronted	FR—fricative	
>, bk	Backed	ST—stop	
		NS—nasal snort	
.	Half-long	SC—stacatto	
:	Long	UN—undefinable noise	

SOURCE: With permission from Allen GD: The PHONASCII System. *Journal of the International Phonetic Association* 1988; 18:21.

TABLE 2.8. English consonants, including the glottal stop by Chomsky–Hall: extended features.

Features	k	q	t	d	p	b	f	v	θ	ð	s	z	ʃ	ʒ	tʃ	dʒ	m	n	ŋ	l	ɹ	h	w	j	ʔ
Vocalic	−	−	−	−	−	−	−	−	−	−	−	−	−	−	−	−	−	−	−	+	+	−	−	−	−
Consonantal	+	+	+	+	+	+	+	+	+	+	+	+	+	+	+	+	+	+	+	+	+	−	−	−	−
High	+	+	−	−	−	−	−	−	−	−	−	−	+	+	+	+	−	−	+	−	−	−	+	+	−
Back	+	+	−	−	−	−	−	−	−	−	−	−	−	−	−	−	−	−	+	−	−	−	+	−	−
Low	−	−	−	−	−	−	−	−	−	−	−	−	−	−	−	−	−	−	−	−	−	+	−	−	+
Anterior	−	−	+	+	+	+	+	+	+	+	+	+	−	−	−	−	+	+	−	+	−	−	−	−	−
Coronal	−	−	+	+	−	−	−	−	+	+	+	+	+	+	+	+	−	+	−	+	+	−	−	−	−
Round	−	−	−	−	−	−	−	−	−	−	−	−	−	−	−	−	−	−	−	−	−	−	+	−	−
Tense	−	+																							
Voice	−	+	−	+	−	+	−	+	−	+	−	+	−	+	−	+	+	+	+	+	+	−	+	+	−
Continuant	−	−	−	−	−	−	+	+	+	+	+	+	+	+	−	−	−	−	−	+	+	+	+	+	−
Nasal	−	−	−	−	−	−	−	−	−	−	−	−	−	−	−	−	+	+	+	−	−	−	−	−	−
Strident	−	−	−	−	−	−	+	+	−	−	+	+	+	+	+	+	−	−	−	−	−	−	−	−	−

Blank = not relevant

  − = binary feature not present

  + = binary feature present

- *Vocalic*—Constriction in the oral cavity is not greater than required for the high vowels /i, u/.
- *Consonantal*—The sound is made with a radical constriction in the midsagittal region of the oral cavity.
- *High*—The body of the tongue is elevated above the neutral position.
- *Back*—The body of the tongue retracts from the neutral position.
- *Low*—The body of the tongue is lowered below the neutral position.
- *Anterior*—The sound is produced further forward in the mouth than /ʃ/.
- *Coronal*—The sound is produced with the blade of the tongue raised from the neutral position.
- *Round*—The lip orifice is narrowed.
- *Tense*—The sound is produced deliberately, accurately, and distinctly.
- *Voice*—During the production of the sound, the larynx vibrates periodically.
- *Continuant*—The vocal tract is partially constricted during the production of the sound.
- *Nasal*—The velopharyngeal valve is sufficiently open during the production of the sound to permit the airsound stream to be directed through the nose.
- *Strident*—The airstream is directed over a rough surface in such a way as to produce an audible noise.

SOURCE: From Owens R Jr: Communication, Language, and Speech. In Shames G, Wiig E: *Human Communication Disorders: An Introduction,* p. 41. Copyright © 1986 by Allyn & Bacon. Reprinted/adapted by permission.

TABLE 2.9. English consonants: manner of articulation, place of articulation, and voicing.

Manner of Articulation	Bilabial		Labiodental		Linguadental		Linguaalveolar		Lingrapalatal		Linguavelar		Glottal	
	−	+	−	+	−	+	−	+	−	+	−	+	−	+
Stop	p	b					t	d			k	g		
Fricative			f	v	θ	ð	s	z	ʃ	ʒ			h	
Affricate							tʃ	dʒ						
Nasal		m						n				ŋ		
Glide	hw	w								r, j				
Lateral								l						

PLACE OF ARTICULATION

SOURCE: From Creaghead NA. Newman PW: Articulatory Phonetics and Phonology. In Creaghead NA. Newman PW. Secord WA (eds.): *Assessment and Remediation of Articulatory and Phonological Disorders*, p. 15. © 1989 by Allyn and Bacon. Reprinted/adapted by permission.

− absence of voicing
+ presence of voicing

	Bilabial	Labiodental	Dental	Alveolar	Postalveolar	Retroflex	Palatal	Velar	Uvular	Pharyngeal	Glottal
Plosive	p b			t d		ʈ ɖ	c ɟ	k ɡ	q ɢ		ʔ
Nasal	m	ɱ		n		ɳ	ɲ	ŋ	ɴ		
Trill	ʙ			r					ʀ		
Tap or Flap				ɾ		ɽ			ɢ̆		
Fricative	ɸ β	f v	θ ð	s z	ʃ ʒ	ʂ ʐ	ç ʝ	x ɣ	χ ʁ	ħ ʕ	h ɦ
Lateral fricative				ɬ ɮ							
Approximant		ʋ		ɹ		ɻ	j	ɰ			
Lateral approximant				l		ɭ	ʎ	ʟ			
Ejective stop	p'			t'		ʈ'	c'	k'	q'		
Implosive	ɓ			t ɗ			c ʄ	k ɠ	q ʛ		

FIGURE 2.6a. **International phonetic alphabet, diacritics, suprasegmentals, and other symbols. Where symbols appear in pairs, the one to the right represents a voiced consonant. Shaded areas denote articulation judged impossible.**

SOURCE: Adapted with permission from Ball MJ, Code C, Rahilly J, and Hazlett D: Non-Segmental Aspects of Disordered Speech: Developments in Transcription, *Clinical Linguistics and Phonetics* 1994;8:68.

DIACRITICS

Voiceless n̥ d̥	More rounded ɔ̹	ʷ Labialized tʷ dʷ	˜ Nasalized ẽ
Voiced s̬ t̬	Less rounded ɔ̜	ʲ Palatalized tʲ dʲ	ⁿ Nasal release dⁿ
ʰ Aspirated tʰ dʰ	Advanced u̟	ˠ Velarized tˠ dˠ	ˡ Lateral release dˡ
Breathy voiced b̤ a̤	Retracted i̠	ˤ Pharyngealized tˤ dˤ	˺ No audible release d̚
Creaky voiced b̰ a̰	¨ Centralized ë	~ Velarized or pharyngealized ɫ	
Linguolabial t̼ d̼	Mid centralized e̽	Raised e̝ ɹ̝ (ɹ̝ = voiced alveolar fricative)	
Dental t̪ d̪	Advanced Tongue root e̘	Lowered e̞ β̞ (β̞ = voiced bilabial appoximant)	
Apical t̺ d̺	Retracted Tongue root e̙	Syllable ɹ̩	Non-syllable e̯
Laminal t̻ d̻	˞ Rhoticity ə˞		

SUPRASEGMENTALS

- ˈ Primary stress
  ˌfoʊnəˈtɪʃən
- ˌ Secondary stress
- ː Long eː
- ˑ Half long eˑ
- ̆ Extra short ĕ
- . Syllable break ɹi.ækt
- | Minor (foot) group
- ‖ Major (intonation) group
- ‿ Linking (absence of a break)
- ↗ Global rise
- ↘ Global fall

LEVEL TONES

˝ or ˥	Extra High
´ or ˦	High
¯ or ˧	Mid
` or ˨	Low
̏ or ˩	Extra low
↓	Downstep
↑	Upstep

CONTOUR TONES

ˇ or ˩˥	rise
ˆ or ˥˩	fall
ˇ or ˦˥	high rise
ˆ or ˩˨	low rise
or	rise fall etc.

FIGURE 2.6b. International phonetic alphabet: diacritics, suprasegmentals, and other symbols.

SOURCE: Adapted with permission from Ball MJ, Code C, Rahilly J, and Hazlett D: Non-Segmental Aspects of Disordered Speech: Developments in Transcription. *Clinical Linguistics and Phonetics* 1994;8:68.

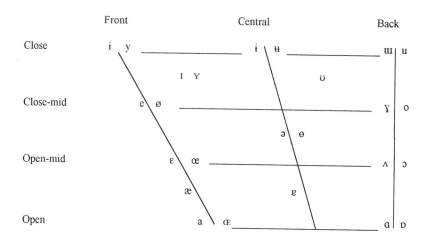

Where symbols appear in pairs, the one to the right represents a rounded vowel.

OTHER SYMBOLS

ʍ	Voiceless labial-velar fricative	ʘ	Bilabial Click
w	Voiced labial-velar approximant	ǀ	Dental click
ɥ	Voiced labial-palatal approximant	ǃ	(Post)alveolar click
ʜ	Voiceless epiglottal fricative	ǂ	Palatoalveolar click
ʡ	Voiced epiglottal plosive	ǁ	Alveolar lateral click
ʕ	Voiced epiglottal fricative	ɺ	Alveolar lateral flap
ɧ	Simultaneous ʃ and x	ɕ ʑ	Alveolo-palatal fricatives
ɜ	Additional mild central vowel		

Figure 2.6c. International Phonetic Alphabet: Vowels.

Source: Adapted with permission from Ball MJ, Code C, Rahilly J, and Hazlett D: Non-Segmental Aspects of Disordered Speech: Developments in Transcription. *Clinical Linguistics and Phonetics* 1994;8:68.

TABLE 2.10. **Phoneme development: age levels according to six studies.**

	Wellman (1931)	Poole (1934)	Templin (1957)	Sander (1972)	Prather (1975)	Arlt (1976)
m	3	3½	3	before 2	2	3
n	3	4½	3	before 2	2	3
h	3	3½	3	before 2	2	3
p	4	3½	3	before 2	2	3
f	3	5½	3	3	2–4	3
w	3	3½	3	before 2	2–8	3
b	3	3½	4	before 2	2–8	3
ŋ		4½	3	2	2	3
j	4	4½	3½	3	2–4	
k	4	4½	4	2	2–4	3
g	4	4½	4	2	2–4	3
l	4	6½	6	3	3–4	4
d	5	4½	4	2	2–4	3
t	5	4½	6	2	2–8	3
s	5	7½	4½	3	3	4
r	5	7½	4	3	3–4	5
tʃ	5		4½	4	3–8	4
v	5	6½	6	4	4	3½
z	5	7½	7	4	4	4
ʒ	6	6½	7	6	4	4
θ		7½	6	5	4	5
dʒ			7	4	4	4
ʃ		6½	4½	4	3–8	4½
ð		6½	7	5	4	5

SOURCE: From Creaghead NA: Articulatory Phonetics and Phonology. In Creaghead NA, Newman PW, Secord WA: *Assessment and Remediation of Articulatory and Phonological Disorders,* 2nd ed. Copyright © 1989 by Allyn & Bacon. Reprinted/adapted by permission.

TABLE 2.11. **Phoneme development: earliest ages (in years) at which sounds were correctly produced, in the word positions indicated for consonants, vowels, and diphthongs, and consonant blends.**

Earliest Age (in years) At Which Sounds Were Correctly Produced, In the Word Positions Indicated, by 75% of 208 Children

Consonants	Beginning position	Middle position	End position
m	2	2	3
n	2	2	3
ng	-	6	3
p	2	2	4
b	2	2	3
t	2	5	3
d	2	3	4
k	3	3	4
g	3	3	4
r	5	4	4
l	4	4	4
f	3	3	3
v	5	5	5
th (uv)*	5	-	-
th (v)**	5	5	-
s	5	5	5
z	5	3	3
sh	5	5	5
h	2	-	-
wh	5	-	-
w	2	2	-
y	4	4	-
ch	5	5	4
j	4	4	6

Vowels and dipthongs	Age
e (beet)	2
i (bit)	4
e (bed)	3
a (cat)	4
u (cup)	2
ah (father)	2
aw (ball)	3
oo (foot)	4
oo (boot)	2
u-e (mule)	3
o-e (coke)	2
a-e (cake)	4
i-e (kite)	3
oy (boy)	3

* (uv) = unvoiced (using only breath to produce the sound, as in the word *th*ree)
** (v) = voiced (using the voice to produce the sound, as in the word *th*e)

(continued)

TABLE 2.11. (*continued*)

Earliest Age (in years) At Which Sounds Were Correctly Produced, In the Word Positions
Indicated, by 75% of 208 Children

Consonants blend	Age	Consonant blend	Age
pr	5	-ks	5
br	5	al	6
tr	5	sw	5
dr	5	tw	5
kr	5	kw	5
gr	5	ngk	4
fr	5	ngk	5
thr	6	-mp	3
pl	5	-nt	4
bl	5	-nd	6
kl	5	spr-	5
gl	5	apl	5
fl	5	str-	5
-ld	6	skr-	5
-lk	5	skw-	5
-lf	5	-ns	5
-lv	5	-ps	5
-lz	5	-ts	5
sm-	5	-mz	5
sn-	5	-nz	5
sp-	5	-ngz	5
st-	5	-dz	5
-st	6	-gz	5
sk-	5		

SOURCE: From Powers MH: Functional Disorders of Articulation/Symptomatology and Etiology.
In Travis LE (ed.): *Handbook of Speech Pathology and Audiology,* p. 842. Prentice-Hall, Englewood Cliffs, NJ, 1971.

TABLE 2.12. **Phonemes: normal aspects of place of articulation, phonetic symbol and key word, manner of articulation, and voicing.**

Place of articulation	Phonetic symbol and key word	Manner of articulation	Voicing
Bilabial	/p/ (pay)	Stop	−
	/b/ (bay)	Stop	+
	/m/ (may)	Nasal	+
Labial/velar	/ʍ/ (which)	Glide (semivowel)	−
	/w/ (witch)	Glide (semivowel)	+
Labiodental	/f/ (fan)	Fricative	−
	/v/ (van)	Fricative	+
Linguadental	/θ/ (thin)	Fricative	−
(interdental)	/ð/ (this)	Fricative	+
	/t/ (two)	Stop	−
	/d/ (do)	Stop	+
	/s/ (sue)	Fricative	−
Lingua-alveolar	/z/ (zoo)	Fricative	+
	/n/ (new)	Nasal	+
	/l/ (Lou)	Lateral	+
	/ɾ/ (butter)	Flap	+
Linguapalatal	/ʃ/ (shoe)	Fricative	−
	/ʒ/ (rouge)	Fricative	+
	/tʃ/ (chin)	Affricate	−
	/dʒ/ (gin)	Affricate	+
	/j/ (you)	Glide (semivowel)	+
	/r/ (rue)	Rhotic	+
Linguavelar	/k/ (back)	Stop	−
	/g/ (bag)	Stop	+
	/ŋ/ (bang)	Nasal	+
Glottal (laryngeal)	/h/ (who)	Fricative	−
	/ʔ/ ---	Stop	+(−)

SOURCE: From Kent R: Normal Aspects Of Articulation. In Bernthal JE, Bankson NW: *Articulation and Phonological Disorders,* 3rd ed., p. 21. Prentice-Hall, Englewood Cliffs, NJ, 1981.

Linguavelar: dorsum or back of tongue and roof of mouth in the velar area

Glottal: the two vocal folds

TABLE 2.13. Phonological development by chronological age and stages.

Stage I (0;9-1;6)	*Nasal plosive* *fricative approximant*					
Stage II (1;6–2;0)	m p b w		n t d			
Stage III (2;0–2;6)	m p b w		n t d			(ŋ) (k g) h
Stage IV (2;6–3;0)	m p b f		n t d s		j	ŋ k g
Stage V (3;0–3;6)	w		(l)			h
Stage VI (3;6–4;0) (4;0–4;6)	m p b f v w		n t d s z l (r)		tʃdʒ ʃ j	ŋ k g h
Stage VII (4;6 <)	m p b f v w	θ ð w	n t d s z l r		tʃdʒ ʃ ʒ j	ŋ k g h

SOURCE: From Grunwell P: *Clinical Phonology,* p. 98. Aspen Systems, Rockville, MD, 1982.

TABLE 2.14. **Phonological processes: basic definitions.**

Assimilation (Assimilatory Process or Consonant Harmony) changes in a speech sound (phone) due to the placement characteristics of another sound with the utterance. Typically, the place of articulation for one consonant affects another consonant within a word so that both consonants are produced at the same place of articulation. Progressive assimilation occurs when an earlier phone in a word affects a later phone. Regressive assimilation occurs when a later phone affects an earlier one.

Backing (Backing to Velars) occurs when posterior consonants are substituted for anterior consonants. Backing to velars is specific to the alteration of any consonant production being replaced by a velar.

Cluster Reduction (Cluster Simplification): One, or more than one, consonant within a cluster is deleted with at least one of the consonants remaining. A cluster, also referred to as blends, consists of two or three consonants. Sometimes the insertion of a schwa between members of a cluster occurs creating an extra syllable. This is also classified as cluster simplification.

Consonant Harmony (Assimilation or Assimilatory Process): changes in a speech sound (phone) due to the placement characteristics of another sound with the utterance. Typically, the place of articulation for one consonant affects another consonant within a word so that both consonants are produced at the same place of articulation. Progressive assimilation occurs when an earlier phone in a word affects a later phone. Regressive assimilation occurs when a later phone affects an earlier one.

Deaffrication occurs when an affricate is produced with only the continuant or fricative feature. The stop feature of the affricate is omitted with the continuant, fricative, feature remaining.

Deletion of Final Consonant (Final Consonant Deletion): The final consonant of a word is deleted and no substitution for the final consonant occurs.

Deletion of Initial Consonant (Initial Consonant Deletion): The initial consonant of a word is deleted and no substitution for the initial consonant occurs. The use of initial glottal stops are not considered deletion of initial consonants. This phonological process is not considered characteristic of normal phonological development.

Devoicing occurs when voiceless consonants are substituted for voiced ones.

Final Consonant Deletion (Deletion of Final Consonant): The final consonant of a word is deleted and no substitution for the final consonant occurs.

Fronting (Velar Fronting) replaces a posterior consonant with an anterior consonant. Typically, a velar consonant is produced as an alveolar consonant in words or syllables.

Glottal Replacement occurs when consonants are replaced with glottal stops.

Initial Consonant Deletion (Deletion of Initial Consonant): The initial consonant of a word is deleted and no substitution for the initial consonant occurs. The use of initial glottal stops are not considered deletion of initial consonants. This phonological process is not considered characteristic of normal phonological development.

Initial Voicing an initial, voiceless consonant is replaced by a voiced consonant. The place and manner of the consonant may or may not be altered. Therefore, this process can occur in conjunction with other phonological processes.

Liquid Simplification occurs when liquids are produced as glides; also referred to as gliding of liquids.

Palatal Fronting: A palatal consonant is produced frontally, usually to the alveolar ridge.

Reduplication occurs when the same sound or syllable is repeated in place of two or more phonemically different units.

Stopping (of Fricatives and Affricates): A stop consonant is substituted for a continuant.

Stridency Deletion occurs when the stridency characteristic of fricative and affricate sounds is deleted or replaced. The strident consonants /s, z, f, v, ʒ, tʃ, dʒ/ lack stridency and are usually replaced with a stop or glide.

(continued)

TABLE 2.14. (*continued*)

Substitution Process modifies the phoneme characteristics resulting in the substitution of one phone for another.

Syllable Reduction occurs when a syllable in a multisyllable word is omitted: The word produced contains fewer syllables than the target production.

Velar Fronting (Fronting) replaces a posterior consonant with an anterior consonant. Typically, a velar consonant is produced as an alveolar consonant in words or syllables.

Vocalization (Vowelization) occurs when a consonant, usually a glide or liquid, is produced as a vowel. This process is the substitution of vowels for consonants.

Voicing is the substituting of voiced sounds for voiceless ones.

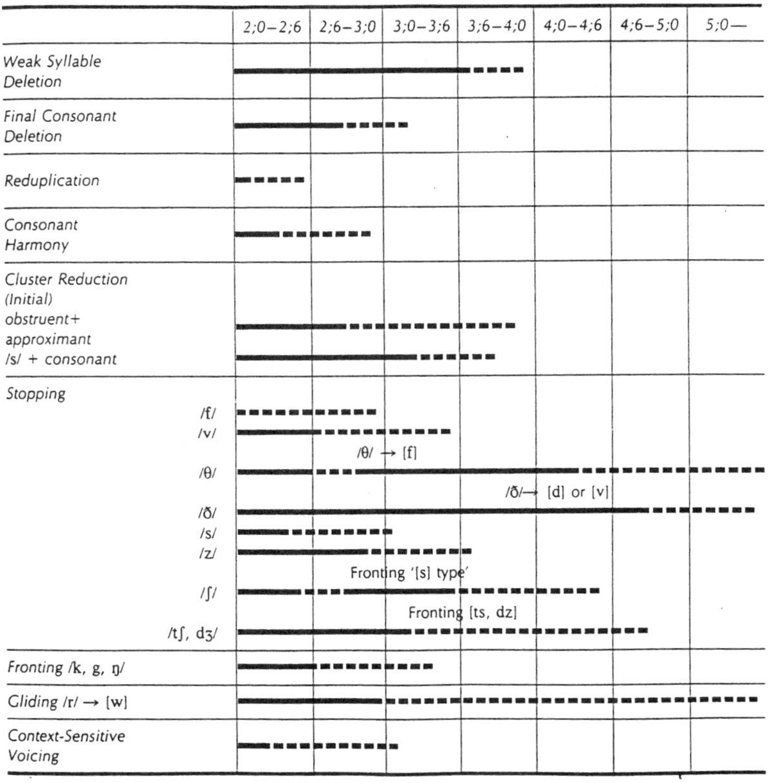

	2;0–2;6	2;6–3;0	3;0–3;6	3;6–4;0	4;0–4;6	4;6–5;0	5;0—
Weak Syllable Deletion							
Final Consonant Deletion							
Reduplication							
Consonant Harmony							
Cluster Reduction (Initial) obstruent+ approximant /s/ + consonant							
Stopping /f/							
/v/							
/θ/		/θ/ → [f]					
/ð/				/ð/→ [d] or [v]			
/s/							
/z/							
/ʃ/		Fronting '[s] type'					
/tʃ, dʒ/			Fronting [ts, dz]				
Fronting /k, g, ŋ/							
Gliding /r/ → [w]							
Context-Sensitive Voicing							

FIGURE 2.7. Phonological processes chronology.

SOURCE: From Grunwell P: *Clinical Phonology*, p. 183. © 1982 by Aspen Publishers, Rockville, MD.

TABLE 2.15. **Phonological processes classifications and examples: structural simplifications and systemic simplifications.**

Structural simplifications	Example	
Developmental		
Weak syllable deletion	/metə/	for *tomato*
Final consonant deletion (including clusters)	/bæ/	for *bad*
	/dɛs/	for *desk*
Vocalization	/wado/	for *water*
Reduplication	/baba/	for *bottle*
Consonant harmony	/gɔg/	for *dog*
Syllable initial cluster reduction	/nek/	for *snake*
Unusual		
Vocalic support of final consonants	/bædə/	for *bad*
Initial consonant adjunction	/wæbu/	for *apple*
Vowel insertion	/pəliz/	for *please*
Dissimilation	/baɪt/	for *pipe*
Perseveration	/lɪptɪp/	for *lipstick*
Metathesis	/æks/	for *ask*

Systemic simplifications	Example	
Developmental		
Fronting	/ti/	for *key*
Stopping	/ti/	for *see*
Gliding	/wo/	for *row*
Context-sensitive voicing	/do/	for *toe*
Glottal replacement	/bæʔ/	for *back*
Glottal insertion	/beʔbiʔ/	for *baby*
Unusual		
Backing	/ko/	for *toe*
Backing in terminations	/mæk/	for *mat*
Tetism	/to/	for *foe*
Labial realizations of fricatives	/fi/	for *see*
Lateral realizations of sibilants	/ɬi/	for *see*
Weakening of plosives	/si/	for *tea*
Affrication of plosives	/tsi/	for *tea*
Denasalization	/do/	for *no*

SOURCE: With permission from Grunwell P: *Phonological Assessment of Child Speech*. College Hill Press, San Diego, 1985.

TABLE 2.16. **Phonological processes of preschool children.**

Processes	Examples
Syllable structure	
Deletion of final consonants	*cu* (/kʌ/ for *cup*
Deletion of unstressed syllables	*nana* for *banana*
Reduplication	*mama, dada, wawa,* (water)
Reduction of clusters	/s/ + consonant (*stop*) = delete /s/ (*top*)
Assimilation	
Contiguous	
Between consonants	*beds* (/bɛdz/), *bets* (/bɛts/)
Regressive VC (vowel alters toward some feature of *C*)	nasalization of vowels: *can*
Noncontiguous	
Back assimilation	*dog* becomes *gog*
Substitution	*dark* becomes *gawk*
Obstruants (plosives, fricatives, and affricates)	
Stopping: replace sound with plosive	*this* becomes *dis*
Fronting: replace palatals and velars (/k/ and /g/), with alveolars (/t/ and /d/)	*Kenny* becomes *Tenny*
	go becomes *do*
Nasals	
Fronting: (/ŋ/ becomes /n/)	*something* becomes *somethin*
Approximants replaced by	
Plosive	*yellow* becomes *yedow*
Glide	*rabbit* becomes *wabbit*
Another approximant	*girl* becomes *gaul* (/gɔl/)
Vowels	
Neutralization: vowels reduced to /ə/ or /a/	*want to* becomes *wanna*
Deletion of sounds	*balloon* becomes *ba-oon*

SOURCE: From Owens RE: *Language Development: An Introduction,* 4th ed., p. 337. Copyright © 1996 by Allyn & Bacon. Reprinted/adapted by permission.

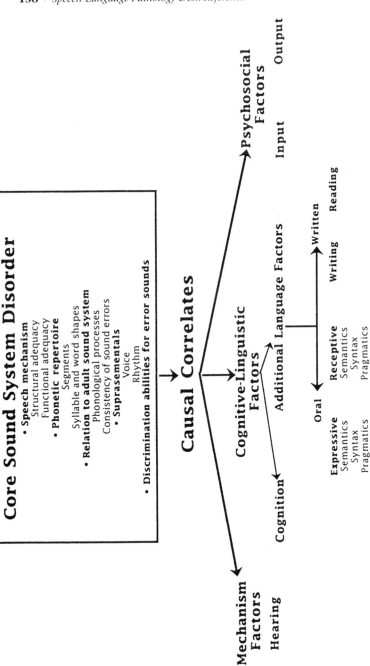

FIGURE 2.8. Speech disorder: core sound system disorder diagram representing factors to be considered in the description of the communicative functioning of a child.

SOURCE: With permission from McCauley RJ: A Comprehensive Phonological Approach to the Assessment and Treatment of Sound System Disorders. *Seminars in Speech and Language* 1993; 14:157.

TABLE 2.17. **Sound system usage: purposes and examples of recommended measures to describe a child's performance.**

Purposes	*Examples of Recommended Measures*
Description of speech mechanism	Standardized oral-peripheral and motor speech evaluation (e.g., St. Louis & Ruscello, 1981)
Description of phonetic repertoire and syllable and canonical shapes	Standardized articulation test or phonological assessment (e.g., Lowe, 1986; Shriberg & Kwiatkowski, 1980)
Phonological process description	Standardized sampling and analysis procedures (e.g., Hodson, 1986; Shriberg & Kwiakowski, 1980)
Description of factors affecting consistency	Stimulability testing (Diedrich, 1983); testing for consistency in differing phonetic environments (Secord, 1981; McDonald, 1964)
Description of suprasegmental phonology	Shriberg & Kwiatkowski (1982c)
Description of discrimination abilities for error sounds	Sound production-perception task (Locke, 1980)

SOURCE: With permission from McCauley RJ: A Comprehensive Phonological Approach to the Assessment and Treatment of Sound System Disorders. *Seminars in Speech and Language* 1993; 14:155.

3

Phonology, Respiration, and Articulation-Adult

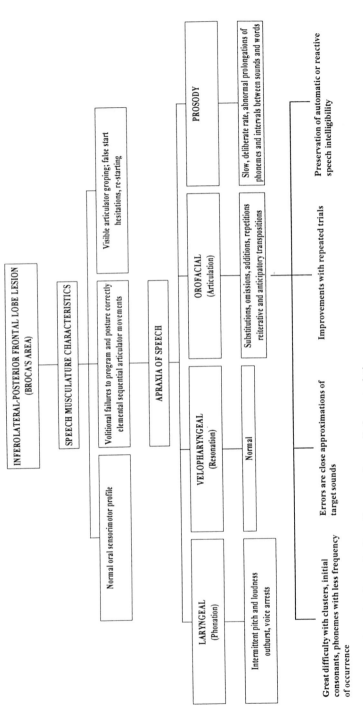

FIGURE 3.1. Apraxia of speech: flow diagram of overall characteristics.

SOURCE: With permission from Dworkin JP: *Motor Speech Disorders: A Treatment Guide*, p. 4. Mosby Year Book, St. Louis, 1991.

TABLE 3.1. **Apraxia of speech (AOS) and conduction aphasia: "traditional" characteristics.**

AOS	Conduction aphasia
Physiology: Absence of (1) muscle weakness, (2) movement slowness, (3) movement incoordination, (4) alterations of muscle tone	Intact movement and muscle physiology
Speech characteristics:	
Groping, off-target, highly inconsistent articulatory errors primarily sound errors of (1) substitution, (2) addition, (3) prolongation, (4) repetition	Repeated trials, attempts at self-correction Sound may be (1) substitutions, (2) omissions, (3) transpositions
Islands of error-free speech	Runs of normally articulated words
Errors especially evident on repetition tasks	More frequently occurring errors on repetition
More errors with increase in word length	Difficulties are linked to the articulatory "planning load"
Preserved auditory language comprehension	Auditory comprehension is relatively well preserved and may be completely normal
Preserved syntax semantics, and morphology	Generally preserved use of grammatical inflections and syntactic structures
Speech error type:	
More consonant than vowel	More consonant than vowel
More substitutions than (1) distortions, (2) omissions, (3) additions	More substitutions than (1) distortions, (2) omissions, (3) additions
More errors in word initial than final position	More errors in word initial than final position
More error of simplification (e.g., consonant cluster reduction) than complication	More error of simplification (e.g., consonant cluster reduction) than complication
More single feature than multiple feature sound substitutions	More single-feature than multiple-feature sound substitutions

SOURCE: With permission from McNeil MR, Robin DA, Schmidt RA: Apraxia of Speech: Definition, Differentiation, and Treatment. In McNeil NM (ed.): *Clinical Management of Sensorimotor Disorders*, p. 317. Thieme, New York, 1997.

TABLE 3.2. **Apraxia of speech (AOS) and dysarthria: "traditional" differentiating characteristics.**

Feature	AOS	Dysarthri
Lesion location	Unilateral/anterior	Bilateral if Cortical, Usually Subcortical
Psychophysiological level/mechanism	Motor programming	Movement Execution
Observed deviant speech behavior	Speech initiation, selection, & sequencing, phoneme substitution; abnormal prosody; infrequent metathetic errors	Sound-level Distortions
Speech processes involved	Essentially normal: 1. Resonance 2. Respiration 3. Phonation	Frequent Disturbance of: 1. Resonance 2. Respiration 3. Phonation
Physiological manifestations	Free from paralysis, paresis, ataxia, involuntary movements	Presence of Paralysis, Paresis, Ataxia, Involuntary Movements
Influence of nonphonologic (phonetic) factors	Effected by word length; error inconsistency	Less effected by word length; errors are more consistent
Oral Nonverbal Apraxia	Frequently present	Absent

SOURCE: With permission from McNeil MR, Robin DA, Schmidt RA: Apraxia of Speech: Definition, Differentiation, and Treatment. In McNeil MR (ed.): *Clinical Management of Sensorimotor Disorders*, p. 314. Thieme, New York, 1997.

TABLE **3.3.** **Apraxia of speech: Tasks and stimuli in the motor speech evaluation for appraisal.***

Task	Stimuli
Vowel prolongation	/a/
Rapid alternating movements	/pʌ/
	/tʌ/
	/kʌ/
	/pʌ-tʌ-kʌ/
Repetition of multisyllabic words	gingerbread
	snowman
	responsibility
	catastrophe
	television
Multiple trials with the same word (5 times)	artillery
	impossibility
	catastrophe
Repetition of words of increasing length	thick-thicker-thickening
	jab-jabber-jabbering
	zip-zipper-zippering
	please-pleasing-pleasingly
	flat-flatter-flattering
Repetition of monosyllabic words	mom, judge, peep, bib, nine, tote, dad, cake, gag, fife
	sis, zoos, church, lull, slush
Repetition of sentences	The valuable watch was missing.
	In the summer they sell vegetables.
	The shipwreck washed up on the shore.
	Please put the groceries in the refrigerator.
Picture description	"Cookie Thief" from the Boston Diagnostic Aphasia Examination (Goodglass and Kaplan, 1983)
Reading aloud	"Grandfather Passage"
Conversation	Biographical Information, Questions About Illness, Speech, and Nonspeech Symptoms

SOURCE: With permission from Wertz RT, Rosenbek JC: Where the Ear Fits: A Perceptual Evaluation of Motor Speech Disorders. *Seminars in Speech and Language* 1992; 13:45.
*Adapted from Wertz, LaPointe, and Rosenbek (1984).

TABLE 3.4. Apraxia of speech (AOS) versus phonemic paraphasia: differentiating characteristics.

Apraxia of speech	*Phonemic paraphasia*

Disturbed prosody:
  Overall rate:
  Slow rate in phonemically "on target" or "off-target" phrases and sentences.
  Inability to increase rate while maintaining phonemic integrity.
	Near normal rate in phonemically "on-target" phrases and sentences.
	Variable *ability to increase rate,* but *within normal ranges,* while maintaining phonemic integrity.

Microsegmental rate:
  Variable, but *overall prolonged movement transitions.*
  Variable, but *prolonged interword intervals* in phonemically "on-target" utterances.
  Variable, but *abnormally long vowels* in multisyllabic words or words in sentences.
  Variable, but *increased movement durations* for individual speech gestures in the production of contextual speech.
  Successive self-initiated trials to repair an error leads *no closer to the target.*
	Variable, but *normal movement transition durations.*
	Variable, but *normal average interword intervals* in phonemically "on-target" utterances.
	Variable, but *normal vowel duration* in multisyllabic words or words in sentences.
	
	Variable, but *average movement durations* within the ranges for normal subjects.
	
	Successive self-initiated trials to repair an error leads *closer to the target.*

Stress assignment: *Presence of errors on stressed syllables.*	*No clear relationship between syllabic stress and error frequency.*

Phonological characteristics:
  With distorted perseverative, anticipatory and exchange phoneme or phoneme cluster errors.
  With phoneme distortions.
  Presence of distorted sound substitutions-primarily of prolonged phonemes and secondarily devoiced phonemes.
	With undistorted perseverative, anticipatory and phoneme exchange or phoneme cluster errors.
	Without phoneme distortions.
	Absence of distorted sound substitutions.

Other kinematic characteristics:
  Inability to track predictable movement patterns with speech articulators.
  Ability to track unpredictable movement patterns with speech articulators.
	Ability to track predictable movement patterns with speech articulators.
	Inability to track unpredictable movement patterns with speech articulators.

Other Characteristics:
  The *location of errors* in the utterance *is consistent* from trial to trial.
  The *types of errors* in the utterance *are not variable* from trial to trial.
	The *location of errors* in the utterance *is not consistent* from trial to trial.
	The *types of errors* in the utterance *are variable* from trial to trial.

Treatment characteristics:
  Positive response to "minimal pairs" treatment.
  Positive response to treatment based on principles of "motor learning."
	Negative response to "minimal pairs" treatment.
	Ineffective response to treatment based on principles of "motor learning."

SOURCE: With permission from McNeil MR, Robin DA, Schmidt RA: Apraxia of Speech: Definition, Differentiation, and Treatment. In McNeil MR (ed.): *Clinical Management of Sensorimotor Disorders,* p. 327. Thieme, New York, 1997.

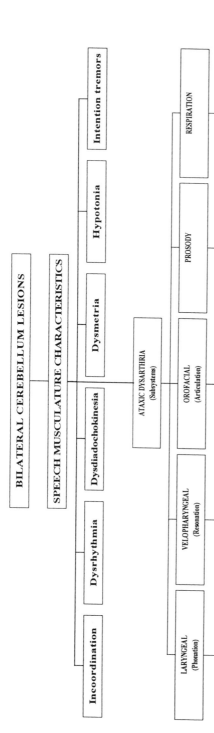

Figure 3.2. Ataxic dysarthria: flow diagram of overall characteristics.

SOURCE: With permission from Dworkin JP: *Motor Speech Disorders: A Treatment Guide*, p. 8. Mosby Year Book, St. Louis, 1991.

TABLE 3.5. Cranial nerve lesions: nerve, distribution, etiologies, and symptoms.

CRANIAL NERVE V (TRIGEMINAL)

Sensory	Distribution
Ophthalmic	Forehead, eyes, nose, temples, and nasal mucosa
Maxillary	Teeth, upper lip, cheeks, hard palate, nasal mucosa
Mandibular	Teeth, lower lip, buccal mucosa, tongue, auditory meatus
Motor	Distribution
Motor root (pons)	Masseter, temporal, internal and external pterygoids
Otic ganglion	Tensor tympani, tensor veli palatini
Mylohyoid	Mylohyoid, anterior belly of digastric
Etiologies	Neuralgias, neuritis, syphilis, tuberculosis, syringobulbia, tumors, basilar meningitis, tic doulourex, para trigeminal
Symptoms	Paralysis or weakness of muscles of mastication with mandible deviation to the affected side

CRANIAL NERVE VII (FACIAL)

Nerve	Distribution
Sensory	
Nervous intermedus	Taste to anterior 2/3 of the tongue
Motor	
Temporal	Frontalis, orbicularis oculi, dilator naris, nasalis
Zygomatic	Zygomaticus, quadrates labii superior, orbicularis oris
Cervicofacial	Risorius, mentalis, quadrates labii inferior, incisivus inferior, buccinator, posterior belly of digastric, stapedius
Etiologies	Bell's palsy, middle ear infections, chilling of the face, tumors
Symptoms	Lesion outside stylomastoid foramen—affected side of mouth droops, buccal stasis of food, no wink, decreased wrinkle of forehead on affected side
	Lesion in facial canal (chords tympani)—reduced taste and salivation
	Lesion in internal auditory meatus—deafness and facial weakness
	Lesion at emergence from pons—facial weakness and other cranial nerve involvement

CRANIAL NERVE IX (GLOSSOPHARYNGEAL)

Nerve	Distribution
Sensory	Pharynx, soft palate, taste posterior 1/3 of tongue, fauces,
Fibers from jugular	tonsils, carotid body, and carotid sinus controlling
ganglia	reflexes for respiration, blood pressure, and heart rate
Motor	Stylopharyngeal
Parasympathetic	Parotid gland
Etiologies	Bonnier's syndrome, Vernet's syndrome, glossopharyngeal neuralgia (paroxysmal pain)
Symptoms	Loss of gag, dysphagia, loss of taste, sensation loss in pharynx and posterior tongue, increased salivation, tachycardia

(continued)

TABLE 3.5. (*continued*)

	CRANIAL NERVE X (VAGUS)
Nerve	Distribution
Sensory	
Auricular	External auditory meatus, dura of posterior fossa
Ganglion nodosum	Pharynx, larynx, trachea, esophageus, abdominal cavity
Internal sup. laryn.	Internal surface of larynx above vocal folds
Motor (nucleus	
ambiguous)	Pharyngeal constrictors, levator veli palatini
Pharyngeal	Cricothyroid
External sup. laryn.	All intrinsic laryngeal muscle except cricothyroid
Recurrent laryngeal	Intramedullary lesions including hemorrhage, thrombosis,
Etiologies	tumors, syphilis, syringobulbia. Peripheral lesions include primary neuritis (alcohol, dipheritic, lead, arsenic), tumors, trauma, surgery, aortic aneurysm
Symptoms	Bilateral recurrent lesions—adductor/abductor paralysis of vocal folds with aphonia, dyspnea, or pseudoasthma, cardiac arrhythmia and death
	Unilateral recurrent lesions—unilateral vocal fold paralysis with dysphonia
	Unilateral pharyngeal nerve—unilateral velar paralysis with hypernasality with deviation to strong side.
	Unilateral superior laryngeal nerve—anesthesia of larynx, fatigue, pitch control problems.
	CRANIAL NERVE XI (SPINAL ACCESSORY)
	Distribution
Nerve	None
Sensory	
Motor	Via Xth cranial nerve contributes to intrinsic laryngeal
Internal medullary	muscle
	Trapezius, sternocleidomastoid
External (spinal)	Meningitis, syphilis, trauma, surgery on tuberculoses
Etiologies	nodes
Symptoms	No rotation of head to healthy side; cannot shrug shoulder
Unilateral	on affected side, affected shoulder droops
	Difficult to rotate head or raise chin, head often drops
Bilateral	forward
	CRANIAL NERVE XII (HYPOGLOSSAL)
	Distribution
Nerve	Intrinsic muscle of tongue, styloglossus, genioglossus,
Hypoglossal	geniohyoid, thyrohyoid, sternohyoid, sternothyroid, omohyoid
Etiologies	Basal skull fractures, dislocation of upper cervical vertebrae, tuberculoses, aneurysm of Circle of Willis, syphilis, and lead, alcohol, arsenic, and carbon monoxide poisonings, brain abscess, syringobulbia

SOURCE: With permission from Hageman C: Flaccid Dysarthria. In McNeil MR (ed.): *Clinical Management of Sensorimotor Disorders*, pp. 196–197. Thieme, New York, 1997.

TABLE **3.6. Dimensions of dysarthria.**

I. Phonation
  A. Pitch
    1. Pitch level
    2. Pitch breaks
    3. Monopitch
    4. Voice tremor
  B. Intensity
    1. Monoloudness
    2. Excess loudness variation
    3. Loudness decay
    4. Alternating loudness
    5. Loudness (overall)
  C. Quality
    1. Harsh voice
    2. Hoarse (wet) voice
    3. Breathy voice (continuous)
    4. Breathy voice (transient)
    5. Strained/strangled voice
    6. Voice stoppages

II. Resonation
  A. Hypernasality
  B. Hyponasality
  C. Nasal emission

III. Respiration
  A. Forced inspiration/expiration

  B. Audible inspiration
  C. Grunt at end of expiration

IV. Articulation
  A. Imprecise consonants
  B. Phonemes prolonged
  C. Irregular articulatory breakdown
  D. Phonemes repeated
  E. Vowels distorted
  F. Intelligibility
  G. Bizarreness

V. Prosody
  A. Rate
  B. Phrases short
  C. Increase of rate in segments
  D. Increase in rate overall
  E. Reduced stress
  F. Variable rate
  G. Intervals prolonged
  H. Inappropriate silences
  I. Short rushes of speech
  J. Excess and equal stress

VI. Other

SOURCE: From Air DH, Wood AS, Neils JR: Considerations for Organic Disorders. In Creaghead NA, Newman PW, Secord WA: *Assessment and Remediation of Articulatory and Phonological Disorders*, p. 276. Copyright © 1989 by Allyn and Bacon. Reprinted/adapted by permission.

Note. The specific characteristics (e.g., pitch level, pitch breaks, monoloudness) are from *Motor Speech Disorders* by F. Darley, A. Aronson, and J. Brown, Philadelphia: W. B. Saunders, 1975.

TABLE **3.7. Dysarthria: lesion site and symptoms for lower motor neuron and motor unit difficulties.**

Lesion site	Symptoms*
Brain stem or peripheral nerve	Loss of muscle contraction of affected units for reflex and voluntary activity; flaccid muscle; reduced reflexes; hypotonia, muscle atrophy, weakness, paralysis, fasciculation
Myoneural junction	Weakness, increased fatiguability over short time periods
Muscle fibers	Muscle hypertrophy or atrophy, failure to relax; failure to contract, fatty infiltration and fibrosis, hypocontraction

SOURCE: With permission from Hageman C: Flaccid Dysarthria. In McNeil MR (ed.): *Clinical Management of Sensorimotor Disorders*, p. 195. Thieme, New York, 1997.
*Chusid (1985).

TABLE 3.8. Dysarthric patients: differential respiration subsystem disturbances.

Dysarthria Type	Poor Posture	Neck and Trunk Rigidity	Reduced Pressure-Generating Capability	Shallow Inhalations	Reduced Exhalation Control	Rapid Breaths	Slow Breaths	Antagonistic Muscular Contractions	Involuntary Muscular Contractions	Irregular Patterns	Sudden Forced Inhalations/Exhalations
Spastic	X	X	X	X	X		X	X			
Ataxic				X	X	X				X	X
Hyperkinetic	X	X		X	X	X		X	X	X	X
Hypokinetic	X	X		X	X	X				X	X
Flaccid	X		X	X	X		X				

SOURCE: With permission from Dworkin JP: *Motor Speech Disorders: A Treatment Guide*, p. 43. Mosby Year Book, St. Louis, 1991.

TABLE 3.9. **Dysarthric patients: differential respiration subsystem treatments, objectives, and methods.**

Sequence of Respiration Subsystem Treatment Exercises	Speech Breathing Objectives	Techniques
Relaxation	Reduce stiffness, tension, and rigidity of head, neck, and trunk musculature	Supine breathing exercises using See Scape device for airflow feedback Alternate tightening and relaxing of respiration subsystem muscular contractions in supine position Passive manipulation of head and neck in sitting position Rag doll exercise Alternatives: drugs, rolfing, meditation, yoga, creative visualization, self-actualization
Postural support	Augment and reinforce respiration subsystem musculoskeletal framework	Adaptive alterations of wheelchair Elastic straps, girdles, slings Alternating sitting and standing positions
Pressure generation	Train low-pressure exhalations, controlled and maintained over time	Adaptive alteration of Sea-Scape device for subglottal air pressure generation practice at 5 cm H_2O/5 seconds
Prolonged inhalation	Improve lung volume Improve strength/ coordination of inhalatory/ exhalatory musculature Maximize no. of syllables/ breath	Manual compressions of abdominal wall as breath is held firmly to combat deflating forces Inverted Sea-Scape device for feedback practice of prolonged inhalations
Prolonged exhalation	Facilitate rate control Modify upper thoracic and clavicular breathing patterns	Prolonged steady exhalations using See-Scape device for feedback practice Variably prolonged exhalations using See-Scape device for feedback

(continued)

TABLE 3.9. *(continued)*

Sequence of Respiration Subsystem Treatment Exercises	*Speech Breathing Objectives*	*Techniques*
Quick breaths	Improve rate alternatives	Multiple quick breaths using See-Scape device for feedback
Inhalatory/exhalatory synchronization	Train cooperative, synchronous contractions of opposing muscle groups	Regularly timed inhalatory/exhalatory maneuvers, using See-Scape device for feedback Repetitions of the consonant /m/ for variably prolonged time intervals, using See-Scape device for feedback
Isolated sounds	Improve coupling of respiration subsystem controls with speech motor output	Isolated vowel prolongations, Fricative prolongations, Real and nonsense word productions ⎱ Using See-Scape device for feedback Vowel and fricative repetitions, CV syllable production at various rates ⎱ Using See-Scape device and metronome for feedback
Connected speech	Increase no. of syllables/breath in connected discourse	Sentence productions, using See-Scape device for feedback Paragraph productions, using See-Scape device for feedback

SOURCE: With permission from Dworkin JP: *Motor Speech Disorders: A Treatment Guide*, p. 76. Mosby Year Book, St. Louis, 1991.

TABLE 3.10. **Dysarthric patients: two types who most commonly exhibit velopharyngeal incompetency—differential resonation subsystems signs, symptoms, and treatments.**

	Flaccid Dysarthric Patient	*Spastic Dysarthric Patient*
Lesion sites:	Unilateral or bilateral ninth and tenth cranial nerves	Bilateral corticobulbar tracts
Medical diagnosis	Bulbar palsy	Pseudobulbar palsy
Pathophysiological velopharyngeal musculature signs and symptoms[1]:	Unilateral or bilateral weakness; unilateral or bilateral paralysis; hypotonicity; hypoactive gag reflex	Bilateral weakness; bilateral paralysis; hypertonicity; variably hyperactive gag reflex
Motor speech effects:	Hypernasality; excess nasal air emission; reduced intraoral air pressure and associated articulatory imprecision	Hypernasality; excess nasal air emission; reduced intraoral air pressure and articulatory imprecision
Treatment considerations[2]:	*Behavioral management:* improve velopharyngeal valving competency and institute speech resonation exercises *Prosthetic appliance:* palatal lift *Surgical intervention:* pharyngeal flap, or muscle implantation	*Behavioral management:* normalize reflex through touch pressure and massage techniques; normalize tone through touch pressure and massage techniques; improve velopharyngeal valving competency through nonspeech and speech exercises *Prosthetic appliance:* palatal lift *Surgical intervention:* pharyngeal flap, or muscle implantation

SOURCE: With permission from Dworkin JP: *Motor Speech Disorders: A Treatment Guide,* p. 86. Mosby Year Book, St. Louis, 1991.
[1]Degree will vary commensurate with extent of neurological involvement.
[2]Sequence and number of applications will vary, depending on the severity of the incompetence and the patient's responses.

TABLE 3.11. **Dysarthric speakers: function component evaluation and diagnostic treatment.**

Component	Tasks
RESPIRATORY STRUCTURES	
Evaluation	Sniff, pant
	Prolong /a/
	Slow and rapid loudness change on /a/
	Counting at different loudness levels
	Shout Short Phrase
Diagnostic treatment	Talk
	Instructions: take lots of air, talk louder, concentrate on speaking clearly
	Provide static support on patient's abdomen
	Vary support on inhalation and exhalation, have patient provide support
	Occlude patient's nose
	Have patient talk in different positions
LARYNGEAL STRUCTURES	
Evaluation	Cough, clear throat
	Prolong /a/
	Slow and fast pitch change on /a/
	Rapid, succinct productions of /i/
	Count down to lowest pitch
	Count up to highest pitch
	Produce lowest, highest, and habitual pitch
	Rapid alternating movements—/pʌ/,/tʌ/,/kʌ/—to detect voicing errors
	Talk
Diagnostic treatment	Instruction: produce speech with more energy
	Produce speech during clinician's manipulation of patient's larynx and respiratory structures
	Produce speech with head forward, turned to the left, turned to the right
	Produce speech while bearing down
VELOPHARYNGEAL STRUCTURES	
Evaluation	Drink from a cup or drinking fountain
	Prolong /a/
	Produce /u-i/
	Produce assimilative sentences, e.g., "Make me a Hong Kong cookie." or "Papa mops."
	Talk
Diagnostic treatment	Compare nares occluded with unoccluded on rapid alternating movements—/pʌ/,/tʌ/,/kʌ/—counting, sentences, e.g., "Buy Bobby a puppy."
	Compare speaking at different rates—slow, normal, rapid
OROFACIAL STRUCTURES	
Evaluation	Rapid alternating movements—/pʌ/,/tʌ/,/kʌ/—at 1, 2, 3, and 4 per second and as fast as possible. All done with urging to be "crisp, even, and as clear as possible."

(continued)

TABLE 3.11. (*continued*)

Component	Tasks
	Repeat performance of rapid alternating movements with bite block
	Word and sentence intelligibility tests
	Talk
Diagnostic treatment	Connected speech under various conditions, including: different rates, increased effort, delayed auditory feedback, binaural masking, gestural reorganization, bite block

SOURCE: With permission from Wert RT, Rosenbek JC: Where the Ear Fits: A Perceptual Evaluation of Motor Speech Disorders. *Seminars in Speech and Language* 1992; 13:48.

TABLE 3.12. Dysarthric speech: perceptual dimensions for rating.

Dimension	Brief Description
Overall severity	Degree of dysarthric impairment across dimensions
Inappropriate voicing	Abnormal cessation, appearance, or continuation of voicing
Intrusive sounds	Extraneous or inappropriate sounds within a word or phrase
Slow rate	Rate of utterance slower than expected for normal production; associated with longer than normal durations
Fast rate	Rate of utterance faster than expected for normal production; associated with shorter than normal durations
Dysrhythmia	Distorted temporal relationships among syllables, pauses and intrasyllabic components; deviant rhythm of stretches of speech
Inappropriate phrasing	Phrases are either too long or too short in relation to breath support for speech.
Consonant omission	Deletion of consonant segments
Consonant distortion	Consonant segments are perceived as inaccurately or imprecisely articulated.
Consonant substitution	Consonant segments are replaced by other consonant segments; phonemic substitutions.
Vowel errors	Deletions, distortions or substitutions of vowel segments
Monoloudness	Phonation as reduced variation in loudness across a multisyllabic utterance.
Reduced stress contrasts	Attenuation of stress or emphasis patterns within utterances; weakening of stress contrasts
Voice quality inconsistency	Changeable or irregular voice quality during an utterance
Breathy voice quality	Voice has breathy quality.
Harsh voice quality	Voice has harsh or rough quality.
Strain-strangle quality	Voice has features of strain–strangle.
Hypernasality	Voice quality has excessive nasalization.
Hyponasality	Voice has less than normal nasality.
Monopitch	Pitch range over an utterance is reduced.
Excessive pitch change	Pitch range over an utterance is variable or extreme in degree.

Each dimension is rated on a 7-point, equal appearing interval scale, as shown by the following example:

OVERALL SEVERITY   1   2   3   4   5   6   7

                                         Least   Most
                                           deviant   deviant
                                           (normal)

SOURCE: With permission from Darley F, Aronson A, Brown J: Differential Diagnostic Patterns of Dysarthria. *Journal of Speech and Hearing Research,* 1969; 12:267–269.

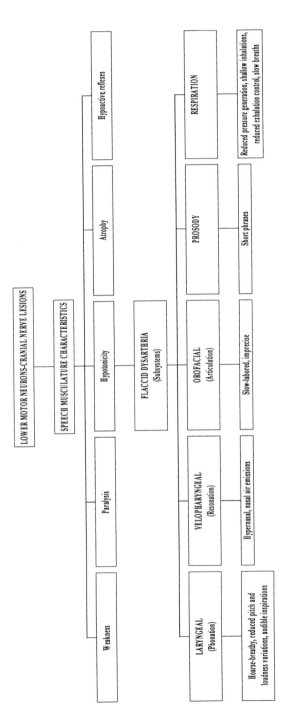

Figure 3.3. Flaccid dysarthria: flow diagram of overall characteristics.

SOURCE: With permission from Dworkin JP: *Motor Speech Disorders: A Treatment Guide*, p. 12. Mosby Year Book. St. Louis, 1991.

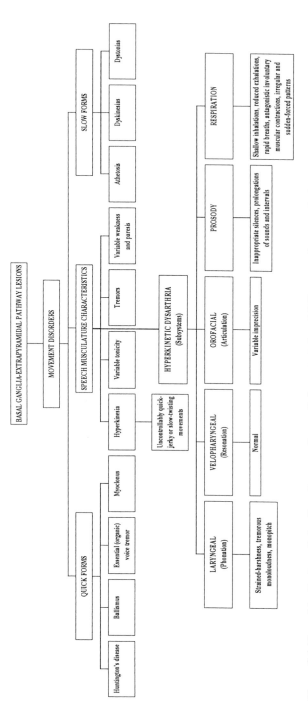

Figure 3.4. Hyperkinetic dysarthria: flow diagram of overall characteristics of different patient populations.

SOURCE: With permission from Dworkin JP: *Motor Speech Disorders: A Treatment Guide*, p. 11. Mosby Year Book, St. Louis, 1991.

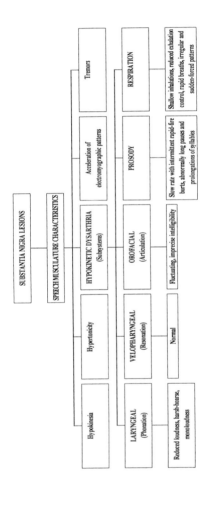

Figure 3.5. Hypokinetic dysarthria: flow diagram of overall characteristics.
SOURCE: With permission from Dworkin JP: *Motor Speech Disorders: A Treatment Guide*, p. 10. Mosby Year Book. St. Louis, 1991.

TABLE 3.13. **Motor examination: nonspeech tasks.**

Pulmonic function
  Maximum expiratory pressure
  Maximum inspiratory pressure
  Flow-volume loops
  Other pulmonic function measures (VC, IC, PEFR, etc.)
  Respiratory maneuvers (e.g., panting, checking, sniffing)
  Pressure regulation (e.g., maintaining a specified intraoral pressure for a prescribed
    duration)
Laryngeal function
  Laryngeal maneuvers (e.g., coughing, adduction of vocal folds)
  Upper airway (articulatory system)
  Compression/contraction force (maximal forces developed by muscles of the tongue, jaw,
    or lip)
  Fine force regulation (e.g., sustaining /s/ production)
  Rapid alternating movement (various structures at maximum rate or prescribed rates)
  Oral nonverbal gestures
  Scoring possibilities:
  Basic response scoring:
    No response / Fragmented / Distorted / Correct
  Elaborated response scoring (detailed description):
    Delay / Self-correction / Perseveration / Nonscorable
  Substitution responses (use of alternative body part):
    Oral / Verbal / Body / Noise
  Augmentation responses (accompanying behaviors)
    Oral / Body / Noise
  Tasks:
  Tongue protrusion
  Baring teeth
  Smile
  Pucker lips
  Cough
  Puff cheeks
  Touch nose with tongue tip
  Touch chin with tongue tip
  Touch corner of mouth with tongue tip
  Blow
  Suck
  Bite lip
  Bite tongue
  Lick lips
  Move tongue from corner to corner of mouth
  Other nonspeech oral motor function
  Mastication
  Swallow (wet and dry, different bolus sizes)

SOURCE: With permission from Kent RD: The Perceptual Sensorimotor Examination for Motor Speech Disorders. In McNeil MR (ed.): *Clinical Management of Sensorimotor Disorders,* p. 30. Thieme, New York, 1997.

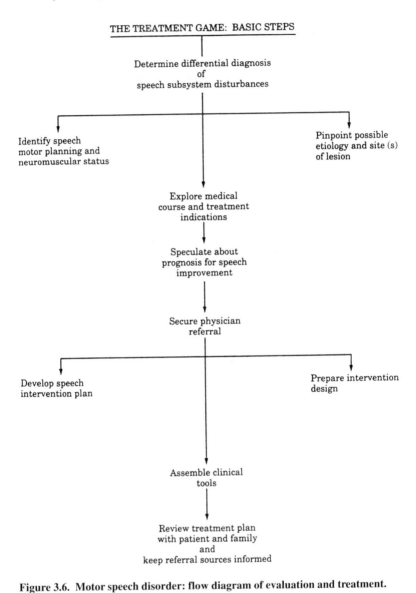

Figure 3.6. Motor speech disorder: flow diagram of evaluation and treatment.
SOURCE: With permission from Dworkin JP: *Motor Speech Disorders: A Treatment Guide,*
p. 21. Mosby Year Book, St. Louis, 1991.

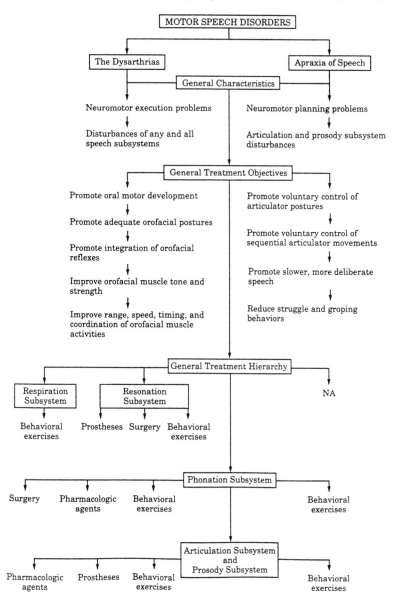

Figure 3.7. Motor speech disorders flow diagram: general characteristics, over-all objectives of intervention, and top-down differential hierarchy of speech subsystem treatments.

SOURCE: With permission from Dworkin JP: *Motor Speech Disorders: A Treatment Guide,* p. 37. Mosby Year Book, St. Louis, 1991.

TABLE 3.14. **Motor speech disorders: differential laryngeal–phonatory features in patients.**

Disorder	Voice Characteristics	Laryngeal Pathophysiology	Lesion Site(s)
Spastic dysarthria	*Relatively constant and predictable:* Strain-strangled quality, periodic arrests of phonation, short phrases, monoloudness, and monopitch	Hyperadduction, weakness and paresis of vocal folds, bilaterally	Bilateral corticobulbar tracts of pyramidal system
Flaccid dysarthria	*Relatively Stable:* Hoarse-breathy quality, reduced pitch and loudness range, short phrases, diplophonia, and inhalatory stridor	Hypoadduction, weakness and paralysis of vocal folds, unilaterally, bilaterally, incomplete or complete	Tenth cranial nerve (Vagus), unilaterally or bilaterally anywhere along its course from brainstem to musculature
Hypokinetic dysarthria	*Predictable:* Harsh–breathy quality, monopitch, and reduced loudness	Rigidity and hypokinesia of vocal folds	Substantia nigra of extrapyramidal system
Ataxic dysarthria	*Variable:* Hoarse–harsh quality, sudden and irregular loudness and pitch outbursts, and coarse tremor	Incoordination and intention tremors of vocal folds	Bilateral, generalized cerebellar structures
Quick (chorea) hyperkinetic dysarthria	*Random:* Harsh–strained quality, intermittent breathiness, irregular pitch alterations, arrests of phonation, monopitch, excessive loudness variations and monoloudness	Involuntary, uncontrollable, jerky, and hyperkinetic vocal fold behaviors	Basal ganglia of extrapyramidal system
Slow (dystonia, dyskinesia, athetosis) hyperkinetic dysarthria	*Unpredictable:* Strained-strangled, hoarse-breathy quality, aperiodic arrests of phonation, excessive loudness variations, monopitch, and stridor	Involuntary, uncontrollable slow, undulating, twisting, writhing, spasmodic vocal fold behaviors	Disseminated extrapyramidal structures

(continued)

TABLE 3.14. (*continued*)

Disorder	Voice Characteristics	Laryngeal Pathophysiology	Lesion Site(s)
Tremor (essential, myoclonous) hyperkinetic dysarthria	*Rhythmic fluctuations or alterations:* in loudness, quavering intonation, monopitch, strained-harsh quality, and episodic laryngospasms with arrests of phonation	Synchronous tremors of abductory-adductory vocal fold musculature	Variable extrapyramidal locations, including cerebral pathways, dentate nucleus, red nucleus, inferior olive, restiform body, and striatum
Apraxia of speech (phonation)	*Inconsistent and intermittent:* Mutism, whispered speech, pitch and loudness outbursts (squeals), and periods of good phonation	Faulty motor planning of vocal fold behaviors during volitional speech efforts	Inferolateral posterior frontal lobe (Broca's area) of language dominant (L) cerebral hemisphere

SOURCE: With permission from Dworkin JP: *Motor Speech Disorders: A Treatment Guide,* p. 136. Mosby Year Book, St. Louis, 1991.

TABLE 3.15. Motor speech disorders: recommended sequence of treatments for commonly co-occurring speech subsystem impairments in patients.

Motor Speech Disorder	Degree of Voice Disturbance	Respiration	Resonation	Phonation	Articulation	Prosody
Spastic dysarthria	Mild	First	First	Second	Second	Third
	Moderate–severe	First	First	Second	Third	Fourth
Flaccid dysarthria	Mild	First	First	Second	Second	Third
	Moderate–severe	First	First	Second	Third	Fourth
Hypokinetic dysarthria	Mild	First	N/A	First	Second	Second
	Moderate–severe	First	N/A	Second	Third	Fourth
Ataxic dysarthria	Mild	First	N/A	First	Second	Second
	Moderate–severe	First	N/A	Second	Third	Fourth
Quick and slow hyperkinetic dysarthria	Mild	First	N/A	First	Second	Second
	Moderate–severe	First	N/A	Second	Third	Fourth
Tremor hyperkinetic dysarthria	Mild	N/A	N/A	First	N/A	N/A
	Moderate–severe	N/A	N/A	First	N/A	N/A
Apraxia of speech	Mild	N/A	N/A	First	Second	Second
	Moderate–severe	N/A	N/A	First	Second	Third

SOURCE: With permission from Dworkin JP: *Motor Speech Disorders: A Treatment Guide*, p. 137. Mosby Year Book, St. Louis, 1991.

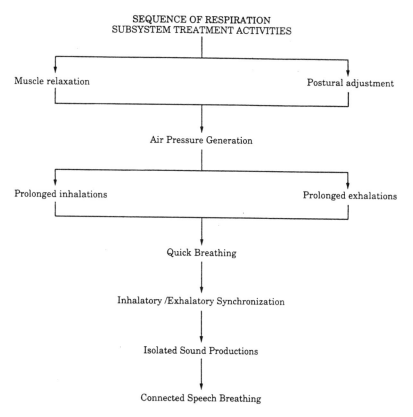

Figure 3.8. Respiration subsystem treatment parameters: recommended treatment activities hierarchy.

SOURCE: With permission from Dworkin JP: *Motor Speech Disorders: A Treatment Guide,* p. 48. Mosby Year Book, St. Louis, 1991.

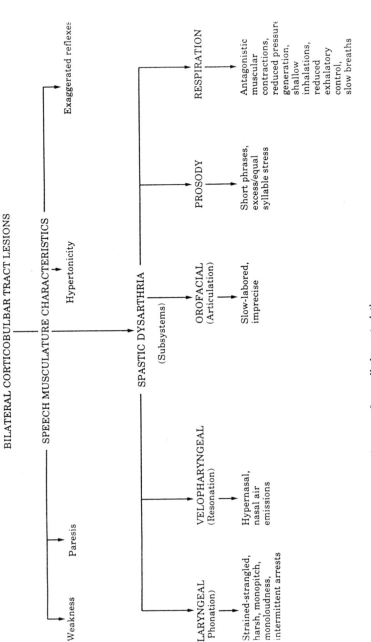

Figure 3.9. Spastic dysarthria: flow diagram of overall characteristics.
SOURCE: With permission from Dworkin JP: *Motor Speech Disorders: A Treatment Guide*, p. 7. Mosby Year Book. St. Louis. 1991.

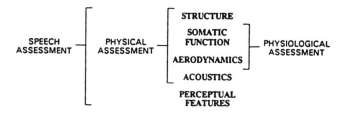

Figure 3.10. Speech assessment: comprehensive structure.*

SOURCE: Orlikoff RF: The Use of Instrumental Measures in the Assessment and Treatment of Motor Speech Disorders. *Seminars in Speech and Language* 1992; 13:26.
*See Table 3.15.

TABLE 3.16. **Speech impairment and disability: information often useful in assessment.**

Assessment	Important Parameters
Structure	Size, symmetry, orientation, shape, color, density, integrity, biomechanical properties (e.g., mass, stiffness)
Somatic function	Neuromuscular activity, structural movement, configuration, placement, contact, speed, duration, force, timing, precision, accuracy, strength, fluidity, regularity
Speech aerodynamics	Air volumes, pressures, and flows
Speech acoustics	Frequency, intensity, timing, duration, transition, periodicity, rate, resonant (i.e., spectral) characteristics
Perceptual features	Speech intelligibility, naturalness, communicative adequacy and efficiency, appropriateness, aesthetic quality

SOURCE: With permission from Orlikoff RF: The Use of Instrumental Measures in the Assessment and Treatment of Motor Speech Disorders. *Seminars in Speech and Language* 1992; 13:29.

TABLE 3.17. **Speech subsystems segregated by disorder type and severity: summary of sequential treatments.**

Disorder/Severity	Respiration	Resonation	Phonation	Articulation	Prosody
FLACCID DYSARTHRIA					
A. Mononeuropathy:					
VIIth nerve	N/A	N/A	N/A	First	Second, if necessary
Xth nerve	N/A	First, if necessary	Second, if necessary	Third, if necessary	Fourth, if necessary
XIIth nerve	N/A	N/A	N/A	First	Second
B. Polyneuropathy:					
VIIth & Xth nerves	N/A	First	Second	Third	Fourth, if necessary
Xth & XIIth nerves	N/A	First	Second	Third	Fourth
VIIth & XII nerves	N/A	N/A	N/A	First	Second
VIIth, Xth, & XIIth nerves	N/A	First	Second	Third	Fourth
SPASTIC DYSARTHRIA					
A. Mild	First	First	Second	Second	Third
B. Moderate/severe	First	Second	Third	Fourth	Fifth
ATAXIC DYSARTHRIA					
A. Mild	First	N/A	First	Second	Third
B. Moderate/severe	First	N/A	Second	Third	Fourth
HYPOKINETIC DYSARTHRIA					
A. Mild	First	N/A	First	Second	Third
B. Moderate/severe	First	N/A	Second	Third	Fourth
HYPERKINETIC DYSARTHRIA					
A. Mild	First	N/A	First	Second	Third
B. Moderate/severe	First	N/A	Second	Third	Fourth
APRAXIA					
A. Speech	N/A	N/A	N/A	First	Second
B. Phonation	N/A	N/A	First	N/A	Second

SOURCE: With permission from Dworkin JP: Motor Speech Disorders: A Treatment Guide, p. 33. Mosby Year Book, St. Louis, 1991.

NOTE: For mixed dysarthria, assume the typical combination of subsystem treatments based on the predominant and secondary components of the composite mixture.

TABLE 3.18. **Speech system: Physical and perceptual aspects of motor speech organized by function.**

	Ventilatory Function	Laryngeal Function	Oropharyngeal Function	Velopharyngeal Function
Salient structures	Thorax/rib cage, diaphragm and abdomen—trunk and neck musculature	Laryngeal cartilages, vocal fold muscular and non-muscular tissues—intrinsic and extrinsic laryngeal musculature	Pharyngeal wall, tongue, velum, hard palate, man-dible, lips, and associated musculature	Pharyngeal wall, tongue, velum, and associated musculature
Speech physiology (kinematics)	Regulation of thoracic cavity dimension/volume	Provision of glottal resistance (valving): a) Modulated b) Static/fixed c) Gross/tran-sient	Provision of oral resistance (valving): a) Occlusions/stoppages b) Major constrictions c) Minor constrictions Provision of an oropharyngeal configuration to effect resonance changes:	Provision of velopharyngeal resistance (valving) Provision of a nasooropharyngeal configuration to effect changes in vocal tract resonance
Speech physiology (aerodynamics)	Generation and regulation of lung volume, generation, control, and maintenance of subglottal pressure	Rapid modulation of the ex-piratory airstream (voice), creation of airflow turbulence (friction), or sudden release of flow under high pressure (plosion)	Generation and regulation of intraoral pres-sure of and oral airflow to create the fricative or plosive sound sources of English speech sounds	Generation and regulation of intraoral pressure and nasal airflow
Speech acoustics	Related to vocal intensity and funda-mental frequency con-trol and regulation, to the intensity of speech sounds, and to phrase length	Vocal intensity and funda-mental fre-quency charac-teristics, voice initiation/ attack, aperiodic noise energy, voic-ing cues/char-acteristics	Various duration, intensity, and the frequency cues relating to the manner and place of artic-ulation formant (and formant transition) energy related to vowel and consonant characteristics	Nasalization of vowels and acoustic cues relating to the manner and place of nasal consonant articulation

(continued)

Table 3.18. (continued)

	Ventilatory Function	Laryngeal Function	Oropharyngeal Function	Velopharyngeal Function
Possible perceptual consequences of pathology	Soft voice, low pitch, restricted pitch and loudness variation, disturbed prosody, inappropriate pauses, hoarseness, harshness, roughness, breathiness, inappropriate voicing, strained–strangled voice, misarticulations, disturbed speech rate and timing, reduced speech intelligibility and naturalness	Inappropriate pitch and loudness, restricted or excessive loudness and pitch variation, voice breaks, dysprosody, hard glottal attack, breathy attack, diplophonia, hoarseness, roughness, breathiness, harshness, inappropriate voicing, tremulousness, strained–strangled voice, reduced speech intelligibility and naturalness	Slurred or imprecise speech, distorted consonants, consonant omissions and substitutions, disturbed prosody, inappropriate pitch and loudness, vowel distortion, reduced vowel differentiation, disturbed speech rate and timing, reduced speech intelligibility and naturalness	Nasal snorting, reduced loudness of high-pressure consonants, hypernasality, hyponasality, distortion, omission or substitution of high-pressure consonants, disturbed prosody, inappropriate pitch and loudness, reduced vowel differentiation, reduced speech intelligibility and natural-ness

SOURCE: With permission from Orlikoff RF: The Use of Instrumental Measures in the Assessment and Treatment of Motor Speech Disorders. *Seminars in Speech and Language* 1992; 13:27.

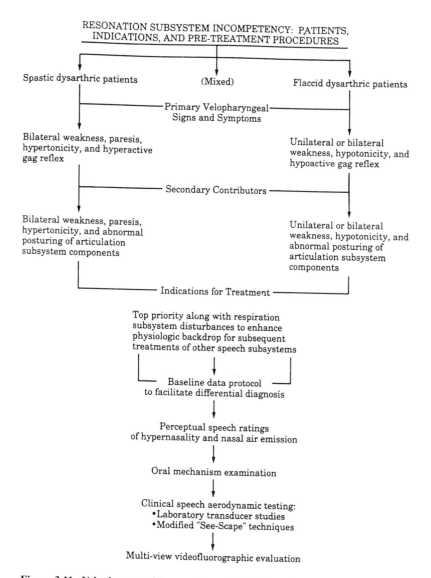

Figure 3.11. Velopharyngeal incompetency (VPI): flow diagram of pretreatment sequential procedures for patients with suspected VPI.

SOURCE: With permission from Dworkin JP: *Motor Speech Disorders: A Treatment Guide,* p. 93. Mosby Year Book, St. Louis, 1991.

4

Child Language

TABLE 4.1. **Attention-deficit/hyperactivity disorder: educational accommodations for children.**

Accommodation type	Examples
Environmental	Modify classroom arrangement
	Decrease environmental distractions
	Highly structured daily routine
	Highly structured transitions
	Organizational aids
	Peer tutor and/or peer behavior managers
Materials	High feedback self-correcting materials
	Introduce novelty
	Advanced organizers
	Interspersed short lessons
	Instructional prompts and cues
Instructional	Structure activities to allow excess energy to be channeled
	Maintain a positive, upbeat, nonthreatening teaching approach
	Teach organization and independent learning skills
	Arrange for an "emergency" signal
Alter criteria or task requirements	Adjust task or lesson lengths commensurate with attentional span
	Eliminate recopying
	Shorten homework assignments
Altered curriculum	Focus on prerequisite skills
	Focus on social skills curriculum

SOURCE: Maag JW, Reid R: Treatment of Attention-Deficit/Hyperactivity Disorder: A Multi-Modal Model for Schools. *Seminars in Speech and Language* 1996; 17:39.

TABLE 4.2. **Attention-deficit/hyperactivity disorder: three core behaviors and 18 behavioral criteria viewed as symptoms in intervention.**

INATTENTION is characterized by difficulty
1. Attending to details
2. Sustaining attention to tasks
3. Listening when spoken to
4. Following through on instructions or finishing tasks
5. Organizing tasks and activities
6. Initiating tasks that require sustained mental effort
7. Keeping track of objects needed for a task
8. Ignoring extraneous stimuli
9. Remembering routine procedures or familiar information

IMPULSIVITY is characterized by
1. Blurting out answers
2. Failing to take turns
3. Intercepting or intruding on others

HYPERACTIVITY is characterized by
1. Fidgeting with hands or feet or squirming in seat
2. Difficulty remaining seated
3. Running or climbing excessively in inappropriate contexts
4. Difficulty engaging in quiet activity
5. Constantly moving or engaging in activity
6. Talking excessively

SOURCE: Norris JA, Hoffman PR: Attaining, Sustaining, and Focusing Attention: Intervention for Children with ADHD. *Seminars in Speech and Language* 1996; 17:61.

TABLE 4.3. **Children with in-place tracheostomies: therapy options to facilitate expressive communication.**

Category	Therapy options
Facilitates oral communication	Speaking valve
	Cannula occlusion
	Electrolarynx
	Buccal speech
	Esophageal speech
	Fenestrated cannula
Facilitates nonoral communication	Manual communication
	Alternative communication systems

SOURCE: Bleile KM, Miller SA: Toddlers with Medical Needs. In Bernthal JE, Bankson NW (eds): *Child Phonology: Characteristics, Assessment, and Intervention with Special Populations,* p. 104. Thieme, New York, 1994.

TABLE **4.4. Communication Bill of Rights.**

1. The right to request desired objects, actions, events, and persons and to express personal preferences or feelings.
2. The right to be offered choices and alternatives.
3. The right to reject or refuse undesired objects, events, or actions, including the right to decline or reject all proffered choices.
4. The right to request, and be given, attention from and interaction with another person.
5. The right to request feedback or information about a state, an object, a person, or an event of interest.
6. The right to active treatment and intervention efforts that will enable people with severe disabilities to communicate messages in whatever modes and as effectively and efficiently as their specific abilities will allow.
7. The right to have communication acts acknowledged and responded to, even when the intent of these acts cannot be fulfilled by the responder.
8. The right to have access at all times to any needed augmentative and alternative communication devices and other assistive devices, and to have those devices in good working order.
9. The right to environmental contexts, interactions, and opportunities that expect and encourage persons with disabilities to participate as full communicative partners with other people, including peers.
10. The right to be informed about the people, things, and events in one's immediate environment.
11. The right to be communicated with in a manner that recognizes and acknowledges the inherent dignity of the person being addressed, including the right to be part of communication exchanges about individuals that are conducted in his or her presence.
12. The right to be communicated with in ways that are meaningful, understandable, and culturally and linguistically appropriate.

SOURCE: Romski MA, Sevcik RA: Communicative Development of Children with Severe Disabilities. In Smith MD, Damico JS (eds): *Childhood Language Disorders,* p. 221. Thieme, New York, 1996.

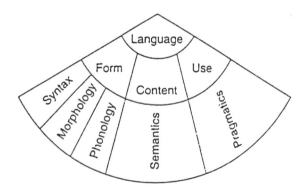

FIGURE **4.1. Components of language**

SOURCE: From Owens RE Jr. *Language Development: An Introduction,* 4th ed. Copyright © 1996 by Allyn & Bacon. Reprinted/adapted by permission.

TABLE 4.5. Communicative temptations.

1. Eat a desired food item in front of the child without offering any to the child.
2. Activate a wind-up toy, let it deactivate, and hand it to the child.
3. Give the child four blocks to drop in a box, one at a time (or use some other action that the child will repeat such as stacking the blocks or dropping the blocks on the floor); then immediately give the child a small animal figure to drop in the box.
4. Look through a few books or a magazine with the child.
5. Open a jar of bubbles, blow bubbles, and then close the jar tightly and give the closed jar to the child.
6. Initiate a familiar and an unfamiliar social game with the child until the child expresses pleasure; then stop the game and wait.
7. Blow up a balloon and slowly deflate it; then hand the deflated balloon to the child or hold the deflated balloon up to your mouth and wait.
8. Hold a food item or toy that the child dislikes out near the child to offer it.
9. Place a desired food item or toy in a clear container that the child cannot open while the child is watching; then put the container in front of the child and wait.
10. Place the child's hands in a cold, wet, or sticky substance, such as jello, pudding, or paste.
11. Roll a ball to the child; after the child returns the ball three times, immediately roll a different toy to the child.
12. Engage the child in putting together a puzzle. After the child has put in three pieces, offer the child a piece that does not fit.
13. Engage the child in an activity with a substance that can be easily spilled (or dropped, broken, torn, etc.), suddenly spill some of the substance on the cable or floor in front of the child and wait.
14. Put an object that makes noise in an opaque container and shake the bag; hold up the container and wait.
15. Give the child the materials for an activity of interest that necessitates the use of an instrument for completion (e.g., piece of paper to draw on or cut; bowl of pudding or soup); hold the instrument out of the child's reach and wait.
16. Engage the child in an activity of interest that necessitates the use of an instrument for completion (e.g., pen, crayon, scissors, stapler, wand for blowing bubbles, spoon); have a third person come over and take the instrument, go sit on the distant side of the room while holding the instrument within the child's sight, and wait.
17. Wave and say "bye" to an object upon removing it from the play area. Repeat this for a second and third situation, and do nothing when removing an object from a fourth situation. These four trials should be presented following four consecutive temptations above.
18. Hide a stuffed animal under the table. Knock, and then bring out the animal. Have the animal greet the child the first time. Repeat this for a second and third time, and do nothing when bringing out the animal the fourth time. These four trials should also be interspersed with the temptations above when presented.

SOURCE: Wetherby AM, Prizant BM: The Expression of Communicative Intent: Assessment Guidelines. *Seminars in Speech and Language* 1989; 10:86.

TABLE **4.6. Ecological communication guidelines.**

OUTCOME **1**: PARTICIPATE IN VARIED SOCIAL AND FUNCTIONAL ROUTINES.

Child Skills:
- Stay with others in play/daily living routines.
- Contact others to initiate a variety of routines.
- Interact/converse for a variety of reasons.

Partner Strategies:
- Contact the child frequently.
- Follow the child's lead.

Measures of Participation:
- Where the child spends time (situations)
- How much time spent in each situation
- With whom the child spends time (partners)
- The frequency and variety of social and functional routines in which the child participates
- Typical amounts of time spent in routines with partners

OUTCOME **2**: BALANCE PARTICIPATION IN ROUTINES.

Child Skills:
- Show a turn-taking play style.
- Imitate others.

Partner Strategies:
- Maintain and balance turn taking in play.
- Maintain and balance turn taking in conversations.
- Wait, signal, and expect.
- Respond with actions and messages.
- Imitate the child at times.

Measures of Balance:
- Ratio of actions each partner contributes to the routine
- Ratio of messages each partner contributes to the routine

OUTCOME **3**: ACT AND COMMUNICATE IN PROGRESSIVELY MATCHED WAYS.

Child Skills:
- Imitate actions and messages partners use.
- Use actions and messages in functional and meaningful ways.
- Use varied messages (gestures, sounds, signs, words, phrases).
- Make self understood.

Partner Strategies:
- Model actions and messages the child can imitate.
- Match child behavior; play in childlike ways.
- Communicate in ways close to the child.
- Comment more than question or command.

Measures of Match:
- Number, range, and functionality of actions each partner contributes to a routine
- Number, range, complexity, and appropriateness of messages each partner contributes to a routine
- Similarity between these measures for each partner

(continued)

TABLE 4.6. (*continued*)

OUTCOME 4: SHARE ENJOYMENT

Child Skills:
• Show enjoyment through face and voice.
• Contact others for fun.

Partner Strategies:
• Be animated.
• Use positive comments.
• Have social, friendly conversations with the child.

Measures of Enjoyment:
• A rating of the pleasure each partner derives from being together in routines

SOURCE: Gillette Y: Early Intervention in Communication Development: A Collaborative Model for Professionals Consulting with Families. In Smith MD, Damico JS (eds): *Childhood Language Disorders,* p. 307. Thieme, New York, 1996.

TABLE 4.7. Environmental assessment guidelines for communication needs of persons with severe disabilities.

1. Identify the familiar and unfamiliar partners for communication in each environment.
2. Describe the opportunities (frequency and type) for communication typically observed in each environment.
3. Compare the opportunities for communication among the different environments and partners within each environment.
4. Determine the proportion of communications that are responded to appropriately and inappropriately in each environment.
5. Identify the specific communicative modes and functions that might be useful in each environment.
6. Identify the partners in each environment who have relatively high rates of permitting, accepting, and responding to the communications of the children.

SOURCE: Romski MA, Sevcik RA: Communicative Development of Children with Severe Disabilities. In Smith MD, Damico JS (eds): *Childhood Language Disorders,* p. 224. Thieme, New York, 1996.

TABLE 4.8. **Higher level thinking skills: language development process.**

KNOWLEDGE—(Recall basic facts and information.) Who—what—where—when which—how many—why (if cause is given)—name—locate—define (if definition is given)—recall—label

COMPRESSION—(Grasp the meaning of information and explain it in own words.) Explain—match—describe—tell in own words—tell main idea—rewrite—illustrate—compare

APPLICATION—(Use learned knowledge in new and concrete situations.) Show—sort—What else?—name some other—Did this ever happen to you?—What's wrong with . . . ?—solve this problem—summarize—apply—think of a synonym for . . .

ANALYSIS—(Take a situation apart to examine or work with the different parts.) Why—How are they alike?—How are they different?—What are the causes?—What are the solutions?—What are the steps?—Which one comes first, last?—What is opposite?—Complete this analogy—Analyze

SYNTHESIS—(Use all previous levels of thinking to form new and creative ideas.) Create—design—predict—think of all the ways—how else—How can you improve?—compose—draw—suppose—What would it be like if?—compose a definition

EVALUATION—(Judge the value of information and justify an answer.) Judge—choose—Which do you like?—Which is best?—recommend—evaluate—decide which—Will it work?—rate from good to poor—select the best meaning of

SOURCE: Based on Benjamin S. Bloom's 1956 works regarding classification of critical thinking domains. Seminar Presentation (March, 1989) by Carolyn Wilson and Janet Lanza.

TABLE **4.9.** Language delay: summary of teaching techniques for children (Simple Summary for Caregivers).

- **START WITH SIMPLE WORDS AND PHRASES**—A strong receptive language base must be built first as a foundation for expressive language which emerges later.
- **USE ACTUAL NAMES OF THINGS WHEN TEACHING LANGUAGE**—Say "bottle" not "ba-ba."
- **USING VARIED REPETITION OF KEY WORDS AND SINGLE CONCEPTS IS CRUCIAL**—This is one of the best ways to pour in all of that extra language that is necessary for learning and is a great tool to aid memory.
- **SPEAK IN SHORT SENTENCES**—Increase sentence length and complexity of meaning as you see your child's language skills improve.
- **PAUSE BETWEEN PHRASES**—This allows your child to process the meaning of each word in the phrase.
- **FOCUS ON ONE TOY OR ACTIVITY AT A TIME TO PREVENT DISTRACTION**—Keep other toys out of sight and keep background noise and activities to a minimum.
- **PLAY WITH YOUR CHILD AT HIS EYE LEVEL**—Sit your child in a high chair or at a table or sit or lie down on the floor when playing with your child and his toys.
- **PLAY FOR A FEW SHORT PERIODS OF TIME**—Five to 10 minutes a day. Increase length and frequency of sessions as your child's attention span increases over time.
- **KNOW WHEN IT IS THE BEST TIME FOR INSTRUCTIVE PLAY**—After naptimes or mornings are the times when children are generally the most refreshed and eager to interact with you.
- **KNOW WHEN TO END PLAY SESSIONS**—If your child grows restless, stops paying attention, or becomes fatigued, it is time to take a break.
- **OFFER PRAISE AND ENCOURAGEMENT**—Children love verbal and physical rewards. Saying "Great job!" or giving a big hug works wonders.
- **MOST IMPORTANT—KEEP THE FUN IN LEARNING! BE ENTHUSIASTIC!**

SOURCE: *The New Language of Toys.* Schwartz S and Miller JH. Published by Woodbine House, 1996. Copyright held by Schwartz and Miller. Used with permission.

TABLE 4.10. **Language development in normally hearing children with average intelligence.**

Vocal Play ← → **Babbling** ← → **Jargon** ← → **Imitation** ← →
  0 months   6 mos.   12 mos.   18 mos.
                    1 word   3 words   22 words

Phrases ← → **Sentences/** ← → **Paragraphs** ← → **Nearly Correct** ← →
                 Questions   **Grammar**
24 months   3 years   4 years   5 years
272 words   896 words   1870 words   2289 words

Full Command of English
6 years
2568 words
Vocabulary numbers taken from Diagnostic Methods in Speech Pathology, p. 192.

SOURCE: *The New Language of Toys,* p. 6. Schwartz S and Miller JH. Published by Woodbine House, 1996. Copyright held by Schwartz and Miller. Used with permission.

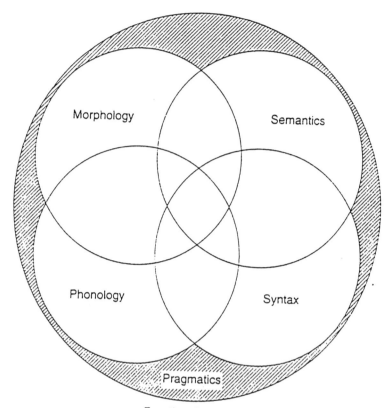

Functionalist Model

Pragmatics is the overall organizing
aspect of language.

Figure 4.2. Language model.

Source: From Owens RE Jr. *Language Development: An Introduction*, 4th ed. Copyright ©
1996 by Allyn & Bacon. Reprinted/adapted by permission.

TABLE **4.11. Language theory summaries: focus and response to errors.**

Theory	Focus	Response to Errors
OPERANT THEORY	Environmental antecedents and consequences to any observable behavior	Withhold or withdraw positive reinforcement.
NATIVISM	Syntax	None, because learning is result of biologic maturation.
INFORMATION PROCESSING THEORIES		
Parallel distributive processing	All cognitive processing, including syntax and morphology	Supply more input of correct pattern. Provide simple input to beginning learners and learners with too much initial auditory memory capacity.
Neuropsychological models	Attention, memory, sensation, processing speed, spatial skills, auditory and visual processing, executive control of resource allocation	Work with child's processing strengths to Foster development of strategies for learning Help child approach problem differently Make compensatory adjustments to learning environments.
Central auditory processing	Not peripheral hearing impairments, but difficulties with processing auditory information, particularly if signal is degraded or if there is noise	Slow down rate of messages; insert more pauses at phrase boundaries. Decrease background noise and/or improve signal-to-noise ratio (accomplished by seat placement, etc.). Supplement auditory messages with visual and other contextual cues. Teach child to monitor listening and ask for clarification.
Attention deficit or attention-deficit/hyperactivity disorder	Deficits in attention resulting in inattention and possibly impulsivity, distractibility, and hyperactivity	Inattention: Alert child prior to sending message or repeat message. Difficulty inhibiting reactions: Reduce extraneous stimuli. Slow processing speed: Reduce length and amount of information, speak more slowly, provide message redundancy, give child longer to respond, or train skill to overlearned level.

(continued)

TABLE **4.11.** (*continued*)

Theory	Focus	Response to Errors
		Difficulty organizing information: Provide supportive organization structure initially and gradually withdraw, model our own organization and planning out loud, mediate problem solving for the child, teach child to recognize own disorganizations, and develop plans for responding to it.
REPRESENTATIONAL THEORIES		
Piagetian theory	Cognitive precursors to symbolic language use Cognitive underpinnings of early semantic relations and later forms expressing time, space causality	Do not correct errors, but provide environment that encourages child's own active exploration.
Event knowledge	Routine events that constitute earliest mental representations	Provide more experience with the routine. Use a routine more familiar to child
Karmiloff–Smith's phase model	Nature of mental representation change over time as skill is better learned.	Depends on phase of mental representation reached for particular skill
SOCIAL THEORIES		
Social constructionist theory	Tutorial skills (mediation, scaffolding) used by adult in teaching child, and how they change as child gains more mastery of that skill	Depends on where skill learning is along the continuum ranging from other-regulation to self-regulation
Social learning theory	Modeling skill for child	Provide correct model

SOURCE: Vigil A, van Kleeck A: Clinical Language Teaching: Theories and Principles to Guide our Responses when Children Miss Our Language Targets. In Smith MD, Damico JS (eds): *Childhood Language Disorders,* pp. 68–69. Thieme, New York, 1996.

TABLE **4.12. Mean length of utterance: Brown's stages of predicted chronological ages and age ranges within one standard deviation of the predicted value.**

Brown's stage	MLU	Predicted chronological age[a]	Predicted age ±1 SD[b] (middle 68%)
Early Stage I	1.01	19.1	16.4–21.8
MLU = 1.01–1.49	1.10	19.8	17.1–22.5
	1.20	20.6	17.9–23.3
	1.30	21.4	18.7–24.1
	1.40	22.2	19.5–24.9
	1.50	23.0	18.5–27.5
Late Stage I	1.60	23.8	19.3–28.3
MLU = 1.50–1.99	1.70	24.6	20.1–29.1
	1.80	25.3	20.8–29.8
	1.90	26.1	21.6–30.6
	2.00	26.9	21.5–32.3
Stage II	2.10	27.7	22.3–33.1
MLU = 2.00–2.49	2.20	28.5	23.1–33.9
	2.30	29.3	23.9–34.7
	2.40	30.1	24.7–35.5
	2.50	30.8	23.9–37.7
Stage III	2.60	31.6	24.7–38.5
MLU = 2.50–2.99	2.70	32.4	25.5–39.3
	2.80	33.2	26.3–40.1
	2.90	34.0	27.1–40.9
	3.00	34.8	28.0–41.6
Early Stage IV	3.10	35.6	28.8–42.4
MLU = 3.00–3.49	3.20	36.3	29.5–43.1
	3.30	37.1	30.3–43.9
	3.40	37.9	31.1–44.7
	3.50	38.7	30.8–46.6
Late Stage IV–	3.60	39.5	31.6–47.4
Early Stage V	3.70	40.3	32.4–48.2
MLU = 3.50–3.99	3.80	41.1	33.2–49.0
	3.90	41.8	33.9–49.7
	4.00	42.6	36.7–48.5
Late Stage V	4.10	43.4	37.5–49.3
MLU = 4.00–4.49	4.20	44.2	38.3–50.1
	4.30	45.0	39.1–50.9
	4.40	45.8	39.9–51.7
	4.50	46.6	40.3–52.9
Poststage V	4.60	47.3	41.0–53.6
MLU = 4.50+	4.70	48.2	41.9–54.5

[a]Age is predicted from the equation Age (in months) = 11.199 +7.857 (MLU)
[b]Computed from obtained standard deviations

(continued)

TABLE 4.12. (*continued*)

Brown's stage	MLU	Predicted chronological age[a]	Predicted age ±1 SD[b] (middle 68%)
Poststage V	4.80	48.9	42.6–55.2
MLU = 4.50+ (cont.)	4.90	49.7	43.4–56.0
	5.00	50.5	42.1–58.9
	5.10	51.3	42.9–59.7
	5.20	52.1	43.7–60.5
	5.30	52.8	44.4–61.2
	5.40	53.6	45.2–62.0
	5.50	54.4	46.0–62.8
	5.60	55.2	46.8–63.6
	5.70	56.0	47.6–64.4
	5.80	56.8	48.4–65.2
	5.90	57.5	49.1–65.9
	6.00	68.3	49.9–66.7

SOURCE: With permission from Miller JF, Chapman RS, Paul R: Procedures for Analyzing Free-Speech Samples: Syntax and Semantics. In Miller JF (ed): *Assessing Language Production in Children*, p. 26. Baltimore: University Park Press, 1981.
[a]Age is predicted from the equation Age (in months) = 11.199 + 7.857 (MLU)
[b]Computed from obtained standard deviations

TABLE **4.13. Mean length of utterance (MLU) calculation: dos and don'ts.**

Once the language sample is transcribed, calculate your client's MLU. The first step is counting the morphemes in each utterance. Lund and Duchan (1988) outline specific *do's and don'ts* for counting morphemes:

EXCLUDE FROM YOUR COUNT:

1. *Imitations* which immediately follow the model utterance and which give the impression that the child would not have said the utterance spontaneously.

2. *Elliptical answers* to questions which give the impression that the utterance would have been more complete if there had been no eliciting question (e.g., *Do you want this? Yes. What do you have? My dolls.*)

3. *Partial utterances* which are interrupted by outside events or shifts in the child's focus (e.g., *That's my—oops.*)

4. *Unintelligible utterances* that contain unintelligible segments. If a major portion of a child's sample is unintelligible, a syllable count by utterance can be substituted for a morpheme count.

5. *Rote passages* such as nursery rhymes, songs, or prose passages which have been memorized and which may not be fully processed linguistically by the child.

6. *False starts and reformulations* within utterances which may either be self-repetitions or changes in the original formulation (e.g., I have one [just like] almost like that; [We] we can't).

7. *Noises* unless they are integrated into meaningful verbal material such as "He went . . ."

8. *Fillers* such as "um, oh, you know" which seem to be nonmeaningful stallers used by the child automatically and not integrated into the meaning of the utterance (e.g., [Well] it was [you know] [like] a party or something).

9. *Identical utterances* that the child says anywhere in the sample. Only one occurrence of each utterance is counted. If there is even a minor change, however, the second utterance is also counted.

10. *Counting or other sequences of enumeration* (e.g., blue, green, yellow, red, purple).

11. *Single words or social phrases* such as "hi," "thank you," "here," "know what?"

COUNT AS ONE MORPHEME:

1. Uninflected lexical morphemes (e.g., run fall) and grammatical morphemes that are whole words (articles, auxiliary verbs, prepositions).

2. Contractions when individual segments do not occur elsewhere in the sample apart from the contraction. If either of the constituent parts of the contraction are found elsewhere, the contraction is counted as two rather than one morpheme (e.g., I'll, it's, can't).

3. Catenatives such as "wanna," "gonna," "hafta" and the infinitive modals that have the same meaning (e.g., *going to* go). This eliminates the problem of judging a morpheme count on the basis of the child's pronunciation. Thus "am gonna" is counted as two morphemes, as is "am going to."

4. Phrases, compound words, diminutives, reduplicated words which occur as inseparable linguistic units for the child or represent single items (e.g., oh boy, all right, once upon a time, a lot of, let's, big wheel, horsie).

5. Irregular past tense. The convention is to count these as single morphemes because children's first meanings for them seem to be distinct from the present tense counterparts (e.g., did, was).

6. Plurals which do not occur in singular form (e.g., pants, clothes), including plural pronouns (us, them).

7. Gerunds and participles that are not part of the verb phrase (*Swimming is* fun; He was *tired;* That is the *cooking* place).

(continued)

TABLE 4.13. (*continued*)

COUNT AS MORE THAN ONE MORPHEME:

1. Inflected forms: regular and irregular plural nouns; possessive nouns; third person singular verb; present participle and past participle when part of the verb phrase; regular past tense verb; reflexive pronoun; comparative and superlative adverbs and adjectives.
2. Contractions when one or both of the individual segments occur separately anywhere in the child's sample (e.g., *It's* if *it or is* occurs elsewhere).

SOURCE: With permission from Lund NJ, Duchan, JF: *Assessing Children's Language in Naturalitic Contexts,* pp. 190–191. Prentice-Hall, Englewood Cliffs, NJ, 1988.

TABLE 4.14. **Mean length of utterance: developmental norms.**

Age (yr.—mo.)	Predicted MLU	Predicted MLU, 1 SD* (middle 68%)	Predicted MLU, 2 SDs (middle 95%)
1—6	1.31	.99–1.64	.66–1.96
1—9	1.62	1.23–2.01	.85–2.39
2—0	1.92	1.47–2.37	1.02–2.82
2—3	2.23	1.72–2.74	1.21–3.25
2—6	2.54	1.97–3.11	1.40–3.68
2—9	2.85	2.22–3.48	1.58–4.12
3—0	3.16	2.47–3.85	1.77–4.55
3—3	3.47	2.71–4.23	1.96–4.98
3—6	3.78	2.96–4.60	2.15–5.41
3—9	4.09	3.21–4.97	2.33–5.85
4—0	4.40	3.46–5.34	2.52–6.28
4—3	4.71	3.71–5.71	2.71–6.71
4—6	5.02	3.96–6.08	2.90–7.15
4—9	5.32	4.20–6.45	3.07–7.57
5—0	5.63	4.44–6.82	3.26–8.00

SOURCE: With permission from Miller JF, Chapman R: The Relation Between Age and Mean Length of Utterance in Morphemes. *Journal of Speech and Hearing Research* 1981; 24:154–161.
*SD is standard deviation

TABLE 4.15. **Metalinguistic skills and awareness: Approximate ages of development.**

Approximate Age	Abilities

1½–2 yrs.	1. Monitor one's own on-going utterances
	  a. Repair spontaneously
	  b. Practice sounds, words, and sentences
	  c. Adjust one's speech to different listeners
	2. Check the result of one's utterance
	  a. Check whether the listener has understood: if not, repair or try again
	  b. Comment explicitly on own utterances and those of others
	  c. Correct others

3–4 yrs.	3. Test for reality
	  a. Decide whether a word or sentence "works" on furthering listener understanding
	4. Attempt to learn language deliberately
	  a. Practice new sounds, words, and sentences
	  b. Practice speech styles of different roles

School age	5. Predict the consequences of using particular forms (inflections, words, phrases, sentences)
	  a. Apply appropriate inflections to "new" words
	  b. Judge utterances as appropriate for a specific listener or setting
	  c. Correct word order and wording in sentences judged as "wrong"
	6. Reflect on the product of an utterance (structure independent of use)
	  a. Identify, specific linguistic units (sounds, syllables, words, sentences)
	  b. Provide definitions of words
	  c. Construct puns, riddles, or other forms of humor
	  d. Explain why some sentences are possible and how to interpret them

SOURCE: From Owens RE: *Language Development: An Introduction,* 4th ed., p. 386. Copyright © 1996 by Allyn & Bacon. Reprinted/adapted by permission.

TABLE 4.16. Morpheme classes and examples.

Morphemes

Free Morphemes			
boy		Bound Morphemes	
girl		Derivational	Inflectional
car	Prefixes	Suffixes	*-s*
idea	*un-*	*-ly*	*-'s*
run	*non-*	*-ist*	*-ing*
walk	*in-*	*-er (painter)*	*-ed*
big	*pre-*	*-ness*	*-er (bigger)*
quick	*trans-*	*-ment*	

SOURCE: From Owens RE: *Language Development: An Introduction,* 4th ed., p. 20. Copyright © 1996 by Allyn & Bacon. Reprinted/adapted by permission.

TABLE 4.17. Pervasive developmental disorder—not otherwise specified (PDD-NOS): resource for assessment of young children.

Resource	Description
Fenson, L., Dale, P., Reznick, S., Thal, D., Bates, E., Hartung, J., Pethick, S., and Reilly, J. (1993). *The MacArthur Communicative Development Inventory.* San Diego: Singular Publishing.	The MacArthur Communicative Development Inventory is comprised of two scales which assess gesture, imitation, lexical acquisition, and the transition to early syntax in young children. The scales are normed for children between 9 and 30 months of age. Parent report.
Schaefer, C. E., Gitlin, K., and Sandgrund, A. (1991). *Play Diagnosis and Assessment.* New York: Wiley.	A cross-disciplinary, applied compilation of developmental play scales, diagnostic play scales, parent-child interaction scales, peer interaction scales, projective play assessments, and play therapy scales.
Weatherby, A., and Prizant, B. (1992). *Communication and Symbolic Behavior Scales (CSBS).* Chicago: The Riverside Publishing Company.	Standardized assessment of communicative and symbolic behaviors of children at a communication age between 8 and 24 months of age but whose chronological age may be 72 months or more. Sampling of the child's communication during natural adult-child interactions and in structured and unstructured contexts.
Greenspan, S.I. (1992). *Infancy and Early Childhood: The Practice of Clinical Assessment and Intervention with Emotional and Developmental Challenges.* Madison, CT: International Universities Press, Inc.	Assessment by history and direct observation of regulatory, relational, organizational, representational, symbolic, communicative, sensory, behavioral, and emotional development in children under 5 years of age.

SOURCE: Kirchner DM: Atypical Cognitive, Linguistic, and Social Development in Children with Pervasive Developmental Disorders of Childhood. In Smith MD, Damico JS (eds): *Childhood Language Disorders,* p. 182. Thieme, New York, 1996.

TABLE 4.18. Pervasive developmental disorders of childhood.

Autistic disorder (infantile autism; Kanner's syndrome)	Rett's disorder	Childhood disintegrativedisorder (Heller'ssyndrome)	Pervasive developmental disorder—NOS (including atypical autism)	Asperger's disorder
Onset: In infancy or early development but always before age 3. A minority of cases report normal development in the first 1–2 years. Ratio 4–5 : 1 males over females. Prevalence is 2–5 in 10,000.	**Onset:** Essential feature is the development of multiple specific deficits following a period of normal functioning after birth. Onset is prior to 5 years and usually in first or second year of life. Females only to date; about 1500 cases worldwide.	**Onset:** Primary difference from autistic disorder is "late onset." Mean age is 3.36 years (range: 1.2–9.0 years); always before 10. Insidious or abrupt. Epidemiological studies are limited but reported more commonly in males.	**Onset:** Infancy and before age 3; typically around age 2. "Subthreshold" classification for children with features of autistic disorder but failing to meet the full criteria for AD. "Atypical autism" includes presentations that do not meet the criteria for autistic disorder in DSM-IV.	**Onset:** Later than autistic disorder at least or recognized later.
Features and Course: Qualitative impairment in social interaction such as use of multiple nonverbal behaviors to regulate social interaction, failure to develop peer relationships at developmental level, lack of spontaneous seeking to share enjoyment, interest, and lack of social/emotional reciprocity. Impaired communication includes delay in or failure to develop spoken language without attempts to com-	**Features and Course:** Apparently normal prenatal and perinatal periods; deceleration of head growth between 5 months and 4 years; loss of acquired purposeful hand skills between 6 and 30 months replaced by stereotypic use of hands; rubbing or mouthing automatisms; severe psychomotor retardation including gait apraxia and truncal apraxia/ataxia between 1–4 years; social with-	**Features and Course:** Marked regression in communication skills, social interaction deficits, stereotypic movements, resistance to change, compulsive behaviors, overactivity, disturbances in affective modulation such as excessive fearfulness or anxiety, and deterioration in adaptive skills. Seizure disorder can be a major complication. Differs from autistic disorder on basis of develop-	**Features and Course:** Sometimes referred to as "atypical autism" or "subthreshold" classification with features similar to but failing to meet full criteria for AD. Range of deficits is similar though children diagnosed with PDD-NOS typically exhibit more differentiated social relatedness, cognitive development, and communicative skills than most autistic children. May or may not have	**Features and Course:** Motor delays or clumsiness in the preschool period, difficulties in social interaction at school, and idiosyncratic interests. No clinically significant delays reported in acquisition of early language milestones, cognition, or adaptive behavior. Dx requires at least 2 criteria in qualitative impairment of social interaction—impairment in use of multiple nonverbal behaviors,

failure to develop peer relationships at developmental level, lack of spontaneous seeking to share enjoyment, interest, and lack of social or emotional reciprocity. At least one criterion must be identified in the category of restricted, repetitive, and stereotyped patterns of behavior, interests, and activities.

restricted range of interests and levels of attachment; eye contact and patterns of affective engagement are usually higher than children with autistic disorder.

mental regression and associated "organicity"; differs from Rett's in that motor function is rarely impaired; regression is between 3–4 years vs. 6–12 months in Rett's. Deterioration is to a much lower level of functioning followed by a plateau of development and limited degrees of recovery.

drawal; some with accompanying clinical seizures or abnormal EEG tracings. "Autistic" features of shorter duration than with the disintegrative disorders of childhood. Dx may be tentative until 4–5 years of age. Dx requires that all criteria are met.

pensate through alternative modes such as gesture or mime, when speech is present impairment in initiation or sustaining conversation, stereotyped and repetitive use of language or idiosyncratic language, lack of spontaneous make-believe play or social imitative play at developmental level. Interests are restricted and may include preoccupation with one or more stereotyped or restricted interests, adherence to specific, nonfunctional routines or rituals, stereotyped and repetitive motor mannerisms, and/or persistent preoccupation with parts of objects. Dx requires at least 6/12 features with at least two in the area of qualitative impairment of social interaction and one in each of the following: qualitative impairment in communication and restricted, repetitive, and stereotyped patterns of behavior, interest, and activity.

(continued)

TABLE 4.18. *(continued)*

Autistic disorder (infantile autism; Kanner's syndrome)	Rett's disorder	Childhood disintegrative disorder (Heller's syndrome)	Pervasive developmental disorder—NOS (including atypical autism)	Asperger's disorder
Linguistic–Cognitive Profile: May have no mode of communication— verbal or nonverbal, higher functioning autistics may have sophisticated expressive language with deficits in form or content of speech, marked deficits in ability to initiate or sustain a conversation, echolalia. Abnormal nonverbal communicative behavior, poor eye contact; poor use of gesture; abnormal prosody; abnormal facial expression. In older children, long-term memory can be excellent; information is repeated again and again regardless of appropriateness. Behavioral disorders range from mild to severe; may have self-injurious behavior. Can be diagnosed with normal	**Linguistic–Cognitive Profile:** Severely impaired expressive and receptive language. Rudimentary language prior to regression; words, but few develop word combinations; poor eye contact; little awareness of others; restricted range of nonverbal expressions of communicative intent. Little or no imitation due to dyspraxia; output constraints may mask higher comprehension.	**Linguistic–Cognitive Profile:** Many reported to have spoken clearly and in sentences prior to onset of regression; more likely than "late onset" autistics to be mute following a prior progression to point of using sentences. Higher IQ late onset autistics never progress past single words of use of phrases. When present, language is characterized by lack of ability to initiate or sustain conversation, stereotyped repetitive use of language, and disorders of syntax, semantics, and pragmatics.	**Linguistic–Cognitive Profile:** Features overlap with those diagnosed with autistic disorder. Early preverbal/gestural systems of communication fail to develop at 12–15 months; oversensitivities to sensory stimuli. Continuum of relationship and affect expression abnormalities. Rigid and idiosyncratic characteristics. Delays in both receptive and expressive language; some have deficits in visual/spatial processing as well. May have well developed rote capacities—reciting numbers, alphabet, colors, recitation of songs and dialogue from books or television pro-grams. Some appear to be hyperlexic.	**Linguistic–Cognitive Profile:** Clinically significant language and cognitive delays are not present in the first 1–3 years. Language and communication deficits are thought to be primarily social rather than linguistic in origin. Syntactic and semantic deficits are not diagnosed in all Asperger's individuals and when present may be an expression of a distinct language disorder. Pragmatic deficits are severe and are observed at the level of appropriateness, nonverbal communication, use of speech acts, and discourse. Communication and social skills covary, evaluate both linguistically and in the social context.

Outcome: Variable severity; long-term prognosis related to language level and overall cognitive level. Behavior may improve or deteriorate during adolescence; 25% may develop a seizure disorder in adolescence.

Outcome: Severe global developmental delay with little or no change in cognitive, motor, or linguistic domains with age.

Outcome: Long-term differences in IQ with CDD children exhibiting lower IQ than "late onset" autistics; limited recovery; progressive in 25% of cases; static in 75% of cases. Loss of skills seems to reach a plateau unless associated with a progressive neurological condition.

Outcome: Variable severity; long-term prognosis related to IQ and development of language and social skills.

Outcome: The duration of the disorder is life-long and contin-uous. As adults, problems with empathy and social interaction persist. May pursue interests privately rather than in social contexts, and social deficits persist. At risk for depression, anti-social behavior, and suicide in severe cases. Social adjustment and eventual outcome depends on levels of support and intervention. Outcome tends to be good.

Source: Kirchner DM: Atypical Cognitive, Linguistic, and Social Development in Children with Pervasive Developmental Disorders of Childhood. In Smith MD, Damico JS (eds): *Childhood Language Disorders*, pp. 161–163. Thieme, New York, 1996.

TABLE 4.19. Piaget's sensorimotor stages.

Stage and age (months)	General	Imitation	Object concept	Causality	Means–Ends
Stage 1 Birth–1	Reflextive	Notion not present.	No differentiation of self from objects.	Egocentric	Notion not present.
Stage 2 1–4	Coordination of sensory schema.	Self-imitation of actions with unexpected results. "Preimitation"	Object followed with eyes until out of view. Change in perspective interpreted as change in object.	No differentiation of self and moving objects.	Notion not present. Intentionality lacking.
Stage 3 4–8	Repetition of actions of others.	Imitation of other's actions already in repertoire.	Anticipation of position of moving objects; no manual search	Self as cause of all events.	Repetition of events with unexpected outcomes; heightened interest in event outcome. Intentionality follows initiation of behavior.
Stage 4 8–12	Known means applied to new problems	**Imitation of behaviors different from those in repertoire.** Facial imitation	**Manual search for object where last seen. Object constancy.**	**Some externalization or causality.** Realization that objects can cause action.	Coordination and integration of schemata. **Establishment of goal prior to initiation of activity.** Anticipation of outcomes.
Stage 5 12–18	Experimentation	Imitation of behaviors markedly different from repertoire	Sequential displacements considered. Awareness of object spacial relations	Realization that he is one of many objects in environment.	New means through experimentation. Tools used.
Stage 6 18–24	Representational thought	**Deferred imitation.**	Representation of displacements. Awareness of unseen movements.	Representation of causality. Able to predict cause-effect relationship.	Language used to influence others. Representation of outcome or end.

Source: From Owens RE: *Language Development: An Introduction*, pp. 139–140. Copyright © 1996 by Allyn & Bacon. Reprinted/adapted by permission.

TABLE 4.20. Piaget's stages of cognitive development.

Stage	Approximate age (years)	Characteristics
Sensorimotor	0–2	Reflexive to proactive behavior
		Ability to represent reality (symbolic function), to invent novel means to desired ends without trial-and-error methodology, to imitate when model not immediately present and to represent absent people and objects
		Symbolic play
Preoperational	2–7	Further development of symbolic function: language, physical problem solving, categorization
		Thinking characterized by centration, irreversibility, and egocentricity
Concrete operational	7–11	Thinking characterized by conservation, decentration, and reversibility
		Logical thought relative to concrete or physical operations
		Categorization into hierarchical and seriational categories
Formal operational	11+	Capability of abstract thought, complex reasoning, flexibility
		Mental hypothesis testing

SOURCE: From Owens RE: *Language Development: An Introduction,* p. 137. Copyright © 1996 by Allyn & Bacon. Reprinted/adapted by permission.

TABLE 4.21. **Prefixes and suffixes with definitions.**

| Prefixes | SUFFIXES | |
	Derivational	Inflectional
a- (in, on, into, in a manner)	-able (ability, tendency, likelihood)	-ed (past)
bi- (twice, two)		-ing (at present)
de- (negative, descent, reversal)	-al (pertaining to, like, action, process)	-s (plural)
ex- (out of, from, thoroughly)		-s (third person marker)
inner- (reciprocal, between, together)	-ance (action state)	-'s (possession)
	-ation (denoting action in a noun)	
mis- (ill, negative, wrong)	-en (used to form verbs from adjectives)	
out- (extra, beyond, not)		
over- (over)	-ance (action, state)	
post- (behind, after)	-er (used as an agentive ending)	
pre- (to, before)	-est (superlative)	
pro- (in favor of)	-ful (full, tending)	
re- (again, backward motion)	-ible (ability, tendency, likelihood)	
semi- (half)		
super- (superior)	-ish (belonging to)	
trans- (across, beyond)	-ism (doctrine, state, practice)	
tri- (three)	-ist (one who does something)	
un- (not, reversal)	-ity (used for abstract nouns)	
under- (under)	-ive (tendency or connection)	
	-ize (action, policy)	
	-less (without)	
	-ly (used to form adverbs)	
	-ment (action, product, means, state)	
	-ness (quality, state)	
	-or (used as an agentive ending)	
	-ous (full of having, like)	
	-y (inclined to)	

SOURCE: From Owens RE: *Language Disorders: A Functional Approach to Assessment and Intervention*, p. 372.Copyright © 1991 by Allyn & Bacon. Reprinted/adapted by permission.

TABLE 4.22. **Storybook reading: eight levels of the semantic continuum from the Situation Discourse-Semantic Model used to focus attention.**

LEVEL VIII: METALANGUAGE
- Words are used to refer to words and their properties, such as their part of speech, number of syllables, or component sounds.
- Communicative intent and meaning are separate from form.
- Specific vocabulary used to refer to metaconcepts.

LEVEL VII: EVALUATION
- Words are distanced from the actual objects or events, instead placing a value judgment or giving significance to them.
- Communicative intent is to influence beliefs or attitudes.
- Word choices have evaluative connotation.

LEVEL VI: INFERENCE
- Words refer to information that integrates background or personal knowledge with information that is present in the context.
- Communicative intent has many layers of meaning.
- Word choice and grammar only suggest implied meanings.

LEVEL V: INTERPRETATION
- Words refer to the manner in which objects, their properties, or relationships are interpreted.
- Communicative intent personal and individualized.
- Functional words (because, wants to) important to the meaning.

LEVEL IV: DESCRIPTION
- Words refer to properties of objects (size, color, volume) or to the relationship between unlike objects related through action.
- Communicative intent explicit.
- Grammatical strategies specify relationships between words.

LEVEL III: LABEL
- Words closely associated with the perception of the object; a concrete label for an object, sound, or other physical entity.
- Communicative intent may extend beyond identifying object.
- Conventional words that may occur within a sentence (I see a ___)

LEVEL II: INDICATION
- Response to the book is used to elicit joint focus or attention.
- Both communicative intent and effect are present.
- Conventional but nonlinguistic gestures, points, and vocalizations.

LEVEL I: REACTION
- Response to the book is a reaction rather than an initiation.
- Reaction has a communicative effect but not produced with a communicative intention.
- Communicative behaviors are not conventional; random gestures, and vocalizations.

SOURCE: Norris JA, Hoffman PR: Attaining, Sustaining, and Focusing Attention: Intervention for Children with ADHD. *Seminars in Speech and Language* 1996; 17:69.

TABLE 4.23. Storybook reading: ten levels of the situational continuum from the Situation–Discourse–Semantic Model used to attain attention.

LEVEL X: LOGICAL
- Book an allegory for truths or generalizations.
- Book viewed as a source of insight or expression.
- Perspective of characters' opinions, actions may be different from interpreted perspective (satire).
- Humor, farce, sarcasm, irony used to expose true meaning.

LEVEL IX: SYMBOLIC
- Book uses words to tell story about unusual or unique event.
- Book viewed as a source of novel, unknown information.
- Perspectives of characters may be culturally or physically different from child's.
- Metaphor and figurative language used to enhance story.

LEVEL VIII: RELATIONAL
- Book uses words to tell stories about events that follow routine scripts (caterpillar ate, spun a chrysalis, became a butterfly).
- Book viewed as a source of authoritative information.
- Perspective of characters are observed by child, not necessarily identified with.
- Examples may be used to clarify or enhance story.

LEVEL VII: DECENTERED
- Book or child uses words to tell stories about commonly observed event.
- Book viewed as a source of mostly known information.
- Perspective of characters and their actions are similar to child's own.
- Sound effects and gestures may be used for support.

LEVEL VI: EGOCENTERED
- Child uses words to tell stories from own experience.
- Story may be dictated and written down.
- All characters, action, changes in location recreated using words.
- Sound effects and gestures may be used for support.

LEVEL V: LOGICAL
- Child uses pictures to infer information not told in the words of story.
- Book viewed as a story enhanced by pictures.
- Words describe character changes through action, location to build plot.
- Props and pretend objects used to reenact story.

LEVEL IV: SYMBOLIC
- Child uses pictures to understand story.
- Book viewed as pictures and words that tell story across pages.
- Pictures of characters that change action, location to build coherent plot.
- Props used to act out story.

LEVEL III: RELATIONAL
- Child looks at picture.
- Book viewed as pages of pictures each showing an action or event.
- Picture of interrelated people, animals, objects.
- Objects used to duplicate pictured actions.

(continued)

TABLE **4.23.** (*continued*)

LEVEL II: DECENTERED
- Child looks at book.
- Book viewed as whole page.
- Picture of many animals or familiar objects.
- Objects used to perform action on pictures.

LEVEL I: EGOCENTERED
- Book brought to child.
- Book viewed as single object.
- Single picture of animal or object.
- Book used to perform action on child's body.

SOURCE: Norris JA, Hoffman PR: Attaining, Sustaining, and Focusing Attention: Intervention for Children with ADHD. *Seminars in Speech and Language* 1996; 17:64.

TABLE 4.24a. **Substance-abuse risk factors and childhood language disorders: behaviors, possible assessment tools, and intervention strategies for premature infants to preschool/school-age children.**

Premature Stage

Goals:
1. Increase infant's ability to self-console and organize states
2. Improve infant's toleration of stimulation and handling
3. Develop visually organized attention
4. Reduce irritability

Behaviors	Possible assessment tools	Intervention strategies

I. Motor
  a. Abnormal muscle tone
  b. Fluctuating muscle tone
  c. Hypertension
II. State
  a. Irritable
  b. Poor self-regulation
  c. Disorganized
  d. Easily overstimulated
  e. Brief, alert periods, no quiet, alert state
  f. Distress cues
    • Color changes
    • Hiccoughs
    • Gaze aversion
    • Yawning
    • Sneezing
    • Frowning
	I. The Neonatal Neurological Examination (Dubowitz & Dubowitz, 1981)
	
	II. Neonatal Individual Development Assessment Program (NIDCAP) (Als, Duffy, & McAnulty, 1982)
	
	Assessment of Preterm Infant Behavior (APIB) (Als, Lester et al., 1982)
		I. • Position prone and sidelying to promote flexion
		  • Swaddle to encourage flexion
		  • Huggel Bunting
		II. • Manipulate the environment (i.e., reduce noise levels, dim lights, etc.)
		  • Provide auditory/ tactile/visual stimulation, using one modality at a time (i.e., voice or face rocking without visual or auditory input)
		  • Swaddle to encourage organization
		  • Vertical rocking
		  • Respond to early distress cues by giving time out
		  • Minimal handling, clustering care, containing limbs when changing positions

III. Feeding
   a. Immature, disorganized sucking/swallowing pattern
   b. Poor coordination between suckling, swallowing, and respiration
   c. Decreased/increased oral motor reflexes
   d. Frantic, disorganized sucking patterns
   e. Vomiting
   f. Regurgitation
   g. Require gavage feedings (i.e., nasogastric/orogastric feeding tubes)
   h. Oral tactile hypersensitivity
   i. Increased exposure to drugs if breastfeeding

IV. Mother–infant interaction
   a. Infant may exhibit distress cues (e.g., gaze aversion, hiccoughs, yawning)

V. Hearing
   a. Neonate may be at risk for hearing loss due to low birthweight, prolonged mechanical ventilation, ototoxic drugs

III. Neonatal Oral Motor Assessment Scale (NOMAS) (Palmer, 1991)

The Mother's Assessment of the Behavior of Her Infant (Field, Dempsey, Mallock, & Shuman, 1978)

Observation of Communicative Interaction (OCI) (Klein & Briggs, 1987)

Auditory Brain Stem Response (ABR)

III. • Place in prone after feeding if baby has been vomiting/regurgitating
   • Swaddle to encourage flexion and organization
   • Short, frequent feedings
   • Experiment with different nipples (e.g., preemie, Nuk, etc.) to regulate flow of formula
   • Provide oral stimulation during gavage feedings to increase frequency of swallowing, weight gain, association of fullness with oral motor sensation, and facilitate transition to oral feedings
   • Burp frequently, and allow frequent breaks during feeding
   • Provide chin and/or cheek support during feedings

IV. • Instruct mother on proper handling, positioning, and calming techniques
   • Instruct mother in reading infants distress cues
   • Educate mother on dangers of breastfeeding while still using drugs

V. • Prevent hearing loss by decreasing noise levels in NICU
   • If hearing loss found immediate fitting of hearing aids to maximize hearing for language acquisition

SOURCE: Maxwell LA, Geschwint-Rabin J: Substance Abuse Risk Factors and Childhood Language Disorders. In Smith MD, Damico JS (eds): *Childhood Language Disorders*, pp. 252–253. Thieme, New York, 1996.

TABLE 4.24b. Newborn stage (0–1 month).

Goals:
1. Increase infant's alertness to enable appropriate parent–child interaction.
2. Decrease irritability and poor self-regulation.
3. Normalize tone.
4. Improve oral feeding skills and decrease oral tactile hypersensitivity.

Behaviors	Possible assessment tools	Intervention strategies
I. Motor a. Hyperextended postures b. Tremors c. Overshooting d. Stiffness or rigidity	I. The Neonatal Neurological Examination (Dubowitz & Dubowitz, 1981)	I. • Encourage flexion, using rolled-up blankets or by swaddling • Position in sidelying • Vertical rocking whle swaddled • Hydrotherapy • Graded auditory and visual stimuli
II. State a. Rapid change from one extreme state to another b. Deep sleep state c. Agitated sleep state d. Vacillation between extremes of state e. Panicked awake state f. Poor transition from one state to another g. Prolonged and/or high-pitched cry h. Inability to sleep	II. Neonatal Behavior Assessment Scales (NBAS) (Brazelton, 1984)	II. • Appropriate positioning and handling (i.e., swaddling and slow vertical rocking) • Appropriate sensory stimulation (i.e., visual/tactile/auditory using multimodal stimulation as tolerated) • Soothe infant by holding snugly and close to body; swaddle if necessary • Aid sleep by reducing environmental stimuli and excessive handling
III. Feeding a. Persistence of immature suckling/swallowing pattern b. Poor oral motor control c. Oral tactile hypersensitivity	III. Prespeech Assessment Scale (Morris, 1982)	III. • Position to encourage flexion • Firm, strong touch to decrease oral/tactile hypersensitivity • Smaller amounts of formula fed more frequently

d. Disorganized suckling/swallowing pattern e. Frantic sucking pattern f. Regurgitation g. Vomiting h. Tongue thrust i. Poor tongue stabilization in midline j. Tongue thrust k. Inadequate nutrition due to long periods of sleep l. Frantic sucking of fists	• Allow more time for feeding, allowing frequent rest periods between suckling • Burp infant gently and frequently • Speak softly and calmly • Experiment with temperature and regulation of liquid flow, using various nipple shapes • Provide chin and/or cheek support to increase sucking ability • Place infant in prone or semiupright position after feeding to avoid aspiration of formula and prevent gastroesophageal-like symptoms • Waken infant for feedings to ensure adequate nutritional intake • To decrease frantic sucking of fists, use infant shirts with sewn-in sleeves for mitts to prevent skin damage or use pacifier

IV. Parent–newborn interaction
  a. At risk due to
    • Gaze aversion
    • Poor state control
    • Abnormal motor behavior
    • Feeding difficulties
	IV. Parent Behavior Progression (Bromwich et al., 1981)
	• Instruct parent on positioning/handling/feeding techniques, through demonstration and teaching
	• Teach parent calming, soothing techniques (i.e., swaddling, vertical rocking, pacifier, etc.)
	• Teach parent to read distress cues (e.g., yawning, frowning, gaze aversion)

V. Hearing Assess hearing if infant is at risk for hearing loss or demonstrates decreased response to sound.	V. ABR • Monitor and screen hearing if warranted (e.g., frequent middle ear infections, family history of hearing loss, etc.) • If hearing loss found immediate fitting of hearing aids to maximize hearing for language acquisition

SOURCE: Maxwell LA, Geschwint-Rabin J: Substance Abuse Risk Factors and Childhood Language Disorders. In Smith MD, Damico JS (eds): *Childhood Language Disorders*, pp. 256–257. Thieme, New York, 1996.

TABLE 4.24c. Infancy (1–12 months).

Goal:
Improve movement patterns to enhance interaction and exploration of environment.

Behaviors	Possible assessment tools	Intervention strategies
I. Motor a. Weak pull-to-sit b. Tremors, trembling, extraneous movement c. Arms in W position d. Increased extensor tone e. Poor antigravity extensor strength	I. Movement Assessment of Infants (MAI) (Chandler, Skillen-Andrews, & Swanson, 1980) Bayley Scales of Infant Development (Bayley, 1969)	I. a. Weak pull-to-sit development: • Move infant from supine to sitting with head support. • Hold infant semireclined, encourage to assist with pull-to-sit b. Decrease tremors: • Swaddle infant and hold close • Hold infant semireclined, keeping arms and shoulders forward. Hold infant's arms and legs close to body • Apply firm, calm touch to tremulous areas c. Arms in W position: • Swaddle infant with arms in midline • Carry infant in semireclined position with shoulders forward • Place infant in cloth, sling-style infant seat • Place infant in Tumble-form feeder chair, assisting in keeping arms midline d. Increased extensor tone: • Lift infant's pelvis up and flex legs toward chest to begin increased kicking movements with lower extremities • Rotate lower extremities side to side • Bring upper extremities down and forward at shoulder girdle, for reaching of objects

Clinical Findings	Assessment	Intervention
II. State a. Poor sleeping patterns b. Hyperirritability c. Difficulty in consoling self d. Poor organization of behavior e. Decreased focused alertness f. Decreased use of adults for solace, play, and object attainment g. Poor self-regulation	II. Test of Sensory Function in Infants (TSFI) (DeGangi & Greenspan, 1989) Receptive-Expressive Emergent Language Scale (REEL-2) (Bzoch & League, 1991)	e. Poor antigravity extensor strength: • Place infant in prone position • Discourage parents from leaving infant in supine or sitting position too long • Discourage supported standing in walkers and jumpers II. • Positioning, handling, and swaddling • Early maternal intervention to teach positioning, handling and reading stress cues • Consistent, loving primary caregiver • Use of rituals, routines, mother-child interactive games • Structure an environment that prevents overstimulation • Use language to organize and explain experiences • Provide appropriate sensory and developmental stimulation using multimodal stimuli
III. Mother–infant interaction At risk for poor mother–infant interaction	III. See Newborn Section	III. • Teach parents appropriate carrying and handling techniques • Teach parents appropriate developmental and motor milestones, and developmentally appropriate activities • Teach parents ways of structuring and organizing environment to prevent overstimulation
IV. Hearing (see Newborn Section) also may be at increased risk if history of frequent middle ear infections	IV. ABR or behavioral audiometry (audiogram/tympanogram)	IV. • Monitor speech sound development • Assess localization to sound and meaningful words

SOURCE: Maxwell LA, Geschwint-Rabin J: Substance Abuse Risk Factors and Childhood Language Disorders. In Smith MD, Damico JS (eds): *Childhood Language Disorders*, pp. 258–259. Thieme, New York, 1996.

TABLE 4.24d. Toddler period (12–30 months).

Goals:
1. Provide early intervention services to monitor and facilitate development skills.
2. Teach caregivers, teachers, and service providers ways to structure environment to enhance child's ability for self-regulation and behavioral control.
3. Provide direct intervention services (e.g., speech therapy) to identify areas of deficit.

Behaviors	Possible assessment tools	Intervention strategies

I. State
  a. Hyperactivity
  b. Poor self-regulation
  c. Impulsivity
  d. Distractibility
  e. Prone to temper tantrums
  f. Poor organization of behavior
	Bayley Scales of Infant Development (Bayley, 1969)	• Structure and organization of the environment
		• Predictable, consistent daily routines
		• Use of language to organize experiences
		• Consistent, loving primary caregiver and service providers
		• Providing environment that avoids overstimulation
		• Use of rituals and mother–child games

II. Social attachment
  a. Bonding difficulties
  b. Difficulty in consoling self
  c. Difficulty in being comforted
  d. Decreased focused alertness
  e. Depressed interactive behaviors
  f. Decreased use of adults for solace, play, and attainment of objects
  g. Less secure attachment to parents		

III. Language
  a. Delayed language
  b. Slow language use
  c. Memory problems
  d. Limited play sequence
  e. Difficulty with processing information
	Sequenced Inventory of Communication Development (Hedrick, Prather & Tobin, 1984)
	
	Rosetti Infant Toddler Language Scale (Rossetti, 1990)
		• Direct speech-language therapy to address deficit areas
		• Provide caregivers with ideas for stimulating language development
		• Structured communication and play activities to stimulate language

IV. Mother-infant interaction
   At risk due to possible behaviors and developmental deficits
V. Hearing
   May be at risk if history of frequent middle ear infection

Behavioral audiometry (audiogram/tympanogram)

- Parent education in managing behavior and providing developmentally appropriate activities to facilitate play and stimulate language
- Ongoing parent education
- Intervene as needed (i.e., pediatrician refers hearing aid fitting, etc.)

SOURCE: Maxwell LA, Geschwint-Rabin J: Substance Abuse Risk Factors and Childhood Language Disorders. In Smith MD, Damico JS (eds): *Childhood Language Disorders*, pp. 258–259. Thieme, New York, 1996.

TABLE 4.24e. **Preschool/school age children.**

Goals:
1. Provide children with early intervention in hopes that they can be transitioned into a regular classroom.
2. Find threshold for loss of behavioral control and teach adaptive self-regulation strategies to mother, teacher, and prenatally exposed child.

Behaviors	Possible assessment tools	Intervention strategies
I. Language	Use norm-referenced tests to assess receptive/expressive/prag-matic language abilities Language: Examples Preschool Language Scale 3 (Zimmerman, Steiner, & Pond, 1992)	• Direct speech/language therapy to enrich vocabulary skills and facilitate overall language abilities • Use whole language • Structured communication activities
a. Delayed acquisition of words b. Difficulty in word-finding preschool level	Expressive One-Word Picture Vocabulary Test-Revised (Gardner, 1990)	• Structured play activities
c. Decreased use of acquired words or gestures to communicate wants and needs d. Language delays	Receptive One-Word Picture Vocabulary Test (Gardner, 1985)	• Use eye contact during interaction
e. Poor pragmatic skills	Clinical Evaluation of Language Fundamentals-Preschool (CELF—Preschool) (Wiig, Secord, & Semel, 1992)	• Remediation of articulation errors
f. Reduced mean length of utterance g. Syntactic disorganization, or syntax limited to simple sentences h. Receptive language impairment		• Provide good language model • Short, direct, clear verbal requests tailored to child's language level • Encourage child to use language and appropriate gesture to communicate
i. Poor/inappropriate pragmatic language abilities (e.g., poor turntaking skills) j. Multiple articulation errors		• Tailor language input to child's level of understanding • Use cuing (visual, tactile) to assist child in understanding requests
k. Auditory processing difficulties		• Use short sentences, and use descriptive comments on activity you or child is engaged in
l. Less spontaneous and developed imitative skills		• Acknowledge child's communication attempts

II. Motor and neurological

a. Possible poor balance

b. Tremulousness, increased startling

c. Poor quality of visual following
d. Fine motor dexterity difficulty
e. Blanking out, bizarre eye movements
f. Problems with auditory/visual processing
g. Poor motor planning

III. Social attachment

a. Decreased/absent stranger separation anxiety
b. Aggressiveness with peers
c. Decreased response to verbal praise
d. Decreased use of adults for solace/comfort

IV. Affective and behavioral

a. Depressed affect, decreased laughter
b. Irritable, explosive, and impulsive behaviors
c. Inability to self-regulate
d. Marked difficulty with transitioning

The Miller Assessment for Preschoolers (Miller, 1982)

Bruininks–Osertsky Test of Motor Proficiency (School Age) Bruininks, 1978)

- Direct occupational therapy to address visual-motor and sensory integrative deficits
- Refer appropriately to occupational or physical therapy
- Use developmentally appropriate activities that promote motor planning strength and balance
- Repetition of directions, comand, provide cuing techniques
-

- Structured play and communication and activities to encourage social interactions among peers
- Encourage attachment through consistency of teachers and service providers
- Small student-to-teacher ratio to allow for individual attention

- Set firm, consistent limits on behavior
- Anticipate and avoid stress
- Use consistent, predictable, daily routines
- Provide opportunity for physical affection during play
- Structure/organize the environment
- Structure transitions
- Structure communication/play activity
- Avoid thresholds of overstimulation
- Teach child to recognize warning signs of over-stimulation
- Movement activities during play to encourage laughing, turn talking, eye contact

(continued)

TABLE 4.24e. (*continued*)

Behaviors	Possible assessment tools	Intervention strategies
V. Problem-solving and attention strategies		• Provide structured organized, predictable environment
a. Poor on-task attention		• Limit distractions
b. Increased distractibility to extraneous sounds and movements		• Teach adaptive, self-regulated strategies
c. Inability to accom-modate in problem-solving situations		• Small student-to-teacher ratio
d. Impulsive responses before "reflecting"		• Help with focusing attention
e. Continuous use of unsuccessful strategies		• Aid in decision making
VI. Mother–child/teacher–child interaction		• Service providers should work with caregivers and teachers on ways to structure environment, avoid overstimulation thresholds, and teach adaptive, self-regulation strategies
VII. Play		• Model appropriate play; participate in play with child
a. Decreased amount of pretend play		• Use descriptive language to comment on what child is doing
b. Does not exhibit the repertoire of play skills that normal peers do		• Limit amount of toys available to decrease overstimulation
c. Difficulty selecting and organizing materials to play with		
d. Easily overstimu-lated by noise and other activities of other children and adults in the play environment		

SOURCE: Maxwell LA, Geschwint-Rabin J: Substance Abuse Risk Factors and Childhood Language Disorders. In Smith MD, Damico JS (eds): *Childhood Language Disorders*, pp. 258–259. Thieme, New York, 1996.

TABLE 4.25a. **Summary of a child's language, motor, and cognitive abilities from birth to 12 months of age.**

SUMMARY OF CHILD'S FIRST YEAR (0–12 MONTHS)*

Developmental Milestones	LANGUAGE		
	Date Achieved	*NOT YET*	*PROGRESSING*
Cries to express needs			
Makes vowel-like cooing sounds			
Responds by smiling to friendly faces			
Turns to sound			
Laughs out loud			
Vocalizes when spoken to			
Uses her voice to express needs			
Babbles several consonants			
"Talks" to toys			
"Talks" to mirror			
Responds to name			
Stops action when "no" is said			
Waves bye bye			
Nods head for "yes"			
Responds to "yes/no" questions			
Enjoys music and rhymes			
One or two words			

Developmental Milestones	PHYSICAL		
	Date Achieved	*NOT YET*	*PROGRESSING*
Follows a moving person			
Follows a moving object			
Focuses on hands			
Brings hand to mouth			
Can hold on to rattles			
Plays with fingers			
Plays with hands			
Can move object from one hand to another			
Can crawl			
Can sit alone			
Can clap hands			
Can drink from a cup			
Can roll a ball			
Can creep upstairs			
Can walk with one hand held			
Can walk alone			
Moves body to music			
Can build a tower of blocks			
how many?			
Can put objects into containers			
Can dump objects out of containers			
Can pick up small objects			

(continued)

TABLE 4.25a. (*continued*)

Developmental Milestones	COGNITIVE		
	Date Achieved	*NOT YET*	*PROGRESSING*
Responds to visual stimulation			
Responds to touch stimulation			
Responds to sound stimulation			
Focuses on faces			
Discriminates between family and strangers			
Enjoys being with people			
Raises arms when told "up"			
Responds to name			
Discriminates between friendly and angry voices			
Understands bye-bye			
Can follow a single direction			
"come here"			
"stand up"			
Has exposure to colors			
red			
green			
blue			
yellow			
black			
white			
Has exposure to facial parts			
Has exposure to vocabulary of textures			
smooth			
scratchy			
bumpy			
rough			
soft			

SOURCE: *The New Language of Toys.* Schwartz S and Miller JH. Published by Woodbine House, 1996. Copyright held by Schwartz and Miller. Used by permission.

*This chart lists skills acquired by babies who have reached the **developmental** age of 12 months. Children who have developmental delays may be chronologically several months to several years older before they acquire these skills.*

TABLE 4.25b. **Summary of a child's second year (12–24 months).**

Developmental Milestones	LANGUAGE		
	Date Achieved	NOT YET	PROGRESSING
Uses jargon			
Names objects			
which ones?			
Uses nouns with adjectives (e.g., big truck; little car, red ball)			
Uses subject–predicate phrases (e.g., Daddy go car)			
Uses two-word sentences			
Can say own name			
Knows at least one family member by name (e.g., Mom or Dad)			
Asks for food at the table			
Follows one direction at a time			
Hums to music			
Imitates your words			
Listens to rhymes			
Uses pronouns			
which ones?			
Comprehends about 300 words			

Developmental Milestones	PHYSICAL		
	Date Achieved	NOT YET	PROGRESSING
Can walk alone			
Can turn pages of book			
Can climb stairs on all fours			
Can pull a toy			
Can climb onto furniture			
Can feed self			
Can undress self			
Can scribble			
Holds crayon in fist			
Can run stiffly			
Can build a tower of blocks how many?			
Can walk up stairs holding hand or rail			
Can walk down stairs holding hand or rail			
Can kick a ball			
Can throw large ball			
Can do single piece puzzles how many pieces?			

(continued)

Table 4.25b. (*continued*)

| Developmental Milestones | COGNITIVE | | |
	Date Achieved	NOT YET	PROGRESSING
Can point to facial features			
eyes			
nose			
mouth			
Follows simple directions			
Give the ball to me			
Sit on the chair			
Can name several nouns that are			
familiar objects			
table			
bed			
toy car			
apple			
Can point to pictures showing			
different action verbs			
Can match colors without necessarily			
knowing the names			
red			
green			
yellow			
blue			
Develops imaginative play			
Has longer attention span			
Can demonstrate understanding of			
prepositions			
in			
out			
up			
down			
Understands math concept of "one			
more"			

Source: *The New Language of Toys*, pp. 116–117. Schwartz S and Miller JH. Published by Woodbine House, 1996. Copyright held by Schwartz and Miller. Used by permission.

TABLE 4.25c. **Summary of a child's third year (24–36 months).**

Developmental Milestones	LANGUAGE		
	Date Achieved	*NOT YET*	*PROGRESSING*
Uses plurals			
Uses noun phrases with articles			
a ball			
an apple			
the door			
Uses three-word phrases			
Mommy bye-bye car			
Uses possessive nouns			
which ones?			
Uses pronoun "I"			
Asks simple questions			
who?			
what?			
when?			
where?			
Adds "ing" to verbs			
Uses past tense for verbs			
Uses 4-word sentences			
Can say whole name			
Can respond to questions with			
choices			
Uses social phrases			
thank you			
please			
Sings along with music			
Outsiders understand his speech			
Knows 800 words			

Developmental Milestones	PHYSICAL		
	Date Achieved	*NOT YET*	*PROGRESSING*
Can walk backwards			
Can walk up stairs			
alternating feet			
holding hands or rail			
Can run without falling			
Can jump; both feet off floor			
Can bounce and catch a large ball			
Can pedal a tricycle			
Can build a tower of blocks			
how many?			
Can hold crayon not fisted			
Can make snips with scissors			
Can hold a glass with one hand			
Can hold fork in fist			

(continued)

TABLE 4.25c. (*continued*)

| Developmental Milestones | COGNITIVE | | |
	Date Achieved	NOT YET	PROGRESSING
Can point to body parts			
hair			
tongue			
teeth			
hand			
ears			
feet			
head			
legs			
arms			
Can name body parts			
mouth			
eyes			
nose			
hair			
hands			
ears			
head			
Can match colors			
orange			
purple			
brown			
black			
Can identify colors			
give me the red car			
blue			
yellow			
green			
Can match shapes			
circle			
square			
triangle			
Can follow directions that include			
prepositions			
put the doll in the box			
put the doll under the box			
Can demonstrate knowledge of			
opposites			
little/big			
short/long			
Can demonstrate knowledge of use			
of common objects			
What do we do with beds?			
Why do we have coats?			
Develops imaginative play more fully			
Able to express feelings			
Understands math concept of "just one"			
Give me just one block			

SOURCE: *The New Language of Toys*, pp. 138–140. Schwartz S and Miller JH. Published by Woodbine House, 1996. Copyright held by Schwartz and Miller. Used by permission.

TABLE 4.25d. Summary of a child's fourth year (36–48 months).

LANGUAGE			
Developmental Milestones	*Date Achieved*	*NOT YET*	*PROGRESSING*
Uses negation			
don't			
won't			
can't			
Uses plurals			
Asks questions			
Can tell of experiences in sequence			
Can say age and sex			
Uses 5-word sentences			
Can deliver a simple message			
Can respond to conversation of others			
Knows some songs			
Knows 1800 words			

PHYSICAL			
Developmental Milestones	*Date Achieved*	*NOT YET*	*PROGRESSING*
Can walk downstairs alternating feet			
Can climb low ladder			
Can run smoothly			
Can jump several times in a row			
how many times?			
Can hop			
how many times?			
Can catch a large ball bounced by			
someone else			
Can bounce a large ball two or three times			
Can wind up a toy			
Can build a tower of blocks			
how many?			
Can do puzzles of 3–5 pieces			
Can put on clothing			
Can pull a wagon			

COGNITIVE			
Developmental Milestones	*Date Achieved*	*NOT YET*	*PROGRESSING*
Can point to body parts			
fingers			
thumb			
toes			
neck			
stomach			
chest			
back			
knee			
chin			
fingernails			

(continued)

TABLE 4.25d. (*continued*)

	COGNITIVE (*continued*)		
Developmental Milestones	*Date Achieved*	*NOT YET*	*PROGRESSING*
Can name body parts			
legs			
arms			
fingers			
thumb			
toes			
neck			
stomach			
chest			
back			
Can match colors			
pink			
gray			
white			
Can show colors when asked			
orange			
purple			
brown			
black			
Can name colors			
red			
yellow			
green			
blue			
Can show shapes when asked			
circle			
square			
triangle			
Can match shapes			
hexagon			
rectangle			
star			
Understands time concepts			
today			
tonight			
last night			
Can point to opposites			
tall/short			
slow/fast			
over/under			
far/near			
Can sort objects by color			
Can sort objects by shape			
Can count to 4			
Understands ordinal numbers			
who goes first?			
whose turn is second?			

(*continued*)

TABLE 4.25d. *(continued)*

	COGNITIVE *(continued)*		
Developmental Milestones	*Date Achieved*	*NOT YET*	*PROGRESSING*
Can tell about the use of household objects			
What do we use a stove for?			
What are dishes for?			
Why do we need houses?			
Can tell what part of the day is for certain activities			
When do we eat breakfast?			
When do we go to sleep?			
Plays with friends own age			
Can express feelings			
Develops more fantasy play			
Can match letters			

SOURCE: *The New Language of Toys,* pp. 168–170. Schwartz S and Miller JH. Published by Woodbine House, 1996. Copyright held by Schwartz and Miller. Used by permission.

TABLE 4.25e. Summary of a child's fifth year (48–60 months).

	LANGUAGE		
Developmental Milestones	*Date Achieved*	*NOT YET*	*PROGRESSING*
Asks for definition of words			
Can define more common words and tell how used			
book, shoe, table			
Almost complete use of correct grammar			
Uses 6–8 word sentences			
Knows town or city			
Knows street address			
Uses social phrases			
excuse me			
Can carry on a conversation			

(continued)

TABLE 4.25e. *(continued)*

	PHYSICAL		
Developmental Milestones	*Date Achieved*	*NOT YET*	*PROGRESSING*
Can walk down stairs carrying object			
Can skip, alternating feet			
Can do a broad jump			
how far?			
Can hop			
how far?			
Can throw a ball			
how far?			
Can play rhythm instruments in time to music			
Can ride small bike with training wheels			
Can do puzzles that are not single pieces			
how many pieces?			
Can hold a pencil in proper position			
Can color within lines			
Can cut with scissors			
Can use knife for spreading			

	COGNITIVE		
Developmental Milestones	*Date Achieved*	*NOT YET*	*PROGRESSING*
Can identify all body parts			
Can name all body parts			
Can name all colors			
Can name all shapes			
Understands directions			
Uses prepositions			
by the			
beside			
below			
behind			
above			
in front of			
Understands time concepts			
yesterday			
tomorrow			
tomorrow night			
Understands opposites			
bottom/top			
go/stop			
low/high			
off/on			
inside/outside			
closed/open			

SOURCE: *The New Language of Toys*, pp. 193–294. Schwartz S and Miller JH. Published by Woodbine House, 1996. Copyright held by Schwartz and Miller. Used by permission.

TABLE 4.25f. Summary of a child's sixth year (60–72 months).

	LANGUAGE		
Developmental Milestones	*Date Achieved*	*NOT YET*	*PROGRESSING*
Can understand a full repertoire of a spoken language			
Has full spoken use of English language			
Continues to ask for definitions of more complex words (e.g., "What does it mean to borrow a book?)			
Uses grammar with a high degree of accuracy			
Can weave several sentences into a spoken paragraph			
Can tell sequence of a simple story (What happened first, next, last) into a short story			

	COGNITIVE		
Developmental Milestones	*Date Achieved*	*NOT YET*	*PROGRESSING*
Can recognize and identify all upper-case letters of the alphabet			
Can recognize and identify all lower-case letters of the alphabet			
Can distinguish between and recite initial consonant sounds of words			
Can distinguish left from right			
Can assemble a simple puzzle (25 pieces)			
Can notice details and patterns of a picture			
Can distinguish missing piece of a picture and/or note "what doesn't belong" in a picture			
Can express feelings of real or imaginary people or animals			
Can explain in detail			
Can follow directions (three items in a sequence; "Please go into the living room, find your book, and put it away in your bedroom upstairs")			
Can turn on a computer, play a familiar game, and turn off computer when finished			

(continued)

TABLE 4.25f. (*continued*)

COGNITIVE (*continued*)			
Developmental Milestones	*Date Achieved*	*NOT YET*	*PROGRESSING*
Can recognize simple words and signs such as "stop," "walk"			
Can read a preprimer with accompanying pictures as a visual cue			
Can memorize and recite a sequence of 7 numbersCan cooperate with peers in a game involving simple rules and turn taking without adult supervision			
Can begin to be less egocentric, and take on another point of view			
Can sort out a group of coins and distinguish pennies from other coins			
Can count to 100, can write to 22			
Can recite ordinal numbers—first through ninth			
Can draw a person figure with up to six body parts			

PHYSICAL			
Gross Motor			
Developmental Milestones	*Date Achieved*	*NOT YET*	*PROGRESSING*
Can hop on one foot for up to 10 seconds			
Can walk on a balance beam			
Can run with greater speed			
Can throw a ball accurately at target (from how many feet away?)			
Can catch a ball (from how many feet away?)			
Can hit a whiffleball with a bat			
Can add speed to running			
Can broad jump a longer distance			
Can kick a ball (how many yards?)			
Can roller skate without holding on for balance			
Can ride a two wheeler with training wheels			

(*continued*)

TABLE **4.25f.** (*continued*)

	PHYSICAL (*continued*)		
	Fine Motor		
Developmental Milestones	*Date Achieved*	*NOT YET*	*PROGRESSING*
Can key in letters and numbers (with increasing speed) at a typewriter or computer keyboard			
Can legibly copy letters and words			
Can copy O, square, triangle, diamond			
Can legibly print first and last names accurately			
Can color a simple picture carefully within the lines			
Can neatly trace letters in a simple picture			
Can use child-sized scissors to neatly cut on a line			
Can tie shoes by himself			
Can button and dress himself			

SOURCE: *The New Language of Toys.* Schwartz S and Miller JH. Published by Woodbine House, 1996. Copyright held by Schwartz and Miller. Used by permission.

TABLE **4.26. Toddlers with medical needs: therapy activities.**

Developmental age range (mo)	Activities
0–6	Shaking rattle
	Listening to music box
	Watching mobile
	Grasping hand-held toy
	Shaking noise-making toy
	Exploring busy box
6–12	Looking in mirror
	Participating in daily living activities
	Blowing bubbles
	Playing with pop-up toy
	Singing gestural song
	Exploring manipulable toy
	Banging toy drum
	Rolling toy car
12–18	Riding in wagon or on tricycle
	Looking at picture book
	Sorting shapes
	Playing music instrument
	Building Mr. and Mrs. Potato Head
18–24	Playing see 'n say
	Playing with doll
	Building blocks
	Making big-piece puzzle

SOURCE: Bleile KM, Miller SA: Toddlers with Medical Needs. In Bernthal JE, Bankson NW (eds): *Child Phonology: Characteristics, Assessment, and Intervention with Special Populations,* p. 96. Thieme, New York, 1994.

TABLE 4.27. Tracheostomies: risk factors for children.

Risk factors	*Causes of disability*
Prematurity with low birthweight	Increased risk of neurologic damage
Respiratory distress syndrome (RDS)	Increased opportunities for oxygen deprivation (RDS may also indicate a more serious underlying condition)
Intraventricular hemorrhage	Increased risk of neurological damage
Birth outside of a hospital	More severe illness and birth trauma
Mechanical ventilation	Increased opportunities for oxygen deprivation (longer ventilation time may also reflect a more serious underlying condition)
Lower socioeconomic status	Poorer developmental outcome due to either lack lack of available developmental services or lack of knowledge regarding how to obtain developmental services
Family history of speech disorders	Possible genetic predisposition for speech problems

SOURCE: Bleile KM, Miller SA: Toddlers with Medical Needs. In Bernthal JE, Bankson NW (eds): *Child Phonology: Characteristics, Assessment, and Intervention with Special Populations,* p. 96. Thieme, New York, 1994.

TABLE 4.28. Vocalization of speech-type sounds: ages of acquisition.

Average age	*Behavior*
Birth to 2 mo	Vegetative sounds
2–3 mo	Begins to produce cooing behaviors
2–4 mo	Begins to produce pleasure sounds such as "mmmm"
3–4 mo	Cooing behavior is well established, babbling behavior (repetition of consonants and vowels) begins to appear
4 mo	Produces some intonation during sound making and may engage in vocal play when playing with toys; vocalizations begin to be dominated by sounds produced at the front of the mouth, including raspberries and trills
6 mo	Reduplicated babbling (repetitions of the same syllable) begins to appear
7–8 mo	Reduplicated babbling well established
9 mo	Produces short exclamations such as "ooh!"
10 mo	Produces nonreduplicative babbling (changes of consonants and vowels within syllables)

SOURCE: Bleile KM, Miller SA: Toddlers with Medical Needs. In Bernthal JE, Bankson NW (eds): *Child Phonology: Characteristics, Assessment, and Intervention with Special Populations,* p. 88. Thieme, New York, 1994.

5

Acquired Neurological Disorders

TABLE 5.1. **Alzheimer's disease: ineffective communication tactics questionnaire.**

As your patient's communication abilities deteriorate, you may find yourself developing some ineffective tactics for dealing with him or her. This happens to people with the best of intentions. Below is a list of responses to your patient that are not unreasonable or unusual. Such responses, however, might actually contribute to a further breakdown in communication between the two of you. Put a check in the column which best describes how frequently you use each tactic. If you have checked "Often" more than five times, it might be helpful to you to seek new responses. Advice on effective communication tactics is available through speech-language pathologists, communication support groups, and several excellent books.

His problem	*Your response*	*Never*	*Sometimes*	*Often*
He doesn't seem to understand conversation.	You say less.			
He doesn't respond to questions the first time you ask.	You yell louder to get through.			
He repeats and repeats.	You just ignore him.			
He asks you a question for the tenth time.	You tell him to be quiet; he won't remember the answer anyway.			
He uses a wrong word.	You correct him immediately, hoping he won't repeat it.			
He needs to have a task explained a dozen times.	You do the job yourself to save you the bother.			
He embarrasses you at your neighbor's house.	You stay home.			
He's dependent like a child.	You talk to him like a child.			
He can't remember names of common objects (e.g., salt, sugar) even though you know he still knows them.	You withhold objects until he says their names, hoping to force him to maintain his vocabulary.			
He "rattles on and on" all day.	You play the radio or TV all day to drown him out.			
He can't stay on the topic of conversation.	You let him go on and on, "tuning him out."			
He is slow to understand and respond.	You "help" him by speaking for him.			
He has difficulty getting idea across.	You distract him by changing the subject or the activity.			
He's driving you crazy.	You call a relative or friend and "vent" within his earshot.			
He gets impatient and frustrated.	You let him know you are just as impatient and frustrated.			

SOURCE: Santo Pietro MJ: Assessing the Communicative Styles of Caregivers of Patients with Alzheimer's Disease. *Seminars in Speech and Language* 1994; 15:254.

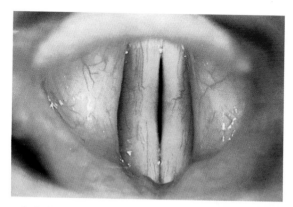

COLOR PLATE 1. Indirect laryngoscopy showing a normal larynx with the vocal cords adducted.

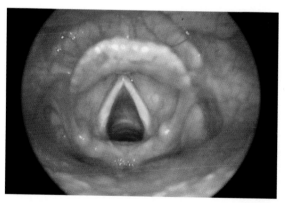

COLOR PLATE 2. Normal larynx showing the vocal cords in the abducted position during inspiration.

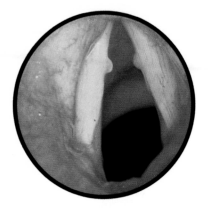

COLOR PLATE 3. Singer's nodes.

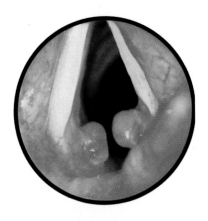

COLOR PLATE 4. Intubation granuloma of both vocal processes.

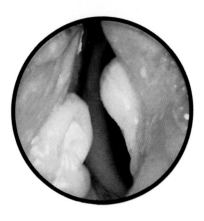

COLOR PLATE 5. Contact ulcer at the typical site on both vocal processes.

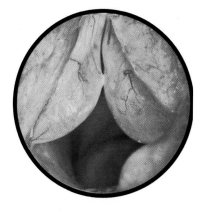

COLOR PLATE 6. Reinke's edema of both vocal cords.

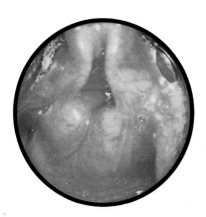

COLOR PLATE 7. Laryngomalacia in a newborn child.

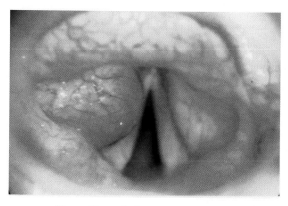

COLOR PLATE 8. Internal laryngocele.

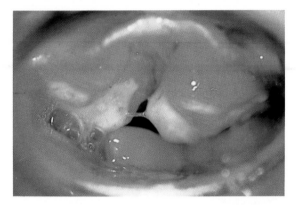

COLOR PLATE 9. Laryngeal fracture with a mucosal hematoma and dislocation of the arytenoid.

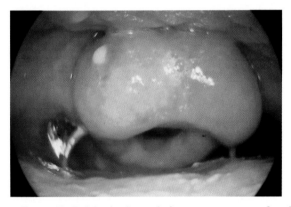

COLOR PLATE 10. Epiglottic abscess before spontaneous perforation.

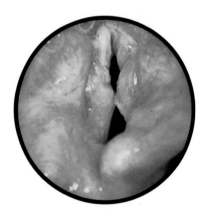

COLOR PLATE 11. Chronic leukoplakia.

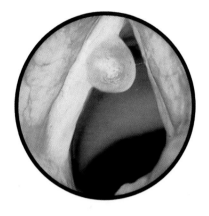

COLOR PLATE 12. Vocal cord polyp.

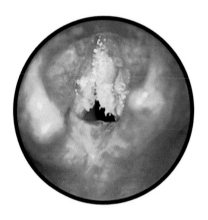

COLOR PLATE 13. Multiple endolaryngeal papillomas.

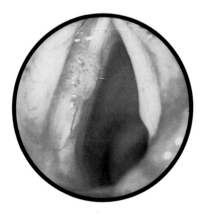

COLOR PLATE 14. Carcinoma in the center of the vocal cord extending to the ventricle.

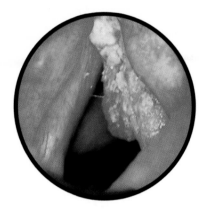

COLOR PLATE 15. Carcinoma of the entire vocal cord, the ventricle and the anterior commissure. The vocal cord is paralysed.

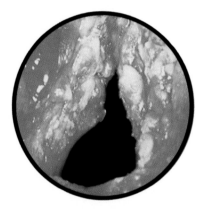

COLOR PLATE 16. Transglottic squamous cell carcinoma.

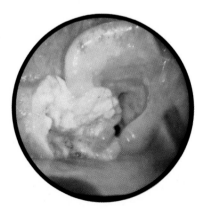

COLOR PLATE 17. Carcinoma of the piriform sinus with invasion of the ipsilateral hemilarynx.

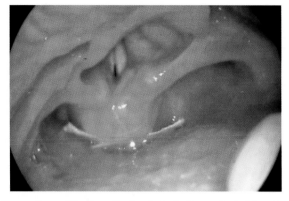

COLOR PLATE 18. Bony foreign body in the postcricoid region.

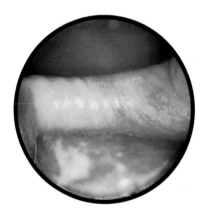

COLOR PLATE 19. Zenker's diverticulum. The bar is in the middle, the esophageal lumen above and the diverticular sac below.

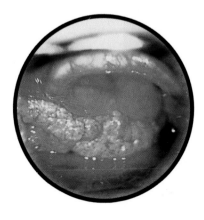

COLOR PLATE 20. Squamous cell carcinoma of the postcricoid space.

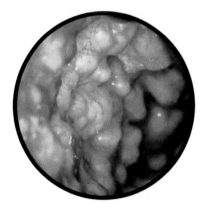

COLOR PLATE 21. Tracheopathia osteo-plastica: view of the left wall of the tra-chea on direct tracheoscopy.

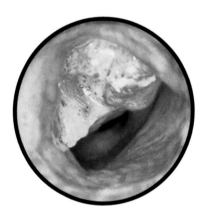

COLOR PLATE 22. Carcinoma of the left main bronchus.

TABLE 5.2. Alzheimer's disease: tough communication situations questionnaire.

In your role as caregiver you face very tough communication situations. This questionnaire lists several encounters in which you are likely to find yourself. Some may be new experiences for you. This chart will help you pinpoint situations that may be especially difficult for you personally. Your counselor or support group can help you develop strategies to handle these communication situations more effectively and with less anxiety.

Rate each situation from 1–5 according to the following scale:

1—Relatively easy, not a problem for me
2—Occasionally difficult, but I do it
3—Moderately difficult, I'd rather avoid it
4—Very difficult, but not impossible
5—Impossible

Rating	*Situation*
_____	Asking for help from family members
_____	Asking for help from professionals
_____	Entering into conflict with other family members
_____	Entering into conflict with the person who has Alzheimer's disease
_____	Exerting influence over others, attempting to get them to agree
_____	Talking about certain subjects such as personal hygiene, details of illness, abusive language, death, autopsy
_____	Sharing information with professionals and people who work for me, such as homemakers, previous acquaintances, other caregivers
_____	Giving support, encouragement, praise out loud to Alzheimer's victim
_____	Seeking support, encouragement, praise from others for myself and for the person with Alzheimer's
_____	Accepting support, encouragement, praise from others
_____	Explaining my decisions and actions to others
_____	Describing my own needs, fears, problems
_____	Talking to my support group
_____	Explaining Alzheimer's disease to children, grandchildren, others
_____	Inviting people to my home

SOURCE: Santo Pietro MJ: Assessing the Communicative Styles of Caregivers of Patients with Alzheimer's Disease. *Seminars in Speech and Language* 1994; 15:253.

TABLE 5.3. **Alzheimer's disease/dementia: caregiver questionnaire to identify feelings that make it difficult to communicate with a patient.**

You might be finding it increasingly difficult to communicate effectively, not only with your Alzheimer's patient, but also with others around you. There are good reasons for this. For one, the difficulties of your situation might be provoking strong negative feelings that you bring with you to communication encounters. That is to be expected. These feelings are normal. You might not even be fully aware that you are carrying them around with you. This questionnaire lists some of these common and expected feelings. Rating yourself honestly on this chart may help you identify feelings that are making positive communication difficult. First put a check in the space that best describes each of your feelings. Then add the numbers of the ratings you chose. If your total score is 75 or higher, you might benefit from talking to other caregivers in a support group or a counselor to work out these feelings.

	Never or rarely 1	Sometimes 2	Often-decreasing 3	Often-increasing 4	All the time 5
Guilty					
Angry					
Confused					
Helpless					
Ready to give up					
Out of control					
Isolated					
Blaming others					
Needy					
Financially strained					
Resigned					
Desperate					
Lonely					
Self-blaming					
Frustrated					
Neglected					
Numb					
Depressed					
Tired					
Uniformed					

SOURCE: Santo Pietro MJ: Assessing the Communicative Styles of Caregivers of Patients with Alzheimer's Disease. *Seminars in Speech and Language* 1994; 15:252.

TABLE 5.4. Anomia: example categories for lexical focus.

First-order	Second-order	Third-order
Fruits and vegetables	Fruits	Citrus fruits
		Berries
	Vegetables	Green vegetables
		Yellow vegetables
Musical instruments	Horns	Brass
		Woodwinds
	String	Played with a bow
		Plucked
	Keyboard	
Sports	Played with a ball	Played with a racket
		Not played with a racket
	Not played with a ball	

SOURCE: Linebaugh CW: Lexical Retrieval Problems: Anomia. In LaPointe LL (ed): *Aphasia and Related Neurogenic Language Disorders*, p. 127. Thieme, New York, 1997.

TABLE 5.5. Anomia: lexical retrieval problems—two representative cueing hierarchies for visual confrontation naming.

Picture
Picture + "Tell me what you do with it."
Picture + "Show me what you do with it."
Picture + Descriptive statement
Picture + Sentence completion
Picture + Sentence completion + Initial phoneme
Picture + "Say _____."

Picture + "Show me what you do with it."
Picture + Functional gesture
Picture + Sentence completion
Picture + Sentence completion +Printed target word and two foils
Picture + Sentence completion +Printed target word
Picture + Sentence completion +Printed target word + Initial phoneme
Picture + "Say _____."

SOURCE: Linebaugh CW: Lexical Retrieval Problems: Anomia. In LaPointe LL (ed): *Aphasia and Related Neurogenic Language Disorders*, p. 126. Thieme, New York, 1997.

TABLE 5.6. **Anomia: tasks for the evaluation of lexical retrieval.**

Visual confrontation naming
Word naming
Responsive naming
Picture-to-word matching
Written confrontation naming
Verbal fluency
Picture description
Story retelling
Story completion
Referential communication
Conversational speech sample

SOURCE: Linebaugh CW: Lexical Retrieval Problems: Anomia. In LaPointe LL (Ed): *Aphasia and Related Neurogenic Language Disorders,* p. 120. Thieme, New York, 1997.

TABLE 5.7. **Anomia: task continuum for facilitating lexical retrieval.**

Picture + Spoken target word
Picture + Spoken target word and two semantically related foils
Picture + Sentence completion with initial phoneme
Picture + Sentence completion
Picture + Descriptive statement
Picture + Functional gesture
Picture only
Descriptive statement only

SOURCE: Linebaugh CW: Lexical Retrieval Problems: Anomia. In LaPointe LL (ed): *Aphasia and Related Neurogenic Language Disorders,* p. 125. Thieme, New York, 1997.

TABLE 5.8. **Aphasia: behavioral patterns of Wernicke's, conduction, and transcortical sensory aphasias.**

	Wernicke's	*Conduction*	*Transcortical sensory*
Auditory comprehension	Severely impaired	Slightly impaired	Severely impaired
Repetition	Impaired	Impaired	Intact
Speech	Fluent, paraphasic	Paraphasic	Fluent, paraphasic
Reading	Impaired	Intact	Impaired
Writing	Impaired	Impaired	Impaired

SOURCE: Graharn-Keegan L, Caspari I: Wernicke's Aphasia. In LaPointe LL (ed): *Aphasia and Related Neurogenic Language Disorders,* p. 46. Thieme, New York, 1997.

TABLE 5.9. **Aphasia: education and counseling considerations for the client and family.**

A major issue that must be addressed early on and continue throughout treatment is counseling and educating the client and family. This should include

1. A general discussion of characteristics of brain damage, possibly with relevant literature and referral to outside sources such as stroke clubs or support groups.
2. Facts on the nature of the disorder with specifics about what is wrong and what is right with the patient.
3. Information on goals and expectations, which includes the aphasic person's input in goal setting and treatment planning.
4. Acquiring information on family interaction, and how their strategies promote or hinder communication.
5. Direct family training in ways to facilitate communication, such as recognizing when to allow the patient more time to elaborate or when to stop and ask for clarification.

SOURCE: Simmons-Mackie N: Conduction Aphasia. In LaPointe LL (ed): *Aphasia and Related Neurogenic Language Disorders,* pp. 78–79. Thieme, New York, 1997.

TABLE 5.10. Aphasia: functional rehabilitation plan for a patient with severe aphasia and right hemiplegia.

Expected Functional Outcome (macro level of function) Related to Living Situation: Mr. P. will live at home with his wife and be independent for up to 10 hours during the day, thus allowing her to return to work.

LONG-TERM GOALS Required functional skill area (middle) level of function	SHORT-TERM GOALS Prerequisite physical and mental skills mental skills (micro level of function) and/or necessary environmental adaptations	Therapeutic methods to be used[1]	Person(s) responsible for shot-term goals[2]	Projected date of achievement[3]	Actual date of achievement[4]
1. Reliable use of an emergency call system	1a. Purchase emergency call system and record appropriate messages. 1b. Motor sequencing skills adequate for operation of system. 1c. Procedural memory adequate for operation of system. 1d. Reading adequate for comprehension of symbols on the emergency call system machine. 1e. Client and family confident that client is able to use system in the event of an emergency.				
2. Leisure-time activities to help fill day	2a. Motor skill with nondominant hand adequate for hammering, sawing, gluing, painting. 2b. Motor-sequencing skills adequate for completion of multiple-step tasks. 2c. Procedural memory adequate for completion of multiple-step project (e.g., building a bird house or child's chair). 2d. Adequate safety awareness when working with tools to assure no safety risks. 2e. Client and family confidence that client is able to entertain himself when he is alone. 2f. Purchase several simple woodworking projects.				

3. Independent preparation of lunch	3a. Motor sequencing skills adequate for preparation of simple lunch (sandwich, soup, microwave meal).
	3b. Motor skill with nondominant hand adequate for opening packages, cutting, etc.
	3c. Adequate safety awareness when working in the kitchen to assure no safety risks.
	3d. Rearrange kitchen cabinets so necessary items are within easy reach.
	3e. Purchase microwave oven.
	3f. Procedural memory adequate for operation of microwave oven.
	3g. Client and family confident that client is able to prepare light meals.
4. Safe ambulation within house and yard	4a. Modify home environment by removing all throw rugs and adding hand railings to all steps.
	4b. Increase client's ability to compensate when he loses his balance.
	4c. Increase client's ability to get up from the floor independently in the event that he falls.
	4d. Client and family confident that client is able to ambulate safely without assistance within the house and yard.

SOURCE: Ramberger G: Functional Perspective for Assessment and Rehabilitation of Persons with Severe Aphasia. *Seminars in Speech and Language* 1994; 15:7.

[1]Treatment plan should include a description of the therapeutic methods to be utilized for the achievement of each short-term goal.

[2]The functional rehabilitation plan is transdisciplinary. Team members from various disciplines work with the patient for the achievement of common goals. Team members assume responsibility or share responsibility for those short-term goals that are within their area of expertise.

[3]Projected dates for the achievement of short-term goals are established at the onset of the rehabilitation program. These dates are used to assess weekly progress toward the achievement of both short- and long-term goals. Should it appear that a patient is not going to achieve a goal within the specified time frame, the team should consider the following possible courses of action: Alter the therapeutic methods being utilized, redefine a more realistic time frame for the achievement of the goal, or reassess the feasibility of ever achieving the goal.

[4]When all of the short-term goals are accomplished, the client will have achieved the corresponding long-term goal. And, when all of the long-term goals are accomplished, the client will have achieved the corresponding functional outcome.

TABLE 5.11. **Aphasia: guidelines for communicating with the severely aphasic person.**

---

1. SIMPLIFY
   Handle only one idea at a time, use short sentences with simple, common words, speak more slowly, but naturally, and do not speak to the patient as if he was a child.

2. CLUE HIM IN
   Be sure you have his attention; use gestures and pointing where possible; facial cues may also help him. Use redundant wording, for example, "Are you hungry enough to eat dinner?" Repeat and reword the idea until he understands.

3. ALLOW TIME
   Allow the patient additional time to understand and to respond. Be patient, unhurried, and accepting of his speech attempts.

4. GUESS
   Determine the subject by asking increasingly specific questions.

5. CONFIRM
   Make statements about what you think he means to make sure you understand. When he responds to a question, ask the opposite also. If the response does not change, you are not communicating.

6. BE CLEAR
   Say "I'm sorry, I don't understand you" when necessary. Do not leave abruptly when attempts fail.

7. REDUCE EXTRANEOUS VARIABLES
   Avoid a noisy environment, additional activities such as television or radio, and talking with more than one person at a time.

8. RESPECT
   Understand that the patient is usually an intelligent adult who is quite aware of his surroundings even though language function is impaired. Include him in the conversation, and do not treat him as though he is not there, deaf, or mentally retarded.

SOURCE: Collins MJ: Global Aphasia. In LaPointe LL (ed): *Aphasia and Related Neurogenic Language Disorders,* pp. 147–148. Thieme, New York, 1997.

TABLE 5.12. **Asphasic syndromes: basic classifications.**

	Auditory Fluency	Comprehension	Repetition	Naming
NONFLUENT				
Broca's	−	+	=	=
Global	−	−	−	−
Transcortical motor	−	+	+	=
FLUENT				
Wernicke's	+	−	−	=
Transcortical sensory	+	−	+	=
Conduction	+	+	−	=
Anomic	+	+	+	−

SOURCE: Kearns KP: Broca's Aphasia. In LaPointe LL (ed): *Aphasia and Related Neurogenic Language Disorders*, p. 14. Thieme, New York, 1997.
Key: (+) Relatively unimpaired; (−) Impaired; (=) Variable impairment across patients.

TABLE 5.13. **Augmentative communication: evolutionary framework for patients with traumatic brain injury.**

	PHASE OF RECOVERY		
	Early	Middle	Late
Status on the Rancho Levels	I–III	IV–V	VI–VIII
Frequency of occurrence of severe expressive communication impairment	Common	Less frequent	Infrequent
Primary reason for lack of speech	Arousal deficits	Cognitive and motor deficits	Persistent motor deficits
Purpose of AAC intervention	Stimulate consistent responses	Provide means for patient to indicate basic needs and to respond to further diagnostic therapy	Improve patient's quality of life and facilitate communication interaction with a variety of partners in a variety of settings

SOURCE: Ladtkow M: Traumatic Brain Injury and Severe Expressive Communication Impairment: The Role of Augmentative Communication. *Seminars in Speech and Language* 1993; 14:63.

TABLE 5.14. **Augmentative communication: example of an evolution of strategies and aids for a nonspeaking traumatic brain-injured patient.**

	Early Phase	*Middle Phase*	*Late Phase*
Patient: David	(0–4 months postonset)	(5 months postonset)	(6–36 months postonset)
Volitional movement (sequential development)	Eye blinks Eye gaze	Eye blinks Eye gaze Minimal R index finger movement Minimal head movement/control Very minimal R arm movement	R arm movement R index finger movement functional for typing Good head movement/control
Speech (sequential development)	None	Very inconsistent ability to initiate phonation Ability to mouth "hi" and "bye"	Fairly consistent ability to phonate spontaneously Ability to vocalize for attention Ability to speak some single words/social greetings in context (e.g., "hi," "bye," "no," "uh huh")
AAC Strategies and Aids	Eye blinks as a consistent response only Eye gaze (at objects/pictures /words)	*Yes/No* 1. Idiosyncratic eye blinks 2. Single switch/tone box 3. Minimally defined head nods *Manual Scanning of Alphabet Board* 1. Signaled with eye blinks 2. Signaled with switch/tone box *Direct Selection— Alphabet/Word/ Phrase Board* 1. Light-pointer (patient rejected) 2. R index finger	Canon Communicator Words + EZ Keys software

SOURCE: Ladtkow M: Traumatic Brain Injury and Severe Expressive Communication Impairment: The Role of Augmentative Communication. *Seminars in Speech and Language* 1993; 14:63.

TABLE 5.15. **Augmentative communication for traumatic brain injury: general assessment parameters for application.**

Cognitive status
Gross motor ability/positioning
Fine motor ability (including handwriting/keyboard skills)
Visual–perceptual abilities (with particular regard to number and type of stimuli presented)
Hearing status
Communication modalities available (facial expressions/eye gaze/gestures/mouthing/vocalizing/speech/writing)
Language comprehension
Reading comprehension
Spelling
Educational history
Symbol recognition (type/number/size/organization)
Transmission technique options (direct selection/scanning/rarely encoding)
Psychosocial status of both patient and family (with particular regard to readiness for and acceptance of AAC)
Communication needs of the patient (with regard to whom/where/what/why/how patient will be communicating)

SOURCE: Ladtkow M: Traumatic Brain Injury and Severe Expressive Communication Impairment: The Role of Augmentative Communication. *Seminars in Speech and Language* 1993; 14:65.

TABLE 5.16. **Augmentative communication: goals for patients with traumatic brain injury and their communication partners.**

Early phase TBI recovery
Patient Develop consistent response to commands
        -Activate a beeper
        -Direct eye gaze
        -Move body pact
      Differentiate/identify familiar objects/people
        -Signal with motor movement
        -Direct eye gaze
        -Signal with beeper
Partner Chart observations of patient
      Create controlled situations
      Provide information to team

Middle phase TBI recovery
Patient Aid Operation and Use
        -Answer yes/no questions
        -Respond to highly structured "wh" questions
      Interaction
        -Signal for attention
        -Initiate basic needs
        -Recognize and respond to structure/feedback from communication partner
Partner Aid Operation and Use
        -Educate others regarding purpose/use of AAC
        -Model use of AAC/provide frequent e-instruction to patient
      Interaction
        -Provide consistent feedback add pause time
        -Make opportunities for patient to initiate/communicate
        -Assist in mode selection and breakdown repair

Late phase TBI recover
Patient Aid Operation and Use
        -Perform basic functions of communication aid (device)
        -Do simple programming with assistance
      Interaction
        -Demonstrate a variety of communication functions
        -Select appropriate mode for situation/partner
        -Establish/maintain topics of conversation
        -Use strategies to increase message speed/efficiency
        -Participate in small groups effectively
Partner Aid Operation and Use
        -Facilitate upkeep/maintenance
        -Facilitate consistency of use
      Interaction
        -Facilitate patient's organization of ideas/topic appropriateness/repair of
         breakdowns
        -Provide pause time and limit questions
        -Create opportunities for social closeness

SOURCE: Ladtkow M: Traumatic Brain Injury and Severe Expressive Communication Impairment: The Role of Augmentative Communication. *Seminars in Speech and Language* 1993; 14:69.

TABLE 5.17. **Augmentative and alternate communication users: transition skills checklists—school to postschool transition.**

5 = able to do entire skill independently and does so whenever needed
4 = able to do entire skill and does so with limited verbal assistance
3 = ble to do all or part of skill, but does so only with verbal assistance
2 = able to do all or part of skill with adaptive devices
1 = able to do all or part of skills with physical guidance
0 = physically unable to do

	Classroom and computer teachers	Speech-language pathologist	Occupational and physical therapist	Student
A. Self-Care Skills				
1. Selects appropriate clothing for weather conditions and work setting				
2. Dresses for school or work				
3. Indicates need for toileting				
4. Transfers to and from toilet				
5. Eats meals neatly with utensils				
6. Drinks neatly from a cup/glass				
7. Orders meals from a restaurant				
8. Brushes teeth				
9. Washes hands				
10. Shaves as needed				
B. Domestic Skills				
1. Launders clothing				
2. Folds and/or hangs clothing				
3. Makes bed				
4. Prepares simple menus and grocery list				
5. Prepares simple meals for self (e.g., sandwiches, frozen dinners)				
6. Loads and unloads dishwasher				
7. Dusts and vacuums				
8. Deals with simple injuries (e.g., cuts, burns)				
9. Maintains and cares for adaptive equipment (e.g., wheelchair)				
10. Knows where to call for replacement or repair of adaptive equipment				

(continued)

TABLE 5.17. (*continued*)

5 = able to do entire skill independently and does so whenever needed
4 = able to do entire skill and does so with limited verbal assistance
3 = able to do all or part of skill, but does so only with verbal assistance
2 = able to do all or part of skill with adaptive devices
1 = able to do all or part of skills with physical guidance
0 = physically unable to do

	Classroom and computer teachers	Speech-language pathologist	Occupational and physical therapist	Student
C. Community Skills				
1. Uses public transportation				
2. Uses handicapped transportation				
3. Uses telephone directory				
4. Uses private/pay telephone				
5. Uses vending machine				
6. Uses money to make purchases				
7. Manages money in a checking or savings account				
8. Budgets money for expenses				
9. Uses community recreation facilities (e.g., theaters, pools)				
10. Engages in leisure activities at home				
11. Tells time				
12. Reads survival words				
13. Reads/looks at magazines, books, etc.				
D. Communication Skills				
1. Asks questions or directions				
2. Asks for wants/needs to be met				
3. Shares information with others				
4. Converses with friends, others				
5. Converses with supervisors, coworkers appropriately				
6. Follows simple commands				

(*continued*)

TABLE 5.17. (*continued*)

5 = able to do entire skill independently and does so whenever needed
4 = able to do entire skill and does so with limited verbal assistance
3 = ble to do all or part of skill, but does so only with verbal assistance
2 = ble to do all or part of skill with adaptive devices
1 = able to do all or part of skills with physical guidance
0 = physically unable to do

		Classroom and computer teachers	*Speech-language pathologist*	*Occupational and physical therapist*	*Student*
	7. Follows 2- to 3-step directions				
	8. Can be understood by unfamiliar people				
E.	Job Performance				
	1. Expresses a desire to work				
	2. Works at a production rate comparable to nondisabled workers				
	3. Comes to work consistently and promptly				
	4. Works attentively for at least 1-hour periods				
	5. Takes breaks and meals appropriately				
	6. Follows a schedule and routine				
	7. Refrains from making negative comments, gestures, etc.				
	8. Demonstrates a willingness to learn new tasks and responsibilities				

SOURCE: Mireda P: School to Postschool Transition Planning for Augmentative and Alternative Communication Users. *Seminars in Speech and Language* 1992; 13:134–135.

TABLE 5.18. **Bodily devices used in clinical lessons.**

Physical mechanism	Nonverbal signals
Body	Orienting, relocating, shifting, tensing
Head	Tilting, turning, lowering, raising
Shoulders	Shrugging, curling, slouching
Torso	Leaning, turning, swaying, rotating
Arms	Raising, reaching, encompassing
Legs	Wiggling, opening closing, crossing
Feet	Tapping, pointing, lifting
Face	Animating, relaxing, talking
Eyebrows	Lifting one, lifting two
Eyelids	Opening, closing, squinting
Eyes	Gazing, staring, shifting, expanding
Cheeks	Smiling, relaxing, flushing
Jaw	Lowering, protruding, tensing
Lips	Pursing, retracting, opening, closing
Voice	Voicing, modulating, silencing
Pitch	Raising, lowering, maintaining
Loudness	Raising, lowering, maintaining
Quality	Slurring, tensing, relaxing
Hands	Gesturing, signing, holding
Palm	Opening, closing, spreading, rotating
Fingers	Pointing, fisting, counting

SOURCE: Panagos JM: Speech Therapy Discourse: The Input to Learning. In Smith MD, Damico JS (eds): *Childhood Language Disorders*, p. 49. Thieme, New York, 1996.

TABLE 5.19. **Broca's aphasia and apraxia of speech compared with conduction aphasia: general characteristics.**

Broca's/apraxia	Conduction
Nonfluent	Fluent
Dysprosody	Intact prosody (with self-corrections and word search)
Agrammatic	Preserved grammar
Comprehension good	Comprehension good
Repetition impaired proportionate to other verbal tasks	Repetition disproportionately impaired
Error recognition	Error recognition
Probably anomic	Probably anomic

SOURCE: Simmons-Mackie N: Conduction Aphasia. In LaPointe LL (ed): *Aphasia and Related Neurogenic Language Disorders*, p. 64. Thieme, New York, 1997.

TABLE 5.20. **Communication opportunities for children with developmental disabilities: format for analysis.**

1. Briefly describe the routine or activity.
2. Listed below are some common types of opportunities to communicate that might occur during typical activities. Circle the term that you feel best describes the frequency of opportunities to communicate that were present during the activity.

Opportunity	*Frequency of Opportunities*			
Requesting	Very often	Often	Occasionally	Never
Making choices	Very often	Often	Occasionally	Never
Imitation	Very often	Often	Occasionally	Never
Greeting	Very often	Often	Occasionally	Never
Responding/commenting	Very often	Often	Occasionally	Never
Positive interaction	Very often	Often	Occasionally	Never
Termination	Very often	Often	Occasionally	Never
Other (list below)	Very often	Often	Occasionally	Never
_____	Very often	Often	Occasionally	Never
_____	Very often	Often	Occasionally	Never

3. How many chances or opportunities did your child have to communicate?

   Many   Many, but   A few   Hardly any   None
              need more

4. How many different reasons to communicate occurred?

   Many   Many, but   A few   Hardly any   None
              need more

5. Did your child usually communicate when an opportunity was available?

   _____ yes
   _____ no

   Please explain, if possible.

6. Is it possible to increase the number of opportunities to communicate?
7. Is it possible to increase the different reasons to communicate?
8. If you feel it is helpful, provide additional comments about this activity or routine. For example, what did your child enjoy? What did your child not enjoy? Would you change any other aspects of this activity or routine?

SOURCE: Wilcox JM: Enhancing Initial Communication Skills in Young Children with Developmental Disabilities Through Partner Programming. *Seminars in Speech and Language* 1992; 13:204.

TABLE 5.21. **Communication skills in young children with developmental disabilities: categories for coding behavioral descriptions.**

1. Eye
    A. Looking toward or away from a person or object/activity: Any reference to behavior involving eye contact, gaze, or orientation toward another person, object, or activity (e.g., "She was watching her mother"). Any reference to behavior involving the termination of eye gaze or orientation with a person or object/activity (e.g., "She stopped looking at the book").
    B. Other eye: Any reference to other behaviors involving the eyes, such as searching, looking up, rolling the eyes, blinking, and so on (e.g., "He blinked," "She rolled her eyes back").
2. Facial expressions
    Any reference to behavior involving a facial expression such as frowning, smiling, grimacing, happy; sad, tired, bored, questioning (e.g., "She looked puzzled," "He made his happy face").
3. Oral motor
    Any reference to behavior involving a specific oral motor movement pattern, excluding behavior involving voice. Examples of descriptions appropriate for this category include kissing, blowing, coughing, thumb sucking, mouthing an object, opening or shutting the mouth, and drooling.
4. Head/neck
    A. Turn toward or away from person/activity: Any reference to behavior involving the orientation of the head/neck toward or away from a person, object, or activity (e.g., "She turned her head toward me" or "He turned his head away from the dog").
    B. Other head/neck movements: Any reference to other behavior involving movements of the head/neck, such as tilting the head, shaking the head, banging the head, raising the head, nodding (e.g., "She nodded," "She shook her head no," "His head went back").
5. Vocal
    A. Sounds, babbling, laughing, and vocal noises: References to speech sound production (e.g., vocalizations, consonant sounds, strings of sounds, syllables (e.g., "She vocalized," "He made the *b* sound"). Any reference to laughing behavior (e.g., "He giggled," "She was laughing"). Any reference to miscellaneous vocal behavior including animal sounds, yawns, environmental noises (e.g., "She made the kitty sounds," "He was imitating the truck sound").
    B. Attempting to talk: References to productions of words, word approximations (e.g., "She was trying to say no," "He said the word," "She was trying to talk").
    C. Crying, protesting, screaming: Any reference to vocal behavior produced to indicate displeasure, boredom, dissatisfaction (e.g., "She was crying," "He was whining," "She sighed," "He whimpered," "She was screaming," "He squealed").
6. Upper extremity
    A. Reach toward a person, object, or activity: Reference to behavior involving use of the arms or hands to reach for or toward a person (e.g., "She was reaching for her mom," "She held her hand out to the teacher"). Reference to behavior involving use of the arms or hands to reach for or toward an object or an activity (e.g., "She held her hand out for the doll," "She reached toward the book"). Reference to behavior involving the use of hands to manipulate or contact people or objects. Descriptions might refer to taking an object, giving or showing an object, picking an object up, or grabbing, touching, dropping, shaking, batting, pushing, rolling, turning, throwing, stacking. Descriptions regarding person contact might include grabbing a person's hand, pushing a person's arm away, or clapping with a person. Some examples include "He took the object when it was offered," "She pushed the teacher's arm way," "She threw the spoon on the floor").

(continued)

TABLE 5.21. (*continued*)

6. Upper extremity (*continued*)
   B. Pointing: Any reference to behavior involving extension of a finger or fingers to point or direct attention (e.g., "She pointed to the picture," "He used his fingers to indicate which one he wanted").
   C. Gesture, signs. Any reference to behavior involving the hands and/or arms to produce a sign or a gesture (e.g., "She made the sign for more," "He made the gesture for going home").
   D. Other upper-extremity movements. References to behaviors involving gross movements of the arms without person contact such as raising the arms, lowering arms, waving, clapping, pulling the arm away (e.g., "She waved hello," "He held his arm up," "She put her arm down"). References to termination of movement involving the hands or arms (e.g., "She quit touching the object," "He stopped moving his arm").
7. Lower-extremity movements
   References to behavior involving the legs or feet (e.g., "She stomped her foot," "He kicked," "She was swinging her legs," "He held his foot out").
8. Total body
   A. Directional movement toward or away from a person, object, or activity: Reference to behavior involving a total body movement (postural shift or moving body from one location to another) toward a person and/or object/activity (e.g., "She moved toward the teacher," "He walked to the chair," "He shifted his trunk forward"). Reference to behavior involving a total body movement (postural shift or moving body from one location to another) away from a person or object/activity (e.g., "He ran away," "She moved her trunk further back," "He rolled away from the teacher").
   B. Other, nondirectional body movement: Reference to behavior involving a total body movement that is neither toward nor away from a person or activity (e.g., "She stretched," "He was squirming," "She sat there," "He was standing patiently," "She rolled over").
9. Cannot assign
   The reported behavior cannot be classified in any of the preceding categories.

SOURCE: Wilcox JM: Enhancing Initial Communication Skills in Young Children with Developmental Disabilities through Partner Programming. *Seminars in Speech and Language* 1992; 13:201.

TABLE 5.22. **Communication skills in young children with developmental disabilities: categories for coding meaning descriptions.**

1. Request: Any reference to solicitation of a service from a listener. Includes descriptions of requests for objects (e.g., "She wants the doll"), actions (e.g., "She wants the cup moved closer"), or information (e.g., "She wants to know if it's time to go").
2. Termination: Any reference to a child's attempts to terminate something. Includes descriptions of disinterest (e.g., "She's bored"), dislike (e.g., "She doesn't like pickles"), refusal ("She doesn't want to get the doll"), frustration ("She's frustrated because she can't reach the cup"), confusion ("She's not sure what's expected of her"), or protest ("She hates to play that game").
3. Comment/response: Any reference to a child's attempt to direct the interactant's attention to some observable referent, or any reference to a child's attempt to respond in some way to a communication that was directed toward him or her. Includes descriptions of acknowledgment (e.g., "She's letting her mom know that she heard her"), answering ("She's trying to answer the question"), naming (e.g., "She's trying to say her brother's name"), providing information ("She's communicating about her new game"), describing (e.g., "She's trying to tell her mother about the picture"), or complying (e.g., "She understood what I asked her to do").
4. Transferring: Any reference to a child giving or receiving an object. Includes descriptions such as "She wants to give her mother the doll" or "She's getting the book from her mother."
5. Greeting: Any reference to a child's noticing another person or family pet in the process of entering or departing from the setting. Includes descriptions such as "She's saying hi to her sister" or "She's watching the cat leave."
6. Imitation: Any reference to a child's attempt to imitate an action or vocalization.
7. Positive interactive expression: Any reference to a child's attempt to express a positive emotional state: Includes descriptions of pleasure (e.g., "She's happy"); excitement (e.g., "She's excited about her new book"); interest or curiosity ("She wonders how the toy works"); anticipation (e.g., "She knows that she's going to get the new toy") or affection ("She loves her dolly").
8. Nonmeaning: No real attempt to interpret meaning of the child behavior, instead the adult focused on further description of the child behavior (e.g., "He was distracted by the noise," "She was responding to her image in the mirror," "He was interacting with mom," "She shifted her attention to mom").
9. Cannot assign: The reported meaning description does not fit in any of the preceding categories, or the partner indicates that he/she didn't know what the meaning might have been.

SOURCE: Wilcox JM: Enhancing Initial Communication Skills in Young Children with Developmental Disabilities through Partner Programming. *Seminars in Speech and Language* 1992; 13:202.

TABLE 5.23. Coping strategies in response to the question "How do people cope?"

PSYCHOLOGICALLY
    Embrace a cause
    Get a new interest, craft, hobby
    Count blessings or accentuate the positive
    List assets
    Proceed one day at a time
    Reduce negative thoughts
    Cultivate and maintain humor
    List strengths of family members
    Realize you are not alone
    Dress up
    Trivialize the trivial
    Treasure little gains
    Keep a journal
    Notice elemental things (sunrise, trees, coffee flavors)
    Plot improvements

PHYSICALLY
    Continue normal routines
    Listen to music, explore new music
    Play the accordion
    Dance
    Exercise
    Fish
    Clean house, tidy-up, and organize
    Cry
    Laugh
    Rest
    Eat cleverly
    Walk the dog
    Take a hike
    Soak in the jacuzzi
    Get a massage
    Play pool
    Plant a garden. Watch it grow.

SPIRITUALLY
    Talk to theologian (priest, minister, rabbi, guru)
    Read spiritual passages
    Read inspirational stories
    Meditate
    Pray
    Spend time at peaceful places (woods, desert, rivers, seashore, mountains)
    Visit house of worship
    Lunch with a monk

(continued)

TABLE 5.23. (*continued*)

SOCIALLY
Interact with old or new friends
Do things with family
Join support groups
Get involved in community activities
Help others
Take a course
Tell a joke
Rent a goofy movie
Go shopping
Play with kids
Visit new places
Get a pet

COGNITIVELY
Read a good book
Read about the disorder or condition
Join local, state, or national organizations or foundations
Talk to other families with similar problems
Attend a workshop
Listen to an audiotape or view video tapes
Ask questions
Surf the Internet
Seek information from many sources

SOURCE: LaPointe LL: Adaptation, Accommodation, Aristos. In LaPointe LL (ed): *Aphasia and Related Neurogenic Language Disorders,* pp. 284–285. Thieme, New York, 1997.

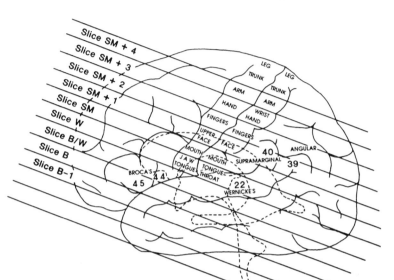

Figure 5.1. Computed tomography (CT) scan: lateral diagram of the location of cortical language areas in relationship to the ventricular system (dotted lines).

Source: Naeser MA, Palumbo CL, Baker EH, Nicholas ML: CT Scan Lesion Site Analysis in Severe Aphasia: Relationship to No Recovery of Speech and Treatment with the Nonverbal Computer-Assisted Visual Communication Program (C-ViC). *Seminars in Speech and Language* 1994; 15:54.

TABLE 5.24. **Dementia: behavior management for decreasing negative thinking—possible guidelines and steps for implementation.**

Steps for implementation

DEFINE AND ANALYZE PROBLEM

Select a specific behavioral outcome, using baseline assessment data to define realistic improvements. Include expected frequency of negative talking and frequency of positive talking (i.e., complaints to be decreased to less than 1 per hour; positive statements increased to at least 2 per hour).

SPECIFY INTERVENTION

With verbalization problems some form of differential attention and reinforcement are most commonly used. Delineate exactly which behaviors are to be ignored and which are to be attended or reinforced. Define and illustrate these behaviors. Specify when the procedure is to be used, by whom, and under what conditions.

TRAIN CAREGIVERS

Introduce caregiver to procedures first through oral and written instructions. Demonstrate how the procedure is used through modeling, illustrating both praise and ignoring. Give family members an opportunity to rehearse the procedures, first acting as the client while the practitioner models and then acting as themselves while the practitioner acts as client. Caregivers then practice the procedure with the client while the practitioner monitors, giving cues or feedback as needed.

EXPLAIN PROCEDURES TO PATIENT AND OBTAIN CONSENT

Inform the patient of the procedure and give him or her opportunities to ask questions and to agree to participate. If the patient objects to the procedure, introduce necessary changes to accommodate the objections.

SET CRITERIA FOR IGNORING AND PRAISING

Specify detail criteria for the use of the intervention; this includes the details of which behavior will be reinforced and which will be systematically ignored.

RECORD

The caregiver records positive and negative behaviors and the praise, ignoring, or reinforcers that follow them.

MONITOR

At least once a week review data and provide verbal praise for using the procedures. Offer additional training as needed.

SOURCE: Pinkston EM: Behavior Management Training for Caregivers of Patients With Dementia. *Seminars in Speech and Language* 1994; 15:287.

TABLE 5.25. **Dementia: behavior management for increasing social behavior—possible guidelines and steps for implementation.**

Steps for implementation

DEFINE AND ANALYZE PROBLEM
Select a specific behavioral outcome, using an analysis of current social behavior to determine the frequency of the desired behavior. Check the behavior with the family and patient to verify its social and clinical relevance. Define the desired outcome in a clear and specific way.

EVALUATE RESOURCES
The primary resource will be the caregiver's desired social contacts and his/her motivation, time, and health to implement the program. Help from relatives or social service agencies to assist in developing response opportunities for the patient.

SELECT TIME, PLACE, AND COMPONENTS OF THE SOCIAL CONTRACT
Choose a time and place that fits into the caregiver's routine and develop a specific set of social behaviors that will solve the problem. Decide what environmental events need to occur in order for the patient to engage in those behaviors. Are special equipment, transportation, cues, etc. needed?

CONTRACT FOR ACTIVITIES
Present one or more possible target activities to the patient, along with discussion and explanation of the time, place, and resources available and the behavioral components. Ask the patient if he or she is willing to participate. Enlist involved relatives in providing resources, participation, and reinforcing patient's agreement to participate.

SPECIFY CONTRACT IN WRITING
Once agreed upon, formalize the contract in verbal and written form. Use either a task assignment contract or an individualized contract to state the specific activity agreed upon, who will do what to achieve it, and when this will occur. Give a copy to each participant.

REHEARSE
Have the family practice the required steps to achieve the social contacts.

PROMPT
Incorporate a variety of possible reminders or prompts including (a) calendar notes/appointment books, (b) reminder telephone calls from practitioner or family members, (c) verbal prompts from those with the patient.

REINFORCE
Teach caregiver(s) to notice, call attention to, and praise social contracts when these occur and to avoid complaining about the patient's not engaging in desired social interaction.

RECORD
Have caregivers note social contacts on recording forms.

MONITOR AND RECORD
Review the data at least once a week and provide verbal praise for task adherence. *Note:* Generally the patient is quite impaired and cannot reinforce caregivers adequately for their efforts and the practitioner should compensate for that to some degree by praise for the caregiver's efforts and specific praise for carrying out prompting and reinforcing tasks.

(continued)

TABLE 5.25. (*continued*)

Steps for implementation

REVIEW

If adherence to the program's task does not occur, there are several possible reasons: (1) you may not have selected a problem that is still important to the caregiver and/or patient; (2) they may not understand how the tasks you asked them to carry out relate to their problem; (3) instructions were not clear; (4) the intervention is more trouble than the problem is worth; or (5) they consider the problem solved or feel satisfied that they can solve it when they want to. Review these items and others that emerge from the conversation.

REVISE

Using the information from the review, revise the program. This may include a small adjustment or it may involve starting at the beginning of this outline and proceeding with new problems.

SOURCE: Pinkston EM: Behavior Management Training for Caregivers of Patients with Dementia. *Seminars in Speech and Language* 1994; 15:286.

TABLE 5.26. **Dementia: specific recommendations for caregivers.**

1. Approach slowly: Dementing patients may get apprehensive or agitated with sudden occurrences. Try to be visible while approaching.
2. Establish eye contact: This enhances readiness to listen and will be helpful in comprehension through reception of visual cues.
3. Be pleasant, monitor, and maximize your coverbal behaviors, such as use of smile, gesture, and posture. Dementing individuals, like most people, respond better to pleasant people.
4. Speak clearly and directly; avoid complex directions.
5. Use referents frequently and avoid pronouns.
6. Speak in short sentences to aid in comprehension and memory.
7. Ask yes/no questions rather than open-ended questions.
8. Be redundant: restate critical facts to compensate for memory loss.
9. Keep topics familiar and observable.
10. Use touch.
11. Maintain structure or routine.
12. Always say goodbye or some other form of departure signal.

SOURCE: Shekim LO: Dementia. In LaPointe LL (ed): *Aphasia and Related Neurogenic Language Disorders*, pp. 246–247. Thieme, New York, 1997.

TABLE 5.27. **Dysgraphia: specific hierarchy of tasks for treatment.**

Task		Input	Output	Stimuli
Copy geometric forms and letters		Visual	Graphic	X, >, T,], V, L, O, H, Z, #.
Copy words		Visual	Graphic	tie, car, bed, pills, comb, money, pants, chair, shoes, glasses
Write single letters to dictation	(List 1)	Auditory	Graphic	i, n, w, h, d, b, u, g, p, m.
	(List 2)			o, y, f, e, s, c, l, r, a, t.
Write words, letter by letter	(List 1)	Auditory	Graphic	top, cat, bad, yes, sit, was, fat, run, pan, fan.
	List 2)			ham, hot, wet, his, dog, bet, bus, let, tin, mop.
Write words to dictation		Auditory	Graphic	Same lists as above.
Write two-letter words and nonwords to dictation	(Words)	Auditory	Graphic	I'm, no, we, hi, do, be, up, go, in, my.
	(Nonwords)			ba, tu, ca, ye, sa, wa, bu, hu, fa, ru.
Write three-letter words to dictation	(Set 1)	Auditory	Graphic	not, wet, his, dog, bet, got, hit, bed, him, nod.
	(Set 2)	Auditory	Graphic	bad, top, cat, yes, sat, was, bus, he's, fat, run.

SOURCE: Tseng CH, McNeil MR: Nature and Management of Acquired Neurogenic Dysgraphias. In LaPointe LL (ed): *Aphasia and Related Neurogenic Language Disorders,* p. 195. Thieme, New York, 1997.

TABLE 5.28. **Dyslexia: principles of treatment.**

---

1. Accurate comprehension of what is read is the primary goal, not accurate oral reading.
2. In selecting or designing the vocabulary or content, the properties or features of words that are known to have an effect on recognition and comprehension should be considered. These features are length, part of speech, frequency of occurrence, concreteness, imageability, and familiarity. Gernsbacher has shown that experiential familiarity has a strong effect on recognition.
3. The individual's interests and functional needs should be of high priority in selecting training material rather than what is readily available in the clinical setting.
4. Reading should be physically facilitated by making certain the print size is large enough, the material is placed in the visual field correctly, and there are no distractions.
5. Difficulty level for contextual reading can be advanced in two major ways: (1) increasing length and (2) increasing vocabulary as well as syntactical complexity. The clinician should consider controlling one or the other as much as possible to be able to analyze reading comprehension failures.
6. If phonemic decoding is chosen as a useful objective, consonants rather than vowels should be targeted.
7. Reading comprehension should be a generative process for understanding. There should be a cognitive interaction with the material. The clinician must facilitate this by the design of the treatment tasks and the selection of stimuli.

SOURCE: Webb WG: Acquired Dyslexias. In LaPointe LL (ed): *Aphasia and Related Neurogenic Language Disorders*, p. 161. Thieme, New York, 1997.

TABLE 5.29. **Dyslexia: suggested comprehension strategies for reading contextual material.**

PREREADING COMPREHENSION STRATEGIES
Overviews
Structural organizers
Setting up a purpose for reading
Client-centered study strategies
Clinician-directed lesson frameworks

DURING READING COMPREHENSION STRATEGIES

Question-answering	Outlining
Inserted questions	Paraphrasing
Immediate oral feedback	Summarizing
Time lines and charts	Study guides
Listing main ideas	Self-monitoring

POSTREADING COMPREHENSION STRATEGIES
Follow-up pre- and during activities
Talk about what has been read
Write about what has been read
Take a test or make up a test on what was read

FIX-UP STRATEGIES (DURING OR AFTER)
Ignore small problems—move on!
Change rate of reading
Suspend judgment
Hypothesize
Reread
Go to another source

SOURCE: Webb WG: Acquired Dyslexias. In LaPointe LL (ed): *Aphasia and Related Neurogenic Language Disorders*, p. 166. Thieme, New York, 1997.

TABLE 5.30. **Family characteristics of healthy and vulnerable families.**

Healthy Families	Vulnerable Families
Open system	Closed system
Permeable boundary	Tight boundary
Many social institution connections religious, school, community)	Few social relationships Weak social supports
Well-defined structure	Restricted access to resources
Strong social supports	Unreceptive to change
Access to resources	Poor communication
Receptive to change	
Good intrafamily communication	

SOURCE: LaPointe LL: Adaptation, Accommodation, Aristos. In LaPointe LL (ed): *Aphasia and Related Neurogenic Language Disorders,* p. 280. Thieme, New York, 1997.

TABLE 5.31. **Functional communication: environmental needs assessment form.**

Client: _____ Date: _____

Source(s) of Information: _____

	LIVING/FAMILY ENVIRONMENT	
	Current	*Projected*

TYPE OF SETTING
  Nursing Home
  Rehab facility (acute or transitional)
  Group home
  Supported living
  Independent living

ACTIVITIES APPLICABLE TO INDIVIDUAL
  Self-care
  Medication/medical condition mgmt
  Meal planning/preparation
  Budgeting, banking, bill payment
  Light or routine housework
  Heavy housework
  Laundry & clothing care
  Home repairs
  Use of telephone
  Time management, scheduling
  Home safety/emergencies
  Yard work
  Child care/parenting
  Correspondence/greeting cards
  Moving arrangements
  Reading magazines/newspaper
  Watching TV/videos
  Card or board games
  Other _____

SOCIAL ROLES EXPECTED OF INDIVIDUAL
  Roommate
  Spouse
  Parent
  Neighbor
  Other _____

	INDIVIDUALS WITH REGULAR CONTACT IN LIVING/FAMILY ENVIRONMENT		
	Name	*Age*	*Relationship*
Current			
Projected			

(continued)

TABLE 5.31. (*continued*)

GENERAL COMMUNITY ENVIRONMENT		
	Current	*Projected*

APPLICABLE ACTIVITIES/SETTINGS
   Community orientation/use of map
   Mobility as a pedestrian
   Use of taxi   Use of public transportation
   Grocery shopping
   Shopping-clothes & personal items
   Pharmacy
   Mall
   Banking
   Post Office
   Restaurants—Fast food
   Restaurants—Sit-down
   Social service agencies
   Church
   Public telephones
   Dry cleaners
   Laundromat
   Lawyer's office
   Insurance companies
   Travel arrangements
   Major transportation terminals
   Support groups/social organizations
   Movie theaters
   Visiting friends in homes

ROLES EXPECTED OF INDIVIDUAL
   Consumer/customer
   Acquaintance
   Stranger
   Citizen
   Friend
   Other _____

INDIVIDUALS WITH WHOM REGULAR CONTACT IS MADE		
Name	*Location*	*Relationship*

SOURCE: Hartley LL: Assessment of Functional Communication. *Seminars in Speech and Language* 1992; 13:278–279.

Codes for Rating Level of Independence in Activities:

NA = Not applicable	V = Can do but needs verbal cues
I = Totally Independent	P = Needs minimal physical assist
S = Needs occasional supervision	D = Totally dependent

TABLE 5.32. Functional communication: informal assessment and behavioral observation form.

Client: _____ Date: _____

	Within normal limits	Not able to judge	Problem area	Comments
ORIENTATION/RECALL				
Person, place, time				
Biographical information				
ATTENTION				
Arousal				
Attention Span				
Distractibility				
Disinhibition				
Perseveration				
Fatigability/endurance				
EXECUTIVE RUNCTIONING				
Awareness of deficits/errors				
Ability to identify goals				
Spontaneous use of strategies				
Ability to accept/use feedback				
Self-correction of errors				
Flexibility in shifting tasks				
Level of effort/cooperation				
RATE OF PROCESSING/RESPONDING				
Motor slowing				
Impulsivity				
Slow rate of processing				
Consistency of responses				
EMOTIONAL CONTROL/AFFECT				
Anxiety				
Emotional lability				
Immaturity/silliness				
Anger				
Frustration tolerance				
Limited range of emotions				

SOURCE: Hartley LL: Assessment of Functional Communication. *Seminars in Speech and Language* 1992; 13:277.

TABLE 5.33. **Global aphasia: communicative writing sequence.**

1. Tracing of single words with necessary assistance.
2. Copying of single words.
3. Prolonged exposure (as long as the patient needs it) of the target word, with several repetitions of the auditory analogue.
4. Brief presentation of auditory and lexical stimulus, with written response.
5. Brief presentation of auditory and lexical stimulus, with imposed delay (5 to 15 seconds), then a written response.
6. Writing to dictation, with a return to previous levels at any point if necessary.
7. Writing to pictured presentation.
8. Writing in response to question, for example, "What would you write if you were thirsty?" or "Write this person's name."

SOURCE: Collins MJ: Global Aphasia. In LaPointe LL (ed): *Aphasia and Related Neurogenic Language Disorders,* p. 145. Thieme, New York, 1997.

TABLE 5.34. **Global aphasia: establishing goals.**

Realistic goals should begin with a needs assessment. All patients need to communicate, but some patients feel the need more than others, and others are less dependent on speech. Part of our understanding what those needs are will come from our data, but we need to rely on our family interview and our covert assessment of the patient as well. Goals will vary, but some realistic goals might include the following:

1. Improving auditory comprehension, supplemented with contextual cues, to permit consistent comprehension of one-step commands in well-controlled situations.
2. Improving production of yes and no to consistent, unequivocal responses in controlled situations.
3. Improving ability to spontaneously produce several written responses, or approximations, of functional or salient words of daily living.
4. Improving production of several simple, unequivocal gestures.
5. Improving drawing so that several simple, unequivocal messages can be conveyed in this modality.
6. Ensuring that a small, basic core of communicative intentions can be conveyed in one or a combination of modalities.

It is realistic to expect that these goals can be attained. They should be minimal goals for all globally aphasic patients. Expanding this repertoire will depend on a number of factors, including availability of the patient, cooperation and motivation, and general health. Enhancing and improving upon them may not always be possible. If new goals beckon, because a person has demonstrated his capacity to reach them, they should be welcomed.

SOURCE: Collins MJ: Global Aphasia. In Lapointe LL (ed): *Aphasia and Related Neurogenic Language Disorders,* p. 141. Thieme, New York, 1997.

TABLE 5.35. **Global aphasia: strengthening the gestural response.**

1. Clinician gestures and says the word simultaneously.
2. Clinician says word, clinician and client gesture simultaneously (clinician assistance with gesture may be required).
3. Client imitates gesture.
4. Client imitates gesture after enforced delay.
5. Client gestures in response to auditory stimulus.
6. Client gestures in response to auditory stimulus after enforced delay.
7. Client gestures in response to written stimulus.
8. Client gestures in response to written stimulus after enforced delay.
9. Client writes word in response to gestural and auditory stimulus.
10. Client gestures in response to appropriate stimuli.

SOURCE: Collins MJ: Global Aphasia. In Lapointe LL (ed): *Aphasia and Related Neurogenic Language Disorders*, p. 144. Thieme, New York, 1997.

TABLE 5.36. **Internal Classification of Impairments, Disabilities, and Handicaps (World Health Organization, 1986).**

Term	Definition	Characteristics
Impairment	In the context of health experience, an impairment is any loss or abnormality of psychological, physiological, or anatomic structure or function.	Impairment is characterized by losses or abnormalities that may be temporary or permanent, and that include the existence or occurrence of an anomaly, defect, or loss in limb, organ, tissue, or other structure of the body, including the systems of mental function. Impairment represents exteriorization of a pathologic state and, in principal, it reflects disturbances at the level of the organ.
Disability	In the context of health experience, a disability is any restriction or lack (resulting from an impairment) of ability to perform an activity in the manner or within the range considered normal for a human being.	Disability is concerned with abilities, in the form of composite activities and behaviors, that are generally accepted as essential components of everyday life. Examples include disturbances in behaving in an appropriate manner, in personal care (such as excretory control and the ability to wash and feed oneself), in the performance of other activities of daily living, and in locomotor activities (such as the ability to walk.)
Handicap	In the context of health experience, a handicap is a disadvantage for a given individual, resulting from an impairment or a disability, that limits or prevents the fulfillment of a role that is normal (depending on age, sex, and social and cultural factors) for that individual.	Handicap is concerned with the value attached to an individual's situation or experience when it departs from the norm. It is characterized by a discordance between the individual's performance or status and the expectations of the individual himself or the particular group of which he is a member. Handicap thus represents socialization of an impairment or disability and as such, it reflects the consequences for the individual—cultural, social, economic, and environmental—that stem from the presence of impairment and disability. Disadvantage arises from the failure or inability to conform to the expectations or norms of the individual's universe. Handicap thus occurs when there is interference with the ability to sustain what might be designated as "survival roles."

SOURCE: Ramberger G: Functional Perspective for Assessment and Rehabilitation of Persons with Severe Aphasia. *Seminars in Speech and Language* 1994; 15:3.

TABLE 5.37. Neurogenic disorders: examples of "pure" clinical characteristics.

	Motor Weakness	Abnormal Reflexes	Vegetative Deficits	Single Movements	Movement Sequences	Motoric Effort	Diadochokinesis	Sound Repertoires	Expressive Language	Receptive Language
Planning apraxia	No	No	No	Intact	Poor	None	Variable	Variable	Variable	Variable
Executive apraxia	No	No	Sometimes	Poor	Poor	Yes	Slow	Limited	Limited	None
Dysarthria	Yes	Yes	Yes	Variable	Variable	Yes	Slow	Related to weakness	Variable	None
Language deficits	No	No	No	Intact	Poor	No	Sequencing problems	Extensive	Deficit	Deficit

TABLE 5.38a. **Pharmacology considerations: drugs known to produce dysarthria, dysphonia, or dyskinesis.***

Class	Generic Name
Antiarrhythmics	Mexiletine
Anticonvulsants	Phynetoin
	Carbamazepine
Antipsychotics	Fluphenazine
	Haloperidol
	Thioridazine
	Chlorpromazine
Antidepressants	Amitriptyline
	Desipramine
	Imipramine
	Lithium salts
Antispasmotics	Baclofen
	Dantrolene
	Botulinium Toxin
Anxiolytics	Alprazolam
	Lorazepam
	Diazepam
Antiviral	Zidovudine (AZT)

*Symptoms may also be produced by a hypersensitivity reaction to any drug.

TABLE 5.38b. **Drugs known to produce dry mouth.**

Class	Generic
Analgesic	Nalbuphine
Antiarrhythmic	Disopyramide
	Nadolol
Antimuscarinic	Atropine
	Scapolamine
	Methscapolamine
	Homatropine
	Ipratroponin
	Cyclopentolate
	Tropicamide
	Propantheline
Anticonvulsant	Carbamazepine
Antidepressant	Amitriptyline
	Desipramine
	Doxepin
	Imipramine
	Maprotiline
	Nortriptyline
	Trimipramine
Antipsychotic	Fluphenazine
	Haloperidol
	Thioridazine
	Chlorpromazine
Antihypertensive	Clonidine
	Methyl Dopa
	Prazosin
Antiparkinson	Amantadine
	Benztropine
	Biperiden
	Bromocriptine
	Levodopa
Anxiolytics	Alprazolam
	Lorazepam
	Diazepam
Appetite suppressant	Diethylpropion
	Mazindol
Bronchodilator	Ephedrine
	Ipratropium
Diuretic	Amiloride
	Triamterene
Other	Allopurinol
	Busulphan
	Dextroamphetamine
	Etretinate
	Isotretinoin
	Ketotifen
	Penicillamine

TABLE 5.38c. Drugs known to alter normal sensation of taste.

Class	Generic Name
Antiarrhythmic	Amiodarone
	Procainamide
Antibiotic	Ceftazidime
	Lincomycin
	Amitriptyline
	Doxepin
Antidepressant	Amitryptyline
	Desipramine
	Doxepin
	mipramine
	Maprotiline
	Nortriptyline
	Trimipramine
Calcium channel blockers	Captopril
	Enalapril
Antileprotic	Ethionamide
Antiprotzoal	Metronidazole
Other	Calcitonin
	Allopurinol
	Aspirin
	Cisplatin
	Clofibrate
	Disulfram
	Ethambutol
	Griseofulvin
	Gold salts
	Levodopa
	Lithium salts
	Penicillamine
	Propantheline

TABLE 5.39. **Pragmatic behavior categories.**

NONVERBAL ASPECTS OF COMMUNICATION
Paralinguistics
Kinesics
Proxemics

INTERACTIONAL ASPECTS OF COMMUNICATION
Turn taking
Conversational repair
Speech acts or social skills

PROPOSITIONAL ASPECTS OF COMMUNICATION
Topic Management
Introduction
Maintenance
Changing
Presupposition
Cohesion
Macrostructure/Discourse grammar

SOURCE: Hartley LL: Assessment of Functional Communication. *Seminars in Speech and Language* 1992; 13:266.

TABLE 5.40. **Pragmatic skills.**

1. Linguistic conversational skills
   A. Speech act use (e.g., comment, request, warn, assert, promise, direct, acknowledge)
   B. Topic skills (e.g., initiation, maintenance, shift, shading)
   C. Turn-taking skills (e.g., initiation, response, interruption/overlap, pause time)
   D. Conversational repair skills (e.g., contingent responses, lexical selection, quantity and conciseness of information, requests for and responses to clarification)
   E. Presuppositional skills (e.g., appropriate use of pronouns, ellipsis, change in register)
2. Nonlinguistic conversational skills
   A. Paralinguistic aspects of communication (e.g., pitch and intensity, fluency, intelligibility)
   B. Extralinguistic aspects of communication (e.g., eye gaze, proximity to conversational partner)

SOURCE: Newhoff M, Apel K: Impairments in Pragmatics. In LaPointe LL (ed): *Aphasia and Related Neurogenic Language Disorders,* p. 252. Thieme, New York, 1997.

TABLE 5.41. **Right-hemisphere deficits:**
                       evaluation procedures for assessing.

INITIAL CONTACT
  Taped interview
  Picture description
  Oral reading: sentences, paragraph

ASSESSMENT OF NONLINGUISTIC DEFICITS
  Tests of Neglect:
    Line bisection
    Cancellation tasks
    Drawing: spontaneous, copy
    Anosognosia testing
    Oral reading: words, sentences, paragraphs
    Writing: spontaneous, copy
  Tests of attention:
    Vigilance tests
    Selective attention tests
    Dual task tests

ASSESSMENT OF EXTRALINGUISTIC DEFICITS
  Story and scene interpretation
  Discourse production and comprehension
  Generating alternative meanings
  Prosodic comprehension and production

SOURCE: Myers PS: Right Hemisphere Syndrome. In
LaPointe LL (ed): *Aphasia and Related Neurogenic Language Disorders,* p. 211. Thieme, New York, 1997.

TABLE 5.42. **Right-hemisphere deficits: extralinguistic disorders associated with RHD.**

MACROSTRUCTURE IMPAIRMENTS
  Reduced number of core concepts
  Reduced accuracy of core concepts
  Reduced number of accurate inferences
  Reduced specificity (increased listener burden)
  Reduced efficiency

IMPAIRED GENERATION OF ALTERNATE MEANINGS
  Reduced recognition of figurative and metaphoric meanings
  Reduced ability to interpret humor, irony, sarcasm
  Reduced capacity to revise original interpretations

REDUCED SENSITIVITY TO COMMUNICATIVE EVENTS
  Reduced awareness of purpose of communicative exchange
  Reduced appreciation of shared knowledge
  Reduced sensitivity to emotional tone
  Reduced eye contact
  Reduced reflection (impulsivity; shallow responses)

IMPAIRED PROSODY
  Reduced sensitivity to emotional prosody (comprehension)
  Reduced use of prosodic features (production)

SOURCE: Myers PS: Right Hemisphere Syndrome. In LaPointe LL (ed): *Aphasia and Related Neurogenic Language Disorders*, p. 203. Thieme, New York, 1997.

TABLE 5.43. **Severe aphasia: guidelines for communicating with the severely aphasic person.**

---

1. Simplify
2. Clue the person in
3. Allow time
4. Guess
5. Confirm
6. Be clear
7. Reduce extraneous variables
8. Respect

SOURCE: Collins MJ: Global Aphasia. In LaPointe LL (ed): *Aphasia and Related Neurogenic Language Disorders*, p. 141. Thieme, New York, 1997.

7 Complete Independence (Timely, Safely) 6 Modified Independence (Device)	NO HELPER

Modified Dependence
  5 Supervision
  4 Minimal Assist (Subject = 75%+)
  3 Moderate Assist (Subject = 50%+)
Complete Dependence
  2 Maximal Assist (Subject = 25%+)
  1 Total Assist (Subject = 0%+)
	HELPER

L E V E L S

	ADMIT	DISCHG	FOL-UP
Self Care A. Eating B. Grooming C. Bathing D. Dressing-Upper Body E. Dressing-Lower Body F. Toileting			
Sphincter Control G. Bladder Management H. Bowel Management			
Mobility Transfer: I. Bed, Chair, Wheelchair J. Toilet K. Tub, Shower			
Locomotion L. Walk/wheel Chair M. Stairs	w/c	w/c	w/c
Communication N. Comprehension O. Expression	a/v v/n	a/v v/n	a/v v/n
Social Cognition P. Social Interaction Q. Problem Solving R. Memory			
Total FIM			

NOTE: Leave no blanks; enter 1 if patient not testable due to risk.

FIGURE 5.2. Severe aphasia: functional independence measure checklist.

SOURCE: Ramberger G: Functional Perspective for Assessment and Rehabilitation of Persons with Severe Aphasia. *Seminars in Speech and Language* 1994; 15:9.

TABLE 5.44. Speech sound error analysis trend comparisons for nonfluent aphasia and apraxia of speech with conduction and fluent aphasia.

Nonfluent/Apraxia	Conduction/Fluent	Reference
Transitionalization or timing errors		Kent and Rosenbek[1]; Canter, Trost, and Burns[2]; Odell et al.[3]
Voice onset time impaired	Voice onset time not impaired	Gandour and Dardaranada[4]
Devoicing of voiced sounds		Nespoulous et al.[5]
Abnormal syllabic stress		Odell et al.[3]
Prevalence of substitutions	Prevalence of substitutions	Monoi et al[6]; Canter et al.[2]; Ardila[7]
Substitutions tend to differ from target by single feature	Substitutions tend to differ by more than one feature	Monoi et al.[6]; Nespoulous et al.[8,5]
Intrusive vowels, prolongations, and artic. hiatuses	Transposition errors, Sequencing errors, Additions	Monoi et al.[6]; Canter et al.[2]; Kent and Rosenbek[1]
	More serial ordering errors	Nespoulous et al.[5]
Primarily consonant errors	Vowel and consonant errors	Monoi et al.[6]
Word initial errors	Initial and noninitial errors	Odell et al.[3]
Errors on word initiation	Errors toward end of word	Canter et al.[2]]
	Disproportionate errors on low probability sentences	Ardila and Rosselli[9]

SOURCE: Simmons-Mackie N: Conduction Aphasia. In LaPointe LL (ed): *Aphasia and Related Neurogenic Language Disorders,* p. 68. Thieme, New York, 1997.

[1]Kent R, Rosenbek J: Acoustic patterns of apraxia of speech. *Journal of Speech and Hearing Research* 1983; 26:231–249.

[2]Canter G, Trost J, Burns M: Contrasting speech patterns in apraxias of speech and phonemic paraphasia. *Brain and Language* 1985; 24:204–222.

[3]Odell K, McNeill M, Rosenbek J, Hunter L: A perceptual comparison of prosodic features in apraxia of speech and conduction aphasia. In Prescott T (ed): *Clinical Aphasiology,* Vol. 19. Austin, TX: PRO-ED, 1991, pp. 295–306.

[4]Gandour J, Dardaranada R: Voice onset time in aphasia: Thai II. Production. *Brain and Language* 1984; 23:177–205.

[5]Nespoulous J, Joanette Y, Ska B, Caplan D, Lecours A: Production deficits in Broca's and conduction aphasia: Repetition versus reading. In Keller E, Gopnik M (eds): *Motor and Sensory Processes of Language.* Hillsdale, NJ: Erlbaum, 1987, pp. 53–81.

[6]Monoi H, Fukusako Y, Itoh M, et al.: Speech sound errors in patients with conduction and Broca's aphasia. *Brain and Language* 1983; 20:175–194.

[7]Ardila A: Phonological transformations in conduction aphasia. *Journal of Psycholinguistic Research* 1992; 21:472–484.

[8]Nespoulous J, Joanette Y, Beland R, et al.: Phonological disturbances in aphasia: Is there a "markedness" effect in aphasic phonemic errors? In Rose F (ed): *Progress in Aphasiology: Advances in Neurology,* Vol. 42. New York: Raven Press, 1984.

[9]Ardila A, Rosslli M: Repetition in aphasia. *Journal of Neurolinguistics* 1992; 7:1–11.

TABLE 5.45. **Traumatic brain injury: anticipated difficulties of the pediatric TBI patient.**

RETURNING HOME
1. Behavioral problems; emotional outbursts, anger, frustration.
2. Inability to follow daily schedule or the rules of the house.
3. Demonstrating a lack of respect for family members.
4. Difficulty in following family activities.
5. Problems completing assigned tasks or chores.
6. Problems understanding written messages or instructions.
7. Difficulties conversing with family and friends.

RETURNING TO SCHOOL
1. Behavioral problems; emotional outbursts, anger, frustration.
2. Inability to follow daily schedule or the rules of the classroom.
3. Demonstrating a lack of respect for authority figures.
4. Difficulty using the appropriate level of language skills.
5. Problems completing assigned tasks.
6. Problems understanding vocabulary and concepts associated with a given subject.
7. Difficulties answering questions.
8. Difficulties asking questions.
9. Problems with following instructions.
10. Inappropriate social interactions.

INTERACTING WITH FRIENDS
1. Behavioral problems; emotional outbursts, anger, frustration.
2. Inability to use or understand slang expressions, puns, jokes or other language forms.
3. Difficulty forming questions.
4. Monopolizing conversations.
5. Problems moving from one social context to the next.
6. Inability to follow rules of a game or social activity.
7. Taking long times to respond and not knowing how close to stand to listeners during conversations.

TABLE 5.46. **Traumatic brain injury: considerations for patients different from other patients.**

Traumatic brain injury is a devastating problem to the individual and their family, since it is acquired after a period of normal development and social interaction. When planning for the reintegration of these individuals, one must remember these individuals:

- Have a successful history of academic, social, and communication outcomes.
- Display discrepancies in the performance ranging from low to high performance.
- Believe they are normal.
- Are variable in performance and will demonstrate unpredictable highs and lows in performance.
- Have difficulties regulating their emotions
- Experience difficulty integrating, structuring and generalizing old and new information.
- Demonstrate patterns of performance that are unique to the brain injury and not similar to other disabilities.
- Have difficulty learning new information and necessitating compensatory and adaptive strategies.
- Experience difficulty with low-level tasks while being able to accomplish related higher level tasks.

TABLE 5.47. Traumatic brain injury: developmental history of communication training within a rehabilitation facility.

STAGE 1: THE 45-MIN INSERVICE FOR DIRECT CARE STAFF

Target group: Nurses (or other direct care staff) and therapists

Content: Nature of cognitive, communicative, and behavioral impairments after TBI

Do's and don'ts of communication

Teaching procedures: Lecture (verbal presentation of information) with role played or videotaped illustrations.

Supervisory follow-up: None

Problems:

1. With the goal of *communicative competence* (vs. acquisition of knowledge), a lecture is a poorly conceived training tool
2. 45 min is insufficient to cover the territory
3. Often the people most in need of help are not present at the inservice
4. Supervisors lack the authority to insist that employees acquire and regularly use the desired competencies

STAGE 2: THE 2-HR INTERACTIVE INSERVICE FOR ALL STAFF

Target group: All staff, not just direct care staff. This includes housekeeping staff, maintenance staff, administrative staff, and others not normally thought to be on the clinical team, but who interact with patients in the facility

Content: The nature of cognitive, communicative, and behavioral impairments is covered, but the main focus is brainstorming about practicing positive ways of communicating

Teaching procedures: Minimal presentation of information; most of the 2 hrs is devoted to defining difficult communication situations and practicing (in dyads or triads) positive ways to negotiate those situations. These practice interactions are observed and coached by the trainer. The focus is acquisition of behavioral *competence,* not declarative knowledge

Supervisory follow-up: None

Problems:

1. The people most in need of help may still not be present
2. People who truly lack communicative competence with challenging partners need more than 2 hrs to become adequately competent
3. Supervisors still have no authority to enforce the competencies. They are not part of job descriptions.
4. Important everyday people like family members and friends are not yet included in the training

STAGE 3: INTERACTIVE TRAINING FOR STAFF AND FAMILY MEMBERS COMBINED WITH ADMINISTRATIVE SUPPORT

Target group: All staff and family members who are frequently present

Content: Same as Stage 2

Teaching procedures: Same as Stage 2

Supervisory follow-up: Communicative competencies are now included as part of all staff members' job descriptions.

Therefore, communicative skill becomes as much a part of the ongoing supervisory process as any other critical job skill

Problems: Individuals (staff or family members) who have the serious gaps in their communicative competencies require more than 2 hrs of inservice training to acquire the needed competencies

(continued)

TABLE 5.47. (*continued*)

STAGE 4: INTERDISCIPLINARY COMPETENCY-BASED TRAINING PLUS ONGOING SITUATIONAL COACHING
  Target group: Same as Stage 3
  Content: Same as Stage 3
  Teaching procedures: Inservice procedures are the same as Stage 3. However, now individualized coaching is offered to those few individuals who require intensive training
  Problems:
    1. This requires a substantial administrative commitment
    2. The coach (often a speech-language pathologist or a behavioral psychologist) must be talented, flexible, and highly respected. It is a difficult job.
    3. Some staff identified in need of help may feel threatened. However, most staff with potential to be positive contributors can come to see the training as a valuable opportunity for them

SOURCE: Ylvisaker M, Feeney TJ, Urbanczyk B: A Social-Environmental Approach to Communication and Behavior after Traumatic Brain Injury. *Seminars in Speech and Language* 1993; 14:83.

TABLE 5.48. Traumatic brain injury: discussion questions to aid the TBI child in coping with situations.

1. What four skills would you improve?
2. What are the three best things about you?
3. How do you act when you have trouble at school or at home?
4. What are the problems you have at school or at home?
5. What do you think other people could do to help you?
6. How are others trying to help you now?
7. What things at school or at home frustrate you?
8. How should others help you with these frustrating things?
9. What situations at home or school give you the most difficulty?

TABLE 5.49. **Traumatic brain injury: guidelines for speech-language pathologists to build collaborations for management.**

1. Identify key personnel involved in the management of the child and the child's integration into society.
2. Highlight the obstacles the child will face in re-entering his environment.
3. Provide accurate information regarding the child's current capabilities and anticipated problems of reentry.
4. Investigate the legal policies pertaining to the child and what resources are needed by the child.
5. Prepare workshop and materials designed to inform professional colleagues about the needs of the child, how transitions should be made, pitfalls associated with transitions, and the treatment goals.

TABLE 5.50. **Traumatic brain injury: impacts on learning.**

Impairments	*Observed behaviors*
Attention deficits	Limited understanding of tasks Inability to complete tasks Distractable
Denial	Limited recognition of change in abilities Resistance to new ideas Desire to return to old life
Inflexibility	Resistance Confusion Inability to cope with real or perceived stress
Memory problems	Uncertainty about new or old material
Poor organization and overload	Comprehension problems Reasoning problems Inability to problem solve Inability to complete tasks Confusion Quits long or complicated tasks Inability to cope without structure
Lack of independence or initiation	Inability to complete tasks in classroom Can't keep up with others Frustration Inactivity is not equal to inability
Orientation difficulties	Gets lost Unable to follow schedule Unable to connect people or events

TABLE 5.51. **Traumatic brain injury: long-term consequences.**

SOCIAL BEHAVIORS
- Loneliness
- Unrealistic plans
- Stubborn
- Impulsivity
- Outbursts of anger
- Dependency
- Poor judgments
- Apathy of lethargy

- Restlessness
- Sexually inappropriate
- Perseveration
- Poor motivation
- Denial
- Depression
- Inability to seek help
- Disinhibition

PHYSICAL CONDITIONS
- Seizures
- Pain
- Bladder and bowel problems
- Strength and stamina reduced
- Visual neglect
- Visual field deficits

- Sensory deficits
- Balance problems
- Mobility
- Coordination hampered
- Motor apraxia
- Sequencing and speed problems

COMMUNICATION DEFICITS
- Expressive language
- Articulation
- Confabulation
- Reading and writing problems

- Receptive language
- Resonance
- Word finding problems
- Abstractions

COGNITIVE PROBLEMS
- Memory
- Concentration
- Unable to plan or meet goals

- Problem solving
- Self-assessment of capabilities
- Egocentric thinking

PATIENT MAY:
- Get lost in familiar settings
- Get distracted in noisy settings
- Not learn from other people or settings

- Be easily influenced by others
- Misperceive actions and events
- Be bossy and assertive
- Withdraw

TABLE 5.52. Traumatic brain injury: organization and memory intervention.

Organizational schema (means for attaining) goal	Tasks & goal	Activity	Reflection*
Perceptual similarity (e.g., color, shape, size, texture, rhyme)	"The shop asked us to organize these leftover pieces of sandpaper so they can be found easily. Let's find a good way to do this."	1. Label small boxes for different grains (extra fine, fine, medium, etc.). 2. Sort the pieces according to their "texture" and put them into the labeled boxes. 3. Call out the textures and time how quickly they can be found.	How did you sort? Why this way? Was it "good"? In what other situations might one sort by texture? What would have happened if you had sorted by size? How could this help you remember where your tools or other possessions are kept or at least help you always locate them?
Semantic similarity (e.g., superordinate category, opposites)	"We were given a job to set up the layout of a new department store. We have to make it easy for customers to find what they want."	Make a floor plan specifying the location of departments. Place labeled items into the departments, grouping them by similarity, in one area, but subgrouped within the area (e.g., Electronic Equipment—TV's, stereos, radios). Make displace arrangement to entice people to buy (e.g., comfortable chair, flowers, glass of wine, and stereo).	How did you arrange the store? Why did you use that arrangement? In what other situations would you group things this way? When would this arrangement be inconvenient? How could knowing this arrangement help your memory of a visit to a store? How did the display arrangement differ from the floor arrangement?
Function (use)	"We are moving furniture into a new house. We have to arrange the living room for watching TV and conversation."	Make a floor plan and arrange labeled blocks representing the furniture. Then arrange them for special occasions, such as a cocktail party, Tupperware party, etc.	How were the items arranged for each activity? Why did you have to change them? How is this different from a department store arrangement?

(continued)

TABLE 5.52. *(continued)*

Organizational schema (means for attaining goal)	Tasks & goal	Activity	Reflection*
Main idea and topic (discourse structure)	"We will present today's news to the orientation group." (Watch a videotaped news item or listen to an audiotaped news item.)	Listen to the tape. Fill in a form answering Who, What, When, Where, Why, and What Happened questions and identifying the main idea. Relate the news item to another person using the diagram as notes. Watch the videotape of a TV show or listen to an audiotape of a radio show.	How did the form help you remember? When wouldn't the form help? How did you stay so organized and coherent when you related the news item?
Story schema	"We will share a short story or TV show with _____, who was unable to see it or hear it."	Fill out a schema diagram, including characters, setting, and episodes. Retell the story using the organizational diagrams as a cue.	How did this form help you remember? How is the information arranged? Why is this arrangement good for a story? Would it be good for a math book? Why not?
General life scripts (abstracted common life events)	"We will write our autobiographies and present a 'This is Your Life' program."	Fill out a form with labeled boxes of common life events (birth, school, marriage, job) and uncommon significant events (e.g., head injury). Using the form as a guide, write the autobiography and then present it formally in a radio program format.	How did this form make your writing more organized? How could the form help reconstruct the past? How is your autobiography organized (e.g., chronologically)? How did the written preparation help the oral presentation?

Specific-event scripts (e.g., going to a restaurant, going to the dentist)	"We will explain to _____ (a small child) what it will be like when he has to go to the dentist."	Fill in a form with relevant information about the situation, to prepare what you are going to say to the child: • Who will be there • Equipment • Sequence of expected events and actions • Expected layout of the room and some variations Then, using the guide, explain to a child or explain in a role-playing situation.	How did this form help you? Why wouldn't a general life script help you? How is your explanation to the child organized? Why would this help you remember what happened to you?

SOURCE: Szekeres SF: Organization as an Intervention Target after Traumatic Brain Injury. *Seminars in Speech and Language* 1992; 13:302–303.
*Possible probe questions to develop metacognition, understanding, and awareness

TABLE 5.53. Traumatic brain injury: stages of recovery for individuals with severe brain injury and their communication partners.

EARLY STAGES OF RECOVERY

INDIVIDUAL WITH TBI
Gradual emergence from coma
Minimal responsiveness to environmental events
Minimal recognition of people, things, and events
Minimal communication
—Comprehension: ranges from no comprehension of language to inconsistent comprehension of simple and contextually supported acts of communication
—Expression: ranges from reflexive acts (e.g., crying out, withdrawing) to deliberate use of eye gaze, reaching, and other gestures to indicate wants and needs

COMMUNICATION PARTNER: FREQUENTLY OBSERVED COMMUNICATION DEFICITS
Failing to talk to or communicate nonverbally with the injured individual
Failing to prepare the injured individual for nursing or therapy procedures with natural gestures and physical prompts in combination with simple verbal cues
Failing to use physical contact to communicate security and acceptance
Failing to notice, interpret, or respond to the individual's natural communication gestures
Failing to prompt communication gestures in appropriate contexts
Attempting to establish yes/no communication before the individual is cognitively ready
Talking about the individual in his or her presence
Creating an environment that is overstimulating and confusing
Misinterpreting negative behavior as intentionally communicative

MIDDLE STAGES OF RECOVERY

INDIVIDUAL WITH TBI
Increasing alertness and responsiveness to environmental events
Gradually decreasing confusion, disorientation, and shallow processing of information
Possibly significant disinhibition, lack of initiation, or both
Comprehension adequate for normal interaction, but inadequate given increases in processing demands
Expressive communication possibly characterized by adequate speech, but disorganized and tangential language that may be contextually inappropriate, perseverative, confabulatory, and bizarre

COMMUNICATION PARTNER: FREQUENTLY OBSERVED COMMUNICATION DEFICITS
Trying to communicate in a confusing environment
Saying too much; saying too little
Failing to provide nonverbal cues
Failing to provide sufficient routine and regularity for individuals to feel oriented and secure
Misinterpreting negative behavior as intentional; taking inappropriate or aggressive language personally
Showing frustration with the injured individual's unsuccessful performance
Ridiculing bizarre utterances
Failing to decipher the communicative intent underlying unusual or aggressive behavior
Failing to provide choices
Not understanding or using the individual's augmentative communication system
Expecting that a person capable of using an augmentative communication system will initiate functional communication with the system and transfer its use to functional settings (thereby frustrating both parties)
Labeling people by their behavior

(continued)

TABLE 5.53. (*continued*)

LATE STAGES OF RECOVERY

INDIVIDUAL WITH TBI

Typically, speech and language that are adequate for ordinary purposes

Possibly inefficient comprehension and expression given increasing processing demands

Often socially ineffective interaction in context, possibly related to some combination of disinhibition, lack of initiation, difficulty reading social cues, difficulty organizing interaction over several turns

COMMUNICATION PARTNER: FREQUENTLY OBSERVED COMMUNICATION DEFICITS

Speaking too fast; saying too much

Not giving injured individuals the opportunity to communicate

Overcompensating by speaking too slowly and simply, speaking for the individual, or in other ways infantilizing people capable of interacting at a higher level

Failing to provide natural consequences for communication successes or failures

Failing to encourage new strategies (e.g., word finding strategies or alternative communication systems if the individual is unable to speak intelligibly)

Failing to encourage new communication strategies in natural environments

Addressing the individual in a patronizing or disrespectful manner

SOURCE: Ylvisaker M, Feeney TJ, Urbanczyk B: A Social–Environmental Approach to Communication and Behavior after Traumatic Brain Injury. *Seminars in Speech and Language* 1993; 14:77.

TABLE 5.54. **Traumatic brain injury stress indices: posttrauma family concerns for children.**

INTAKE ASSESSMENT QUESTIONS

1. Are the medical conditions affecting your child distressing to you?
2. Are you able to obtain the medical information you need to know about your child?
3. Is your child reacting differently to you and your family?
4. Are other children or members of your family acting differently?
5. Are you or your spouse missing work?
6. Has your family schedule been affected in any way?
7. Are you experiencing difficulty managing your child's behavior?
8. Are you experiencing difficulty in managing the behavior of your other children?
9. Are your other children coping with your child's injury or hospitalization?
10. Are you experiencing difficulty in arranging care for your other children or family members?
11. Are you experiencing difficulty with everyday activities?
12. Are you able to talk with your spouse about your child's condition?
13. Are you disagreeing with your spouse or other family members regarding how to care for your child?
14. Are you concerned about how other members of your family are coping with your child's injury?

ONGOING FOLLOW-UP ASSESSMENTS

1. Is there any change to how your child is reacting to you and your family?
2. Are you distressed regarding your child's condition?
3. Are you experiencing difficulty in controlling your child's behavior?
4. Are you experiencing difficulty in controlling the behavior of other children in your family?
5. Are you concerned about the recovery of your child?
6. Do you worry about your child's future?
7. Has your home or work schedule been affected in any way?
8. Are you able to manage all your activities at home?
9. Is it difficult for you to accept your child's injury?
10. Do you worry how your child is accepted by his friends?

TABLE 5.55. **Right-hemisphere syndrome: nonlinguistic deficits associated with RHD.**

Left-neglect
Anosognosia
Attentional impairments
    Arousal
    Vigilance
    Maintenance
    Selective attention

SOURCE: Myers PS: Right Hemisphere Syndrome. In LaPointe LL (ed): *Aphasia and Related Neurogenic Language Disorders*, p. 203. Thieme, New York, 1997.

TABLE 5.56. Word retrieval: sample of verbal tasks of varying association strength.

Task	Example
1. Paired associates.	"Shoes and _____."
2. Contrastive associates.	"Hot and _____."
3. Complete a spoken sentence with the written word provided.	"You drive a _____." (Show written word CAR.)
4. Complete a spoken sentence with a picture provided.	"You drive a _____." (Show picture of car.)
5. Complete a spoken sentence.	"You drive a _____."
6. Answer a structured question.	"What do you drive?"
7. Answer a question.	"You drive this. What do you call it?"
8. Answer a low-association question.	"What do you call this?" (Show picture of car.)
9. Semantic category.	Name a mode of transportation.

SOURCE: Simmons-Mackie N: Conduction Aphasia. In LaPointe LL (ed): *Aphasia and Related Neurogenic Language Disorders*, p. 80. Thieme, New York, 1997.

6

Fluency

TABLE 6.1. **Cluttering and stuttering compared.**

	Stuttering	*Cluttering*
Interpretation	Functional; secondary	Hereditary; primary central
Underlying disturbance	Neurovegetative dysfunctional	language imbalance (lack of maturation of CNS mostly absent)
Awareness of disorder	Strong	Mostly absent
Speech characteristics		
Specific symptoms	Clonic and tonic inhibition	Hesitation, repetition (without inhibition)
Rate of delivery	Rather slow	Mostly quick
Sentence structure	Mostly correct	Often incorrect
Fear of specific sounds	Present	Absent
Heightened attention	Worse	Better
Relaxed attention	Better	Worse
Foreign language	Worse	Better
Gesturing	Stiff, inhibited	Broad, uninhibited
Reading allowed		
Well-known text	Better	Worse
Unknown text	Worse	Better
Writing characteristics	Compressed; high-pressure strokes	Loose, disorderly
School performance	Good to superior	Underachiever
Psychological attitudes	Embarrassed, inhibited	Carefree, sociable
	Painstaking, compulsive	Impatient, impulsive
	Grudge-bearer	Easily forgetting
	Penetrating	Superficial
Experimental responses:		
Alcohol	Better	Worse
Lee effect	Better	Worse
EEG	Borderline normal	Often deviant
Chlorpromazine	Worse	Better
Dexfenmetrazine	Better	Worse
Course	Fluctuating; spontaneous improvements and relapses	Persistent
Therapy	Attention should be diverted from details; psychotherapy	Concentration on details
Prognosis	Depends on emotional adjustment	Depends on acquiring concentration

SOURCE: From Weiss DA: Similarities and Differences between Stuttering and Cluttering. *Folia Phoniatrica* (Basel) 1967; 19:98–104.

TABLE 6.2. **Cluttering characteristics.**

Varied symptoms are typical of cluttering. The literature reports that as many as 62 separate characteristics of cluttering have been described. Other data list three obligatory symptoms that were pathognomonic and essential for diagnosis: (1) excessive repetitions of speech, (2) short attention span and poor concentration, and (3) lack of complete awareness of the problem. Over a dozen facultative symptoms are often present but not mandatory. Review of the literature and integration of information that supports or clarifies Weiss's listing may be helpful. Weiss later presented a revised list of 21 symptoms, which are listed below. The first five symptoms are obligatory and must be present in every case.

OBLIGATORY SYMPTOMS:
1. Repetitions are excessive (8 to 10 repetitions).
2. Lack of awareness (does not believe his or her speech deviates).
3. Weakness of concentration and shortness of attention span.
4. Perceptual weakness.
5. Poorly organized thinking (speaks before clarifying thoughts).

FACULTATIVE SYMPTOMS:
1. Excessive speech rate (tachylalia most conspicuous symptom).
2. Interjection (long, drawn-out vowels occur frequently).
3. Vowel stops (pauses before initial vowel).
4. Articulatory and motor disabilities (deletes phonemes/dyslalic).
5. Grammatical difficulties (inattentive to details and grammar).
6. Vocal monotony lack of speech melody or intonation.
7. Respiration (jerky).
8. Delayed speech development (late talkers).

ASSOCIATED SYMPTOMS:
1. Reading disorder (a frequent problem that Weiss suggests may be used for diagnostic confirmation).
2. Writing disorder (motor and imagination difficulties).
3. Lack of rhythmical and musical ability (poor singing).
4. Restlessness and hyperactivity (fidgeting is typical).
5. Electroencephalographic (EEG) findings (deviations on EEG common).
6. Lag in maturation (occurs often).
7. Hereditary (familial factor/organic flavor).
8. Subgroups (eg, receptive versus expressive; or a grouping of overhurried speech, hesitation and repetition, and talking in circles).

SOURCE: Adapted from Daly DA: Cluttering: Another Fluency Syndrome. In Curlee RF (ed) *Stuttering and Related Disorders of Fluency,* p. 182. Thieme, New York, 1993.

TABLE 6.3. Disfluency classifications and types.

Silent Periods
  Pauses: speaking interruptions of quiet that break the rhythm of the phrase or sentence.
Speaking Disruptions
  Revisions: alterations made before or after an utterance is completed.
  Prolongations: lengthening a syllable or sound.
  Interjections: Adding an extraneous sound before the phrase, within a word, or between words of a phrase.
  Phonatory: abnormalities of phonation (such as pitch breaks, changes in pitch, or vocal fry) disturbing the rhythm.
Repetitions
  Phrase: at least one or more repetitions of a portion of a phrase.
  Whole-word: at least one or more repetitions of a word.
  Part-word: at least one or more repetitions of a sound or a syllable in a word.

TABLE 6.4. Disfluencies normally observed in children and typically not considered true stuttering.

Usually Normal	*Example*
Silent pauses	Child casually hesitates before the first word of a sentence or within the sentence as he/she processes the correct manner to articulate a sound, word, phrase, or sentence. There is typically no accompanying evidence of the symptoms listed in Table 6.9.
Whole-word repetitions	Child casually repeats the first word of the sentence 1–3 times using normal rhythm and stress as he/she searches for the next word or words to follow. There is typically no accompanying evidence of the symptoms listed in Table 6.9.
Interjections of sounds, syllables, or words	Child casually interjects sounds, syllables, or words using normal rhythm and stress before or during the production of a phrase or sentence as he/she searches for the next word or words to follow. There is typically no accompanying evidence of the symptoms listed in Table 6.9.
Revisions of word, phrase, or sentence	Child casually attempts to revise the word or words, he/she has started to say using normal rhythm and stress as he/she searches for the correct word or pronunciation. There is typically no accompanying evidence of the symptoms listed in Table 6.9.

SOURCE: From Ramig PR: Parent–Clinician–Child Partnership in the Therapeutic Process of the Preschool- and Elementary-Aged Child Who Stutters. *Seminars in Speech and Hearing* 1993; 14:228.

TABLE 6.5. Speaking rates of children in words and syllables per minute: Means and standard deviations.

Grade	Words per Minute	Standard Deviation	Syllables per Minute	Standard Deviation
1	124.92	12.17	147.66	13.47
2	130.44	12.05	156.72	17.14
3	133.44	10.01	158.94	14.86
4	139.32	16.33	165.66	24.58
5	141.84	16.24	170.04	23.19

SOURCE: Runyan CM, Runyan SE: Therapy for School-Age Stutters: An Update on the Fluency Rules Program. In Curlee RF (ed) *Stuttering and Related Disorders of Fluency,* p. 103. Thieme, New York, 1993.

TABLE 6.6. Stutterer's reactions to selected speaking situations.

Situation	Frequency*	Level of difficulty*	Level of confidence*
Talking on the telephone to a friend or family member.			
Talking on the telephone to a stranger.			
Using the telephone to purchase a ticket.			
Talking to a stranger in a social situation.			
Introducing myself.			
Placing an order in a restaurant.			
Talking to a close friend.			
Talking with parents.			
Talking with a sales clerk.			
Meeting someone for the first time.			
Asking for information.			
Being interviewed for a job.			
Talking with teachers.			
Making an appointment.			
Making introductions.			
Speaking before a group.			
Asking a question or making a comment in class.			
Giving my name in a classroom situation.			
Giving a prepared speech.			
Talking to someone of the opposite sex.			
Participating at a meeting.			
Reading aloud to others.			
Conversation at the dinner table:			
with family.			
with friends.			
with strangers.			

*SCALE VALUES:		
Frequency	*Level of Difficulty*	*Level of Confidence*
I encounter this situation:	This situation is:	In this situation I have:
1. More than once per day	1. Not difficult	1 Total lack of confidence
2. Daily	2. Slightly difficult	2. Very little confidence
3. Several times per week	3 Somewhat difficult	3. Some confidence
4. Less than once per week	4. Very difficult	4. Considerable confidence
5. Rarely	5. Almost impossible	5. Complete confidence

SOURCE: From Johnson W, Darley FL, Spriesterbach DC: *Diagnostic Methods in Speech Pathology*, pp. 317–319. Harper & Row, New York, 1963.
*Patterned after the Iowa Stutterer's Self-Ratings of Reactions to Speech Situations.

TABLE 6.7. **Stuttering: measurement strategies.**

1. Percentage of syllables stuttered (%SS)

$$\%SS = \frac{\text{total number of stutterings}}{\text{total number of syllables spoken}}$$

   The total number of stutterings is determined by counting all moments of stuttering in the talking sample. When more than one stuttering occurs in a word, each moment is counted. The total number of syllables spoken is determined from the total amount of client talking time (CTT) in the sample and the average number of syllables spoken per minute. Total CTT is determined by cumulating the durations of client talking in the session to be analyzed. The timing record is discontinued for client pauses greater than 2 sec (e.g., when turning pages of a book, when another person is talking, or when the speaker pauses between sentences or thoughts).

   A precise calculation of the average number of syllables spoken per minute depends on a count of the total number of syllables spoken during the entire sample. In the interest of saving analysis time, a less precise method is to select talking intervals randomly selected from the entire sample for a total CTT of at least 2 min. The estimated number of syllables spoken per minute (Est[syl/min]) is then determined by dividing the number of syllables spoken by the accumulated CTT. The total number of syllables spoken in the entire sample is then estimated as the product of Est(syl/min) and the total CTT.

$$\text{Total Syl} = \text{Est(syl/min)} \times \text{Total CTT}$$

2. Average duration of stutterings is estimated by timing the duration of 10 stutterings selected for representativeness. ("Random" selection cannot be used in view of the representativeness criterion.) The total of the 10 durations then is divided by 10 to give an estimate of the average duration.
3. Duration of the three longest stutterings is determined simply by timing what are judged to be the three longest stutterings in the entire sample.
4. Overall speaking rate (approximate) in syl/min is calculated by dividing the number of syllables spoken in 2 min (or other duration N used in #1 above) by 2 (or N other than 2).
5. Articulatory rate (AR) in syl/min is calculated as

$$\text{AR(syl/min)} = \frac{\text{total number of nonstuttered syllables}}{\text{total talking time for fluent sample}}$$

   An appropriate synonym for articulation rate is syllable rate (or, better yet, fluent syllable rate).

   Articulatory rate is based on a count of the number of syllables produced during at least 10 randomly selected intervals of speech that are free of stuttering or disfluencies and from which pauses greater than 2 sec have been eliminated. (If necessary, fewer than 10 intervals may be used, but the accuracy of the estimate will be reduced.) The accumulated talking time for these intervals is used in the denominator of the formula shown above.

6. Average duration of nonstuttered intervals also is based on the 10 or more samples of nonstuttered speech used in #5 above. The total talking time for these intervals is divided by the number of intervals (10 or more) to give the average duration of nonstuttered intervals.
7. Duration of the three longest nonstuttered intervals is determined by timing what are judged to be the three longest intervals of talking that are free of stuttering.
8. Average length of nonstuttered intervals is calculated by dividing the total number of syllables determined in #5 above by the number of intervals (10 or more). The quotient is an estimate of the length in syllables of the typical nonstuttered interval.
9. Length of the three longest nonstuttered intervals is the length in syllables of the three samples selected in #7 above.
10. Naturalness rating is the examiner's overall impression of the naturalness of the complete speech sample registered on a 9-point scale where 1 = highly unnatural.

Source: With permission from Costello-Ingham, J. Department of Speech and Hearing Sciences, University of California–Santa Barbara.

TABLE 6.8. **Stutterer's reaction to self-descriptive statements.**

By placing an "X" in the appropriate space, indicate the extent to which each of the following statements holds true for you. (The actual questionnaire format shows the scale values after each statement.)

Statements:

Feeling embarrassed about my speech.
Fear of a word I can't say fluently.
Avoiding words and sounds I have trouble with.
Fear of talking before a group.
Feelings of nervousness and tension before speaking.
Fear of being asked my name.
Feeling that I should be able to speak better.
Fear of talking on the telephone.
Not talking because I may have trouble.
Feeling helpless about the way I speak.
Hiding the fact that I have a speech problem.
Feeling that stuttering is the most significant factor in my life.
Not being able to say what I feel.
Inability to talk to strangers.
Feeling that my speech is uncontrollable.
Feeling that people react to the way I talk, not the way I am.
Feeling that if I didn't stutter, my other problems would be insignificant.
Feeling ill at ease with people.
Unwillingness to assume responsibility.
Worrying about the impression I will make.
Feeling that I am socially inadequate.
Feeling that I am less capable than other people.
Feeling that other people have more important things to say than I do.

Scale:

:_____	:_____	:_____	:_____	:_____
Never or rarely true	Seldom true	Some-times true	Usually true	Almost always or always true

---

SOURCE: Prins D: Management of Stuttering: Treatment of Adolescents and Adults. In Curlee RF (ed) *Stuttering and Related Disorders of Fluency*, p. 137. Thieme, New York, 1993.

TABLE 6.9. **Stuttering symptoms (true disfluency): One or more evident in approximately 1 out of 30 children.**

Symptom	Example
Within-word repetitions	Child repeats first letter or syllable of a word, such as t-t-t-table or ta-ta-ta-table, etc.
Prolongation of sound or syllable	Child stretches out a sound or syllable, such as r-------abbit or ra-------bbit.
Insertion of the schwa vowel	Child inserts a weak, neutral vowel, such as buh-buh-buh-baby in place of bay-bay-bay-baby.
Struggle and tension	Child struggles and forces in his/her attempt to speak, especially at the beginning of sentences. Tension may be apparent in the lip, neck, and/or jaw area as child attempts to talk. In addition, ongoing speech may sound disrythmic due to tension.
Rise in pitch and loudness	Child may increase his/her pitch and volume as he/she repeats and/or prolongs sounds and/or syllables.
Evidence of tremors	Rapid and fleeting quivering or "vibration" of the lips, tongue, or jaw may occur as the child blocks, repeats, or prolonges sounds or syllables.
Avoidance and revision	As the child becomes more concerned and frustrated by his/her speech, he/she may display an unusual number of pauses, substitutions of words, interjection of extraneous sounds, words, or phrases, and avoidance of talking.
Evidence of fear	As the child becomes more aware, embarrassed, and shameful of his/her speech, he/she may begin to display expressions of fear as he/she anticipates or experiences stuttering.
Difficulty starting and/or sustaining airflow and voicing	Breathing may be irregular, and speech may occur in spurts as the child struggles to initiate and/or maintain his/her voicing.

SOURCE: Ramig PR: Parent–Clinician–Child Partnership in the Therapeutic Process of the Preschool- and Elementary-Aged Child Who Stutters. *Seminars in Speech and Hearing* 1993; 14:228.

7

Voice

TABLE 7.1. **Amyotrophic lateral sclerosis—mixed dysarthria: laryngeal–phonatory characteristics.***

	Findings
PERCEPTUAL	
Phonation	Hoarseness or harshness having a strained–strangled quality; "wet" or "gurgly" components; rapid tremor or "flutter" on vowel prolongation. Breathy if strong flaccid component; pitch is abnormally low. Monopitch. Loudness is reduced. Monoloudness. Inhalatory stridor if severe. Reduced sharpness of cough. Inappropriate crying or laughter may be present.
Resonation	Hypernasality; nasal emission.
Articulation	Imprecise consonants; abnormally slow rate.
Language	Normal.
PHYSICAL	
Larynx	Vocal folds appear normal in structure. If major component is spastic, vocal folds appear to adduct normally or may hyperadduct, along with false vocal folds. Adduction may be bilaterally symmetric, or one vocal fold may adduct less fully than the other. If there is a major flaccid component, vocal folds may adduct and abduct with less than normal excursions.
Velopharynx	Bilateral velopharyngeal insufficiency, possibly asymmetric. Hyperactive gag reflex.
Tongue	Topographically abnormal. Furrowed and reduced in size owing to atrophy. Fasciculations. Weakness. Slow alternate motion rate (AMR) on lateral movements on /tʌ/ and /kʌ/ syllable repetitions.
Lips	Weak. Slow movements on AMR for /pʌ/.
Teeth	Normal.
Hard palate	Normal.
Mandible	Slow AMR.
GENERAL MEDICAL	Nonspecific.
OTHER NEUROLOGICAL SIGNS	
Peripheral nervous system	Signs of flaccid paralysis.
Central nervous system	Signs of spasticity.
PSYCHIATRIC/PSYCHOLOGICAL	Nonspecific. Pseudobulbar crying and laughter may give erroneous impression of emotional lability and intellectual deterioration.

SOURCE: Aronson AE: *Clinical Voice Disorders,* p. 95. Thieme, New York, 1990.

*Basically same as in any other nervous system disease affecting both pyramidal and lower motor neuron tracts bilaterally.

TABLE 7.2. **Apraxia of speech: laryngeal-phonatory characteristics.**

Findings

PERCEPTUAL

Phonation
Varies, from normal in some patients to mutism in others. Phonation may be impossible because of apparent loss of recall for integration of respiratory and laryngeal movements, resulting in trial-and-error efforts to phonate, but silent nevertheless. Aphonic (whispered) speech can occur. Inability to cough volitionally or clear throat.

Resonation
Normal.

Articulation
Phoneme omissions, substitutions, reversals, and additions; stuttering-like blocking.

Language
May be relatively normal or aphasic.

PHYSICAL

Larynx
Vocal folds appear normal in structure and function.

Velopharynx
Normal.

Tongue
Topographically normal. May have associated dysarthric signs. Trial-and-error nonspeech volitional movements (oral nonverbal apraxia).

Lips
Trial-and-error nonspeech volitional movements may be present. Sequential motor rates, the rapid sequencing of sounds from /pʌ/ to /tʌ/ to /kʌ/, may be mildly to severely impaired.

Teeth
Normal.

Hard palate
Normal.

Mandible
Normal.

GENERAL MEDICAL
Nonspecific.

OTHER NEUROLOGICAL SIGNS

Peripheral nervous system
Normal.

Central nervous system
A wide variety of dysarthric, apraxic, and other abnormal signs may coexist.

PSYCHIATRIC/PSYCHOLOGICAL
Nonspecific.

SOURCE: Aronson AE: *Clinical Voice Disorders,* p. 107. Thieme, New York, 1990.

TABLE 7.3. **Arthur.**

Once, a long time ago, there was a young rat named Arthur who could never make up his flighty mind. Whenever his swell friends used to ask him to go out to play with them, he would only answer airily, "I don't know." He wouldn't try to say yes, or no either. He would always shirk from making a specific choice.

His proud Aunt Helen scolded him: "Now look here," she stated, "no one is going to aid or care for you if you carry on like this. You have no more mind than a stray blade of grass."

That very night, there was a big thundering crash, and in the foggy morning some zealous man, with 20 boys and girls, rode up and looked closely at the fallen barn. One of them slipped back a broken board and saw a squashed young rat, quite dead, half in and half out of his hole. Thus, in the end the poor shirker got his just dues. Oddly enough, his Aunt Helen was glad. "I hate such oozy, oily sneaks," she said.

324 • *Speech-Language Pathology Desk Reference*

TABLE 7.4. Artificial larynges.

Bruce Medical Supply
411 Waverly Oaks Road,
Department 10266
Waltham, MA 02254-9166
(800) 225–8446
Fax (617) 894–9519

The Servox speech aid takes the place of vocal cords. Small, light, and comfortable, the dual button unit allows greater flexibility in pitch, volume, and intonation. When pressed against the neck, it generates sound vibrations that are conducted into mouth and throat cavities to create speech.

HARC Mercantile Ltd.
(delivery address)
111 West Centre Avenue
Portage, MI 49024
(800) 445–9968
(mailing address)
P.O. Box 3055
Kalamazoo, MI 49003-3055
(800) 438–4272
(616) 324–1615
Fax (800) 413–5248
Web site: http://www.harcmercantile.com

Wide range of assistive devices for hearing impaired and accessories for laryngectomees, including artificial larynges. Voice amplifiers and products for visually impaired individuals.

HITEC Group International, Inc.
8160 Madison Avenue
Burr Ridge, IL 60521
Linda Gallas, Nancy Lilley, Diane Comparone
(630) 654–9200
Fax (630) 654–9219
E-mail: snp@hitec.com
Web site: http://www.hitec.com

Supplies artificial larynges, voice amplifiers, and accessories, featuring Servox, Nuvois, and Amplicord. A wide assortment of assistive devices. Free catalog containing nearly 1000 products.

INHEALTH Technologies
1110 Mark Avenue
Carpinteria, CA 93013
Jobeth Seder, Product Specialist
(805) 684–8594
E-mail: jseder@inhealth.com
Web site: http:.//www.inhealth.com

INHEALTH features the Bloom–Singer line of voice restoration products and other accessories for laryngectomees.

Luminaud, Inc.
8688 Tyler Boulevard
Mentor, OH 44060
Tom Lennox
(216) 255–9082
Fax (216) 255–2250

Cooper–Rand intraoral and other models of artificial larynges. Various models available for hand and arm mobility limitations and quadriplegics.

Siemens Professional Products Division
16 East Piper Lane
Prospect Heights, IL 60070-1799
(800) 333–9083
Fax (847) 808–1299
Web site: http//www.siemens-hearing.com

Sole U.S. agent for Servox electrolarynx, batteries, chargers, and accessories. Wide assortment of auditory trainers, assistive listening devices, and audiometric equipment.

TABLE 7.5. **Ataxic dysarthria: laryngeal–phonatory characteristics.**

	Findings
PERCEPTUAL	
Phonation	Frequently normal. Others have harsh voice quality, monopitch, monoloudness, excess and equal stress on ordinarily unstressed words or syllables, excess loudness, bursts of loudness, and coarse voice tremor.
Resonation	Normal.
Articulation	Imprecise consonants; irregular articulatory breakdown; distorted vowels; slow rate.
Language	Normal.
PHYSICAL	
Larynx	Vocal folds appear normal in structure and function.
Velopharynx	Normal.
Tongue	Topographically normal. Irregular and slow AMRs on /tʌ/ and /kʌ/ and on lateral tongue movements.
Lips	Irregular and slow AMRs for /pʌ/.
Teeth	Normal.
Hard palate	Normal.
Mandible	Normal.
GENERAL MEDICAL	Nonspecific. *Note:* Ataxic dysarthria may be a sign of moderate to severe hypothyroidism, and drug and alcohol abuse.
OTHER NEUROLOGICAL SIGNS	
Peripheral nervous system	Normal.
Central nervous system	Signs of ataxia.
PSYCHIATRIC/PSYCHOLOGICAL	Nonspecific.

SOURCE: Aronson AE: *Clinical Voice Disorders,* p. 98. Thieme, New York, 1990.

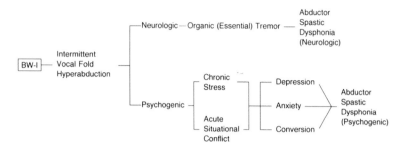

FIGURE 7.1. Breathy, whispered voice (intermittent): analysis schema.
SOURCE: Aronson AE: *Clinical Voice Disorders,* p. 301. Thieme, New York, 1990.

TABLE 7.6. **Cervical dystonia: acoustic voice–speech parameters significantly different from normal individuals.***

Parameter	Gender
Lower habitual fundamental frequency	Females
Lower ceiling fundamental frequency	Females
Restricted frequency range	Females
Shorter /s/ duration	Both
Shorter /z/ duration	Both
Shorter maximum phonation duration	Both
Slower sequential movement rates	Both
Slower alternate movement rates	Both
Longer phonatory reaction time	Both
Slower reading rate (WPM)	Both
Lower overall intelligibility rating	Both
Increased jitter values	Both
Increased shimmer values	Both
Decreased harmonic-to-noise ratio	Females

SOURCE: Zraick RI, LaPointe LL: Hyperkinetic Dysarthria. In McNeil MR (ed): *Clinical Management of Sensorimotor Disorders,* p. 254. Thieme, New York, 1997.

*From Case, LaPointe, & Duane, 1991; LaPointe, Case, & Duane, 1993; Zriack, LaPointe, Case, & Duane, 1993.

TABLE 7.7. Chorea–Hyperkinetic dysarthria: laryngeal–phonatory characteristics.

	Findings
PERCEPTUAL	
Phonation	Intermittently harsh, strained–strangled voice quality, transient breathiness; distorted vowels, monopitch; excess loudness variations; monoloudness, excess, equal stress on ordinarily unstressed words or syllables; reduced stress; sudden, forced inspiration/expiration.
Resonation	Intermittent hypernasality.
Articulation	Imprecise consonants; distorted vowels; prolonged intervals between syllables and words; variable rate; inappropriate silences; prolonged phonemes; short phrases; irregular articulatory breakdown.
Language	Normal. Defective in patients who have undergone intellectual deterioration.
PHYSICAL	
Larynx	Vocal folds appear normal in structure, intermittent hyperadduction.
Velopharynx	Normal in appearance.
Tongue	Topographically normal. Quick unpatterned movements at rest and during (AMRs) for /tʌ/ and /kʌ/, which are irregular.
Lips	Quick unpatterned movements at rest and during AMRs for /pʌ/.
Teeth	Normal.
Hard palate	Normal.
Mandible	Quick asymmetric movements at rest and during speech.
GENERAL MEDICAL	Nonspecific.
OTHER NEUROLOGICAL SIGNS	
Peripheral nervous system	Normal.
Central nervous system	Choreic movements elsewhere in the body.
PSYCHIATRIC/PSYCHOLOGICAL	Intellectual and behavior changes associated with dementia, if present.

SOURCE: Aronson AE: *Clinical Voice Disorders,* p. 95. Thieme, New York, 1990.

TABLE 7.8. Cleft lip and palate classifications by the American Cleft Palate Association.

CLEFTS OF PREPALATE		
Cleft lip	Unilateral	Right, left
		Extent in thirds
	Bilateral	Right, left
		Extent in thirds
	Median	Extent in thirds
	Prolabium	Small, medium, large
	Congenital scar	Right, left, median
		Extent in thirds
Cleft of alveolar process	Unilateral	Right, left
		Extent in thirds
	Bilateral	Right, left
		Extent in thirds
	Median	Extent in thirds
Cleft of prepalate	Any combination of foregoing types	Submucous right, left, median
	Prepalate profusion	
	Prepalate rotation	
	Prepalate arrest (median cleft)	
CLEFTS OF PALATE		
Cleft soft palate	Extent	Posteroanterior in thirds
		Width (maximum in mm)
	Palatal shortness	None, slight, moderate, marked
	Submucous cleft	Extent in thirds
Cleft hard palate	Extent	Posteroanterior in thirds
		Width (maximum in mm)
	Vomer attachment	Right, left, absent
	Submucous cleft	Extent in thirds
Cleft of soft and hard palate		
Clefts of prepalate and palate	Any combination of clefts described under clefts of prepalate and clefts of palate.	

SOURCE: Aronson AE: *Clinical Voice Disorders*, p. 208. Thieme, New York, 1990.

TABLE 7.9. **Congenital disorders of the larynx: classifications.**

CARTILAGINOUS ANOMALIES
Laryngomalacia (congenital laryngeal stridor)
Epiglottic anomalies
  Absent
  Bifid
  Tubular
Thyroid cartilage anomalies
  Nonfusion of ala
Absence of superior or inferior cornua
Arytenoid cartilage anomalies
  Atavistic
Cricoid cartilage anomalies
  Subglottic stenosis
  Fusion of entire ring
  Failure of dorsal function (cleft)

SOFT TISSUE ANOMALIES
Cysts and laryngoceles
  Internal: ventricular; aryepiglottic fold and arytenoid
  External
  Combined
Webs, stenoses, and atresias
  Supraglottic
  Glottic
  Subglottic
Cri du chat syndrome

NEUROLOGIC LESIONS
Unilateral vocal fold paralysis
Bilateral vocal fold paralysis

VASCULAR ANOMALIES
Hemangiomas
Lymphangiomas

SOURCE: Tucker HM: *The Larynx,* 2nd ed., p. 189. Thieme, New York, 1993.

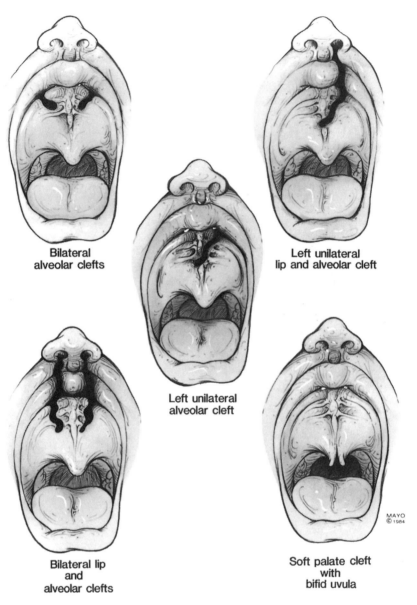

Bilateral
alveolar clefts

Left unilateral
lip and alveolar cleft

Left unilateral
alveolar cleft

Bilateral lip
and
alveolar clefts

Soft palate cleft
with
bifid uvula

MAYO
©1984

FIGURE 7.2a. Cleft varieties of the hard palate, soft palate, and alveolar processes.SOURCE: Aronson AE: *Clinical Voice Disorders*, p-. 214–215. Thieme, New York, 1990.

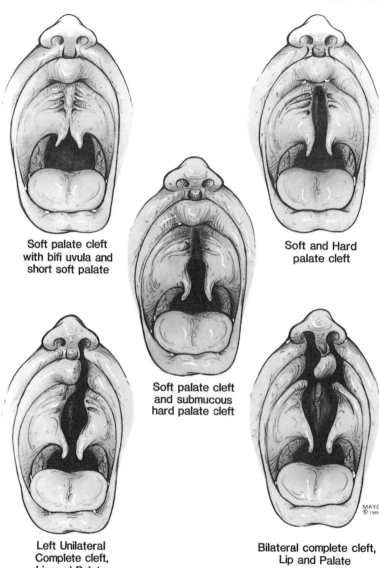

Soft palate cleft
with bifi uvula and
short soft palate

Soft and Hard
palate cleft

Soft palate cleft
and submucous
hard palate cleft

Left Unilateral
Complete cleft,
Lip and Palate

Bilateral complete cleft,
Lip and Palate

MAYO
© 1984

FIGURE 7.2b.

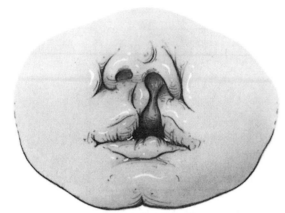

Left unilateral

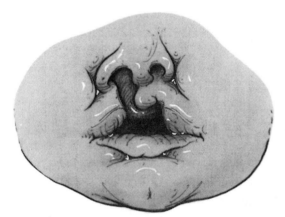

Bilateral R 3/3 L1/3

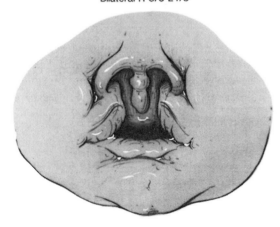

FIGURE 7.3. Cleft varieties of the upper lip.
SOURCE: Aronson AE: *Clinical Voice Disorders,* p. 213. Thieme, New York, 1990.

TABLE 7.10. Cranial nerve assessment techniques.

STATIC ASSESSMENT

Cranial Nerves V and VII
1. Look ahead with mouth closed and a relaxed face.

Cranial Nerves XI, X, XI, and XII
1. Open mouth widely with tongue relaxed on floor of mouth.

DYNAMIC ASSESSMENT: NONSPEECH

Cranial Nerve V
1. Clench teeth tightly.
2. While examiner applies resistance to jaw, lower the jaw.
3. Slowly lower and raise jaw.

Cranial Nerve VII
1. Gaze up and down with frown.
2. Protrude lips into pucker.
3. Pucker lips and smile multiple times.
4. Puff cheeks as if blowing out candle.
5. Smile showing teeth.

Cranial Nerves IX, X, and XI
1. Protrude tongue out of mouth and hold air in cheeks.
2. Shrug shoulders while providing resistance to movement.

Cranial Nerve XII
1. Protrude tongue.
2. Lick lips from corner to corner.
3. Touch upper teeth with tongue and lower tongue.
4. Push tongue against tongue depressor.
5. Push tongue against right and left cheeks while providing resistance to cheeks.

DYNAMIC ASSESSMENT: SPEECH

Cranial Nerve V
1. Repeat /ja/ as rapidly as possible for 10 to 15 seconds.

Cranial Nerve VII
1. Repeat /pa/ as rapidly as possible with bite block in teeth.
2. Repeat /pa/ as rapidly as possible with free-moving jaw.
3. Repeat /u-l-u-l-u-l/ as rapidly as possible.

Cranial Nerves IX, X, and XI
1. Sustain an /a/ sound.
2. Repeat /a/ multiple times.
3. Repeat /u/ while occluding and opening nostrils.
4. Cough, clear throat and produce hard glottal attack.
5. Vary pitch by singing scale.

Cranial Nerve XII
1. Repeat /ta/ as rapidly as possible with bite block in teeth.
2. Repeat /ta/ as rapidly as possible with free-moving jaw.
3. Repeat /ka/ as rapidly as possible with bite block in teeth.
4. Repeat /ka/ as rapidly as possible with free-moving jaw.
5. Repeat /pa-ta-ka/ as rapidly as possible.

(continued)

TABLE **7.10.** (*continued*)

SENSORY ASSESSMENT
Cranial Nerve V
1. Ask about numbness of face.
2. Check face for touch, temperature, and pain sensations.

Cranial Nerve VII
1. Discriminate tastes of sugar and salt placed on anterior two-thirds of tongue.

Cranial Nerves IX, X, and XI
1. Breathe gently while posterior wall of pharynx is stroked to induce gag reflex.

TABLE **7.11.** **Durational characteristics (mean rates and standard deviations) for three speaking tasks (rainbow passage, conversational speech, and reading of conversational speech sample) by 60 male and 60 female subjects.**

	ALL SUBJECTS		MALE SUBJECTS		FEMALE SUBJECTS	
	x	*S.D.*	*x*	*S.D.*	*x*	*S.D.*
Rainbow passage	188.4	19.7	187.6	21.4	190.6	15.3
Conversational speech	172.6	33.4	172.5	33.1	174.2	31.3
Reading of conversational speech	197.4	31.6	196.1	35.1	198.7	27.9

SOURCE: With permission from Walker VG: Durational characteristics of young adults during speaking and reading tasks. *Folia Phoniatr Logop.* 1988; 40:15, Karger, Basel.

TABLE 7.12. Dystonia hyperkinetic dysarthria, laryngeal phonatory characteristics.

	Findings
PERCEPTUAL	
Phonation	Slow, continuous changes in strained–hoarse quality; breathiness; excess loudness variations; voice arrests; monopitch; monoloudness; reduced stress; excess and equal stress on ordinarily unstressed syllables and words.
Resonation	Normal.
Articulation	Imprecise consonants; distorted vowels; short phrases; inappropriate silences.
Language	Normal. May be defective if dysarthria is associated with focal language disorders or diffuse intellectual disorders.
PHYSICAL	
Larynx	Vocal folds appear normal in structure and function; intermittent hyperadduction.
Velopharynx	Normal.
Tongue	Topographically normal. Slow, unpatterned protusive, lateral, and rotatory movements at rest and during speech. AMR's on /tʌ/ and /kʌ/ are slow and highly irregular.
Lips	Slow unpatterned lip rounding and spreading. Alternate motion rates for /pʌ/ are slow and highly irregular.
Teeth	Normal.
Hard palate	Normal.
Mandible	Slow unpatterned depression, lateralization, and elevation.
GENERAL MEDICAL	Nonspecific.
OTHER NEUROLOGICAL SIGNS	
Peripheral nervous system	Normal.
Central nervous system	Signs of dystonia may be confined to larynx or may occur elsewhere in the body.
PSYCHIATRIC/PSYCHOLOGICAL	Nonspecific. Intellectual and behavioral aberrations present if diffuse central nervous system disease is present.

SOURCE: Aronson AE: *Clinical Voice Disorders,* p. 101. Thieme, New York, 1990.

TABLE 7.13. Exhalation (forced): muscles used.

Name	Attachments	Innervation	Action
1. Rectus abdominis	Ribs 5 and 7, xyphoid process of sternum	T7, T8, T9, T10, T11	Compresses abdominal contents
2. Transversus abdominis	From lower six ribs, lumbar fascia, ilium, and fascia of thigh to fellow of opposite side.	Branches from 7th to 12th intercostal, the iliohypogastric, and ilioinguinal nerves	Constricts and compresses abdominal contents
3. Obliquus intemus abdoniinis	Lumbar fascia, ilium, fascia of thigh to cartilages or 8, 9, or 10 ribs	Branches of 8th to 12th intercostal nerves, the iliohypogastric, and ilioinguinal nerves	Compresses abdominal contents
4. Obliquus externus abdominis	From ilium, fascia from thigh, and pubis to lower eight ribs in alternation with those of serratus anterior and latissimus	Branches of 8th intercostal nerves, the iliohypogastric and ilioinguinal nerves	Compresses abdominal contents

SOURCE: Aronson AE: *Clinical Voice Disorders,* p. 357. Thieme, New York, 1990.

TABLE 7.14. Focal dystonia: classification according to distribution of body parts affected.

Type of focal dystonia	Body part affected
Blepharospasm	Eyelid
Oromandibular	Mouth
Adductor dysphonia	Larynx
Writer's cramp	Arm
Spasmodic torticollis	Neck

SOURCE: Zraick RI, LaPointe LL: Hyperkinetic Dysarthria. In McNeil MR (ed): *Clinical Management of Sensorimotor Disorders,* p. 253. Thieme, New York, 1997.

TABLE 7.15. Averages of fundamental and formant frequencies and formant amplitudes of vowels by 76 speakers.

		i	I	ɛ	æ	a	ɔ	ʊ	u	ʌ	3̂
Fundamental frequencies (cps)	M	136	135	130	127	124	129	137	141	130	133
	W	235	232	223	210	212	216	232	231	221	218
	Ch	272	269	260	251	256	263	276	274	261	261
Formant frequencies (cps)											
F_1	M	270	390	530	660	730	570	440	300	640	490
	W	310	430	610	860	850	590	470	370	760	500
	Ch	370	530	690	1010	1030	680	560	430	850	560
F_2	M	2290	1990	1840	1720	1090	840	1020	870	1190	1350
	W	2790	2480	2330	2050	1220	920	1160	950	1400	1640
	Ch	3200	2730	2610	2320	1370	1060	1410	1170	1590	1820
F_3	M	3010	2550	2480	2410	2440	2410	2240	2240	2390	1690
	W	3310	3070	2990	2850	2810	2710	2680	2670	2780	1960
	Ch	3730	3600	3570	3320	3170	3180	3310	3260	3360	2160
Formant amplitudes (db)	L_1	-4	-3	-2	-1	-1	0	-1	-3	-1	-5
	L_2	-24	-23	-17	-12	-5	-7	-12	-19	-10	-15
	L_3	-28	-27	-24	-22	-28	-34	-34	-43	-27	-20

SOURCE: From Peterson GE, Barney HE: Control Methods Used in a Study of Vowels. *Journal of the Acoustical Society of America* 1952; 24:183.

TABLE **7.16. Fundamental frequency (Hz) for females: age ranges.***

Age Range (Years)	No.	Mean Fundamental Frequency (Hz)
20–29	10	227
30–39	10	214
40–49	10	214
50–59	10	214
60–69	10	209
70–79	10	206
80–90	10	197

SOURCE: Aronson AE: *Clinical Voice Disorders,* p. 46. Thieme, New York, 1990.

*From Kelly A: Fundamental frequency measurement of female voices from twenty to ninety years of age. (Unpublished manuscript.) Greensboro, University of North Carolina, 1977.

TABLE **7.17. Fundamental frequency (Hz) for males—comparative studies: means listed as a function of age.**

Age Range (Years)	No.	Mean Fundamental Frequencies (Hz)	Investigators
20–29	175	120	Hollien and Shipp (1972)
	27	119	Hanley (1951)
	157	128	Hollien and Jackson (1973)
	24	132	Philhour (1948)
	6	132	Pronovost (1942)
	103	138	Majewski et al (1959)
30–39	175	112	Hollien and Shipp (1972)
40–49	175	107	Hollien and Shipp (1972)
	39	113	Mysak (1959)
50–59	175	118	Hollien and Shipp (1972)
60–69	175	112	Hollien and Shipp (1972)
70–79	175	132	Hollien and Shipp (1972)
	39	124	Mysak (1959)
80–89	175	146	Hollien and Shipp (1972)
	39	141	Mysak (1959)

SOURCE: Aronson AE: *Clinical Voice Disorders,* p. 45. Thieme, New York, 1990.

TABLE 7.18. Gilles de la Tourette's syndrome—hyperkinetic dysarthria: laryngeal–phonatory characteristics.

	Findings
PERCEPTUAL (*Note:* The following vary among patients; not all are found in a given patient.)	
Phonation	Involuntary grunting, coughing, throat-clearing, barking, squealing, shrieking, screaming, gurgling, moaning.
Resonation	Snorting, sniffing.
Articulation	Whistling; clicking, lip-smacking, spitting, stuttering-like repetitions of sounds.
Language	Echolalia; coprolalia.
PHYSICAL	
Larynx	Vocal folds appear normal in structure and function.
Velopharynx	Normal.
Tongue	Normal.
Lips	Normal.
Teeth	Normal.
Hard palate	Normal.
Mandible	Normal.
GENERAL MEDICAL	Nonspecific.
OTHER NEUROLOGICAL SIGNS	
Peripheral nervous system	Normal.
Central nervous system	Jerky bodily movements.
PSYCHIATRIC/PSYCHOLOGICAL	Emotional, behavioral problems secondary to adverse social effects of above

SOURCE: Aronson AE: *Clinical Voice Disorders,* p. 106. Thieme, New York, 1990.

TABLE 7.19. Inhalation (forced): muscles used.

Name	Attachments	Innervation	Action
1. Sternocleidomastoideus	From mastoid process of skull to front of sternum and inner surface of medial third of clavicle.	Spinal portion of accessory nerve and branches from anterior rami of 2nd and 3rd cervical nerves.	Lifts sternum when both act together and when head held erect; flexes neck; rotates head to opposite side.
2. Serratus posterior superior	From ligament of neck and spinous process of 7th cervical vertebra and first three thoracic vertebrae.	Branches of anterior rami of upper four thoracic nerves.	Exact function not determined; position and attachment would suggest it to be elevator of ribs 2, 3, 4, 5.
3. Pectoralis minor	From outer surfaces of 3rd, 4th, and 5th ribs at point lateral to junction of ribs with costal cartilages, to end of coracoid.	Medial anterior thoracic nerve originating in brachial plexus. Fibers are from 8th cervical and 1st thoracic nerve.	Tends to lift scapula away from ribs, but if scapula is fixed it may lift the middle ribs.
4. Pectoralis major	From anterior border of clavicle, sternum, cartilages of first six ribs, to ridge of outer border or bicipital groove of humerus.	Medial and lateral anterior thoracic nerves from brachial plexus. Fibers from 5th cervical to 1st thoracic nerves.	Is believed that if arms are fixed, will raise ribs. Also flexes, adducts, and rotates arm medially; draws arm or shoulder forward, medially, or downward.
5. Latissimus dorsi	From spinous process of lower six thoracic, lumbar vertebrae, back of sacrum, crest of ilium, and lower three ribs.	Thoracodorsal nerve from brachial plexus; fibers come from 6th, 7th, and 8th cervical nerves.	Is believed to elevate lower ribs if arm fixed; also extends, adducts, and rotates arm medially; draws shoulder downward and backward.

SOURCE: Aronson AE: *Clinical Voice Disorders*, p. 356. Thieme, New York, 1990.

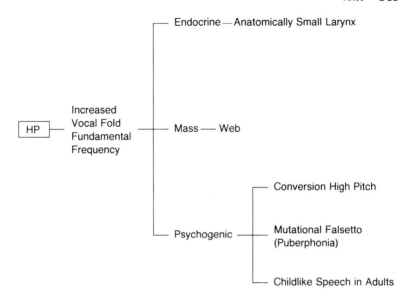

Figure 7.4. High-pitch voice: analysis schema.
SOURCE: Aronson AE: *Clinical Voice Disorders,* p. 306. Thieme, New York, 1990.

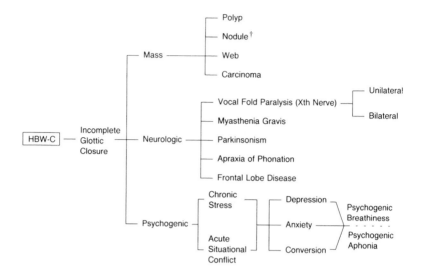

FIGURE 7.5. Husky, breathy, whispered voice (continuous): analysis schema.

†Important to note that chronic stress is a causative factor in the developmenet of vocal nodule.

SOURCE: Aronson AE: *Clinical Voice Disorders,* p. 277. Thieme, New York, 1990.

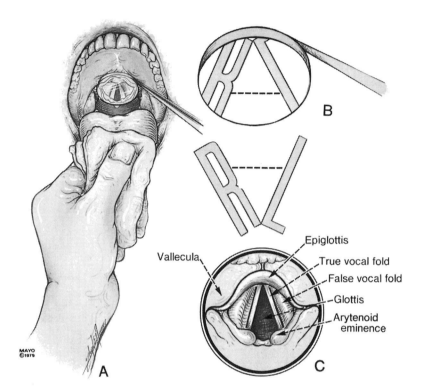

FIGURE 7.6. Indirect laryngoscopy: illustration with mirror reversal of vocal folds and key anatomic landmarks.

SOURCE: Aronson AE: *Clinical Voice Disorders,* p. 242. Thieme, New York, 1990.

TABLE 7.20. Inhalation (quiet): muscles used.

Name	Attachments	Innervation	Action
1. Diaphragm	1. Sternal: dorsal surface of lower part of sternum. 2. Costal: cartilaginous and bony portions of ribs 7–12. 3. Lumbar: Lumbar vertebrae. All converge and insert into central tendon.	Phrenic nerve from cervical plexus; contain fibers from 3rd, 4th, and 5th cervical nerves.	Draws central tendon down; increases volume, decreases pressure in thoracic cavity; presses against abdominal viscera protruding anterior abdominal region.
2. Scalenus anterior	From anterior tubercles of transverse processes of 3rd, 4th, 5th, 6th cervical vertebrae to scalene tubercle on inner border of first rib.	Branches of lower cervical nerves.	Fixes and raises first rib; bends and slightly rotates the neck.
3. Scalenus medius	From posterior tubercles of transverse processes of lower six cervical vertebrae to upper surface of first rib.	Branches of lower cervical nerves.	Fixes and raises first rib; bends and slightly rotates the neck.
4. Scalenus posterior	From posterior tubercles of transverse processes of lower two or three cervical vertebrae to outer surface of second rib behind attachment of serratus anterior.	Phrenic nerve from cervical plexus; contain fibers from 3rd, 4th, and 5th cervical nerves.	Fixes and raises second rib; bends and slightly rotates neck.

5. Intercostales Externi	From lower borders of first 11 ribs to upper borders of last 11 ribs.	Intercostal nerves	Maintains constant distance between ribs in order to prevent bulging or retraction during changes of intrathoracic pressures. Alter distances between ribs during postural changes.
6. Intercostales interni	From ridge on inner surface of a rib or the corresponding costal cartilage to upper border of rib below.	Intercostal nerves	Maintains constant distance between ribs in order to prevent bulging or retraction during changes of intrathoracic pressure. Alter distances between ribs during postural changes.

SOURCE: Aronson AE: *Clinical Voice Disorders*, p. 356. Thieme, New York, 1990.

TABLE 7.21. **Iowa Pressure Articulation Test items.**

Single items	Two-element items	Three-element items
s−	sk−	str−
−k−	sm−, −sm, sn−	−mps
ʃ−, −z−	−kɚ, st−	
−s−, −ʃ−	kr−	
−g−, −s	sp−, tr−, gr−, −gɚ,	
k−, g−, −g	−ɚk, −pt, kl−, gl−	
−ʃ, dʒ−	−ʃɚ, bl−, −ks	
−k	br−, dr−, tw−	
t−, −f−, −f	−pɚ, pl−, −lf	

SOURCE: With permission from Morris HL, Spriestersbach DC, Darley FL: Assessing Competency of Velopharyngeal Closure. *Journal of Speech and Hearing Research* 1961; 4:54.

Note. These 43 items constitute the Iowa Pressure Articulation Test. Items are arranged in descending order of group differences. *Certain Language Skills in Children* by M.C. Templin, 1957, Minneapolis: University of Minnesota Press. From "Articulation Test for Assessing Competency of Velopharyngeal Closure" by H.L. Morris, D.C. Spriestersbach, and F.L. Darley, 1961, *Journal of Speech and Hearing Research, 4,* p. 54.

TABLE 7.22. **Laryngeal dimensions.***

	Infancy (mm)	Puberty (mm)	ADULT Male (mm)	ADULT Female (mm)
VOCAL CORD—LENGTH	6–8	12–15	17–23	12.5–17
Membranous portion	3–4	7–8	11.5–16	8–11.5
Cartilaginous portion	3–4	5–7	5.5–7	4.5–5.5
GLOTTIS—WIDTH AT REST	3	5	8	6
Maximum	6	12	19	13
INFRAGLOTTIS—SAGITTAL	5–7	15	25	18
Transverse	5–7	15	24	17

SOURCE: Aronson AE: *Clinical Voice Disorders,* p. 44. Thieme, New York, 1990.

*From Ballenger JJ: *Diseases of the Nose, Throat and Ear.* Philadelphia, Lea & Febiger, 1969, p. 275.

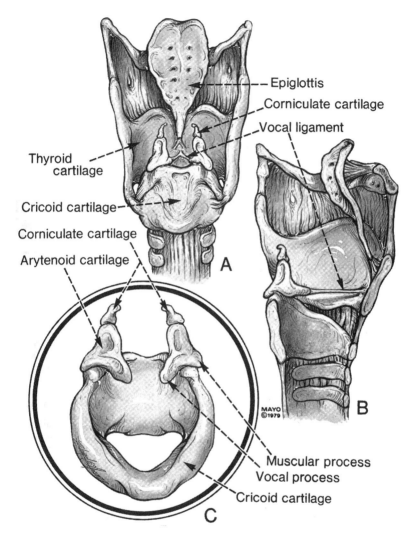

FIGURE 7.7. Laryngeal cartilages: diagram (without cuneiform cartilages shown).
SOURCE: Aronson AE: *Clinical Voice Disorders,* p. 15. Thieme, New York, 1990.

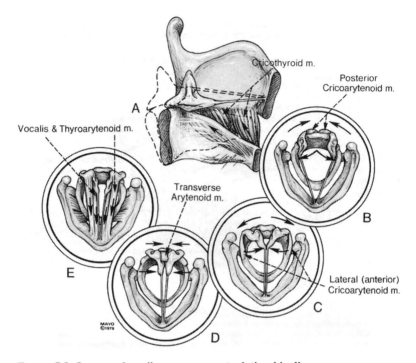

FIGURE 7.8. Laryngeal cartilages: movement relationship diagram.
SOURCE: Aronson AE: *Clinical Voice Disorders,* p. 24. Thieme, New York, 1990.

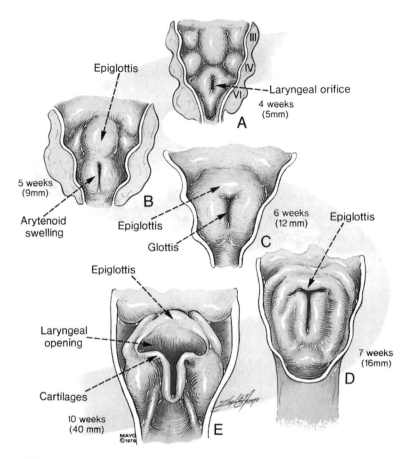

FIGURE 7.9. Laryngeal development: embryological stages.
SOURCE: Aronson AE: *Clinical Voice Disorders,* p. 22. Thieme, New York, 1990.

TABLE 7.23. **Myasthenia gravis–flaccid dysarthria: laryngeal–phonatory characteristics.**

	Findings
PERCEPTUAL	
Phonation	Breathy voice quality, weak intensity. Deterioration of phonation during stressful counting or other prolonged speaking activities; reduced sharpness of cough after stressful speaking. Can exist in the absence of remaining signs of dysarthria.
Resonation	Initially normal; hypernasality develops after stressful speaking.
Articulation	Initially normal; articulatory imprecision develops after stressful speaking.
Language	Normal.
PHYSICAL	
Larynx	In milder cases, vocal folds may appear normal in structure and function despite dysphonia; absence of positive laryngologic findings does not exclude presence of milder degrees of bilateral adductor weakness of vocal folds. In more severe cases, folds may fail to adduct and abduct completely, bilaterally. Bowing may be present.
Velopharynx	Initially normal; velopharyngeal insufficiency after stressful speaking. Hypoactive gag reflex.
Tongue	Initially normal; tongue weakness after stressful speaking.
Lips	Initially normal; lip weakness after stressful speaking; lateral smile.
Teeth	Normal.
Hard palate	Normal.
Mandible	Initially normal; mandibular muscle weakness after stressful speaking.
GENERAL MEDICAL	Patient may complain of general fatigue, particularly after exercise. Findings can be nonspecific, leading to erroneous diagnosis of functional illness.
OTHER NEUROLOGICAL SIGNS	
Peripheral nervous system	Weakness of bulbar musculature; positive Tensilon test.
Central nervous system	Normal.
PSYCHIATRIC/PSYCHOLOGICAL	Patient may complain of fatigue, loss of energy, or loss of interest, which may be erroneously diagnosed as signs of primary depression. Patients may become secondarily depressed about lack of energy.

SOURCE: Aronson AE: *Clinical Voice Disorders,* p. 88. Thieme, New York, 1990.

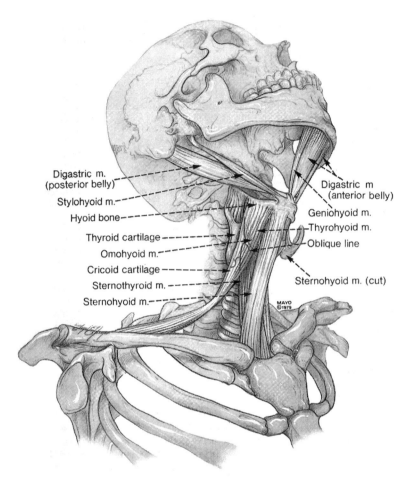

FIGURE 7.10. Laryngeal muscles (extrinsic): diagram (without mylohyoid and stylopharyngeal muscles shown).

SOURCE: Aronson AE: *Clinical Voice Disorders,* p. 17. Thieme, New York, 1990.

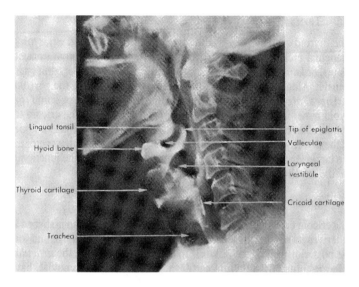

FIGURE 7.11. Larynx and hyoid bone in relationship to cervical vertebrae: lateral radiograph of the head and neck.

SOURCE: Aronson AE: *Clinical Voice Disorders,* p. 14. Thieme, New York, 1990.

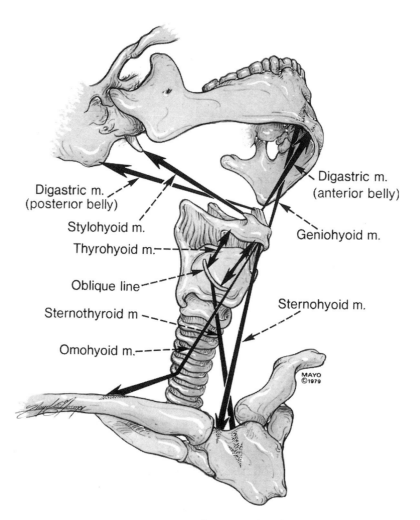

Digastric m.
(posterior belly)

Stylohyoid m.

Thyrohyoid m.

Oblique line

Sternothyroid m

Omohyoid m.

Digastric m.
(anterior belly)

Geniohyoid m.

Sternohyoid m.

MAYO
©1979

FIGURE 7.12. Larynx and hyoid bone: sling suspension diagram.
SOURCE: Aronson AE: *Clinical Voice Disorders,* p. 23. Thieme, New York, 1990.

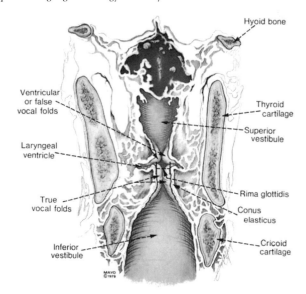

FIGURE 7.13. Larynx: coronal section.
SOURCE: Aronson AE: *Clinical Voice Disorders,* p. 19. Thieme, New York, 1990.

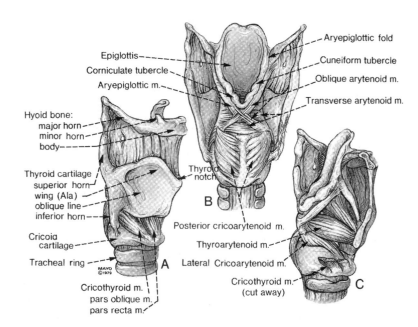

FIGURE 7.14. Larynx: lateral and posterior views.
SOURCE: Aronson AE: *Clinical Voice Disorders,* p. 14. Thieme, New York, 1990.

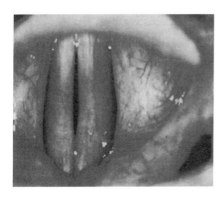

FIGURE 7.15. Larynx: normal view during phonation.
SOURCE: Aronson AE: *Clinical Voice Disorders,* p. 19. Thieme, New York, 1990.

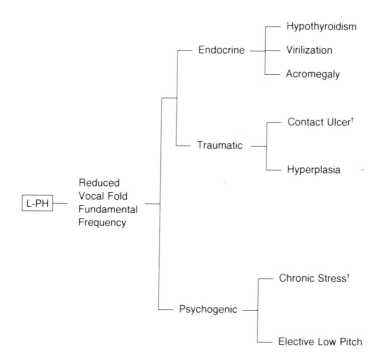

FIGURE 7.16. Low-pitch hoarse voice: analysis schema.
*Important to note that chronic stress is a causative factor in the development of contact ulcer.
SOURCE: Aronson AE: *Clinical Voice Disorders,* p. 304. Thieme, New York, 1990.

TABLE 7.24. **My grandfather.**

You wish to know all about my grandfather. Well, he is nearly 93 years old; he dresses himself in an ancient black frock coat, usually minus several buttons; yet he still thinks as swiftly as ever. A long, flowing beard clings to his chin, giving those who observe him a pronounced feeling of the utmost respect. When he speaks, his voice is just a bit cracked and quivers a trifle. Twice a day, he plays skillfully and with zest upon our small organ. Except in the winter when the cold or snow or ice prevents, he slowly takes a short walk in the open air each day. We have often urged him to walk more and smoke less, but he always answers, "Banana oil." Grandfather likes to be modern in his language.

TABLE 7.25. **Nasal resonatory disorders: etiology.**

HYPERNASALITY AND NASAL EMISSION
    Organic
        Anatomic
            Overt cleft palate with or without cleft lip.
            Submucous cleft palate.
            Congenitally short soft palate or large nasopharynx.
            Traumatic structural damage.
        Neurological (dysarthria)
            Lower motor neuron (flaccid).
            Unilateral upper motor neuron (flaccid).
            Bilateral upper motor neuron (spastic).
            Mixed lower-upper motor neuron (flaccid–spastic).
            Hyperkinetic (dystonic–choreic).
        Psychogenic
            Conversion reaction
            Immature personality
            Poor motivation
            Imitative
HYPONASALITY
    Organic
        Hypertrophied adenoids
        Tumors
        Inflammations
        Postsurgical repair
        Patulous eustachian tube
        Nasal deformity
MIXED NASALITY
    Combinations of organic etiologies of hypernasality and hyponasality.

SOURCE: Aronson AE: *Clinical Voice Disorders,* p. 199. Thieme, New York, 1990.

Voice • 357

TABLE 7.26. Palatopharyngolaryngeal myoclonus–hyperkinetic dysarthria: Laryngeal–phonatory characteristics.

	Findings
PERCEPTUAL	
Phonation	Momentary voice arrests during contextual speech if severe, but often undetectable under this condition. On vowel prolongation, momentary voice arrests occur rhythmically, ranging from 60 to 240 beats per minute (1 to 4 c./sec). *Note:* Because often undetectable during contextual speech, vowel prolongation must be tested in all suspected cases.
Resonation	Normal
Articulation	Normal. Patient may have articulatory defects of flaccid, spastic, or ataxic dysarthria.
Language	Normal
PHYSICAL	
Larynx*	Vocal folds adduct rhythmically and momentarily on vowel prolongation, synchronously with voice arrests. Myoclonic movements of larynx and pharynx can be seen observing the movements beneath the skin of the neck.
Velopharynx*	Soft palate elevates and falls, and lateral pharyngeal walls adduct and abduct synchronously with laryngeal movements.
Tongue	Normal. May enter into myoclonic movements in synchrony with above structures.
Lips	Normal
Teeth	Normal
Hard palate	Normal
Mandible	Normal
GENERAL MEDICAL	Nonspecific
OTHER NEUROLOGICAL SIGNS	
Peripheral nervous system	Normal
Central nervous system	Other signs of brain stem lesion may be present or absent.
PSYCHIATRIC/PSYCHOLOGICAL	Normal

SOURCE: Aronson AE: *Clinical Voice Disorders*, p. 105. Thieme, New York, 1990.

*In order to detect presence of this syndrome, observation of the oral musculature while patient is quiet and holding mouth open as steadily as possible is imperative; *myoclonic* movements are present at rest as well as during phonation.

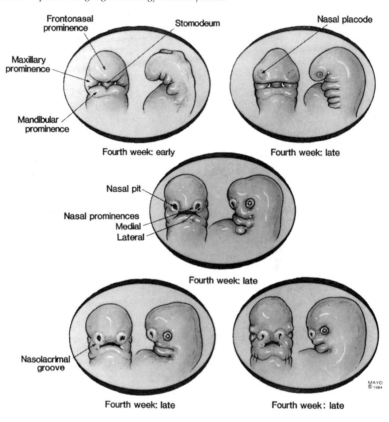

FIGURE 7.17a–d. Palate and face development during embryonic and fetal stages.
SOURCE: Aronson AE: *Clinical Voice Disorders,* pp. 209–211. Thieme, New York, 1990.

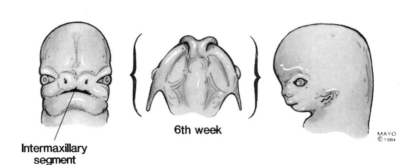

FIGURE 7.17b.

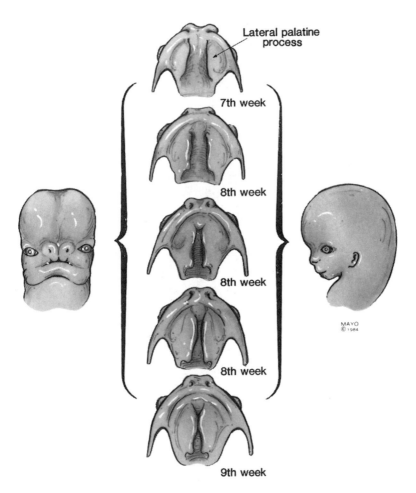

Lateral palatine process

7th week

8th week

8th week

8th week

9th week

MAYO
© 1984

FIGURE 7.17c.

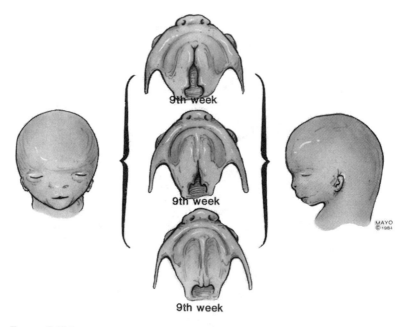

FIGURE 7.17d.

TABLE 7.27. **Parkinsonism–hypokinetic dysarthria: laryngeal–phonatory characteristics.**

	Findings
PERCEPTUAL	
Phonation	Monopitch, reduced stress, monoloudness, reduced loudness, harsh quality. *Note:* Reduced loudness and breathiness in the absence of other neurologic signs can indicate early parkinsonism.
Resonation	Normal
Articulation	Imprecise consonants; short rushes of speech; accelerated rate; stuttering-like repetitions of syllables, words, or phrases (palilalia).
Language	Usually normal. Language functions may be decreased as part of overall slowing of general intellectual processes.
PHYSICAL	
Larynx	Vocal folds appear normal in structure. Adductor, abductor movements are bilaterally symmetric, but there may be incomplete closure of vocal folds accounting for breathy voice quality.
Velopharynx	Normal
Tongue	Topographically normal. AMRs for /tʌ/ and /kʌ/ sound rapid and are reduced in amplitude of movement.
Lips	AMRs for /pʌ/ sound rapid and are reduced in amplitude of movement.
Teeth	Normal
Hard palate	Normal
Mandible	Reduced range of motion during articulation.
GENERAL MEDICAL	Nonspecific
OTHER NEUROLOGICAL SIGNS	
Peripheral nervous system	Normal
Central nervous system	Signs of hypokinesia elsewhere in the body. *Note: Hypokinetic dysarthria in the form of dysphonia only can be the first sign of early parkinsonism.*
PSYCHIATRIC/PSYCHOLOGICAL	Nonspecific. Masked facies may give the erroneous impression of flatness of affect or of depression.

SOURCE: Aronson AE: *Clinical Voice Disorders*, p. 97. Thieme, New York, 1990.

TABLE 7.28. Pseudobulbar (spastic) dysarthria: laryngeal–phonatory characteristics.

	Findings
PERCEPTUAL	
Phonation	Hoarseness or harshness having a strained–strangled quality. Pitch is abnormally low. Monopitch. Loudness is reduced. Monoloudness. Almost never occurs without accompanying signs of dysarthria. Inappropriate crying or laughter may be present.
Resonation	Hypernasality
Articulation	Imprecise consonants; abnormally slow rate.
Language	Normal, provided language areas are spared.
PHYSICAL	
Larynx	Vocal folds appear normal in structure. Normal to hyperadduction of true and false vocal folds may occur bilaterally.
Velopharynx	Bilateral velopharyngeal insufficiency. Hyperactive gag reflex.
Tongue	Topographically normal. May be smaller, more contracted than normal. Tongue weakness. Slow AMR on lateral movements and on /tʌ/ and /kʌ/ syllable repetitions.
Lips	Weak, slow movements on AMR for /pʌ/.
Teeth	Normal
Hard palate	Normal
Mandible	Slow AMR
GENERAL MEDICAL	Nonspecific
OTHER NEUROLOGICAL SIGNS	
Peripheral nervous system	Normal
Central nervous system	Signs of spasticity
PSYCHIATRIC/PSYCHOLOGICAL	Nonspecific. Pseudobulbar crying and laughter may give erroneous impression of emotional lability and intellectual deterioration.

SOURCE: Aronson AE: *Clinical Voice Disorders*, p. 92. Thieme, New York, 1990.

TABLE 7.29. Rainbow passage.

When the sunlight strikes raindrops in the air they act like a prism and form a rainbow. The rainbow is a division of white light into many beautiful colors. These take the shape of a long round arch, with its path high above, and its two ends apparently beyond the horizon. There is, according to legend, a boiling pot of gold at one end. People look, but no one ever finds it. When a man looks for something beyond his reach, his friends say he is looking for the pot of gold at the end of the rainbow.

SOURCE: With permission from Fairbanks G: *Voice and Articulation Drillbook*, p. 127. Addison-Wesley Educational Publishers, New York, 1960.

TABLE 7.30. /s/ and /z/ maximum duration data and s/z ratio information.*

Source	Subjects	MAXIMUM /s/ DURATION			MAXIMUM /z/ DURATION			s/z RATIO	
		M	SD	Range	M	SD	Range	M	Range
Tait et al (1980)	Girls, 5 years	8.3	4.0	4.8–18.3	10.0	3.3	5.2–16.0	0.83	0.50–1.14
	Boys, 5 years	7.9	1.4	5.4–9.8	8.6	2.1	6.6–13.0	0.92	0.82–1.08
	Girls, 7 years	10.2	2–6	7.3–16.0	13.1	4.0	9.1–20.0	0.78	0.51–1.10
	Boys, 7 years	9.3	1.7	7.4–12.5	13.2	3.6	9.2–19.6	0.70	0.52–0.97
	Girls, 9 years	14.4	3.1	9.3–20.9	15.8	5.2	8.5–24.2	0.91	0.75–1.26
	Boys, 9 years	16.7	8.5	7.1–44.0	18.1	6.8	10.1–33.1	0.92	0.41–2.67
Eckel & Boone (1981)	Mixed ages, both sexes	17.7	7.6	5–38	18.6	7.0	5–37	0.99	0.41–2.67
Young & Bless (1983)	Sedate geriatrics	14.7	4.4	7.7–21.6	19.3	8.4	10.2–35.6	0.76	—
	Active geriatrics	20.2	13.4	6.4–51.3	24.5	8.0	14.7–36.6	0.82	—

SOURCE: Kent RD: The Perceptual Sensorimotor Examination for Motor Speech Disorders. In McNeil MR (ed): *Clinical Management of Sensorimotor Disorders*, p. 36. Thieme, New York, 1997.

*Normative data on maximum /s/ and /z/ duration and the s/z ratio (all values in seconds). Reprinted from Kent et al (1987, p. 372), with permission from the American Speech–Language Hearing Association. See original article for sources.

TABLE 7.31. Tremor of organic (essential) origin hyperkinetic dysarthria: laryngeal–phonatory characteristics.

	Findings
PERCEPTUAL	
Phonation	Quavering or intermittent voice arrests during contextual speech. Rhythmic tremor and/or voice arrests on vowel prolongation ranging from approximately 4–7 c./sec. *Note:* In severe organic voice tremor the voice arrests take the form of severe laryngospasm that may be mistaken for the syndrome of spastic (spasmodic) dysphonia with voice arrests may show a smoothing out of these arrests into ordinary tremor when sustaining a vowel at a high pitch level. Fluctuating strained–hoarseness along with tremor in more severe cases.
Resonation	Normal
Articulation	Normal. May have irregular articulatory breakdowns reminiscent of ataxic dysarthria.
Language	Normal
PHYSICAL	
Larynx	Vocal folds appear normal in structure. On vowel prolongation, adductor–abductor oscillations synchronous with voice tremor can be seen as well as pharyngeal wall movements. Tremor movements of larynx can be seen under skin of neck, with the larynx oscillating vertically. Voice arrests occur at the maximum laryngeal height of each oscillation.
Velopharynx	Normal. Soft palate may move synchronously with laryngeal and pharyngeal tremor.
Tongue	Topographically normal. On vowel prolongation, tremor movements of tongue may be seen synchronously with laryngeal tremor.
Lips	Normal. May be tremorous.
Teeth	Normal
Hard palate	Normal
Mandible	Normal. May be tremorous.
GENERAL MEDICAL	Nonspecific
OTHER NEUROLOGICAL SIGNS	
Peripheral nervous system	Normal
Central nervous system	Head and hand tremor, unilateral or bilateral may be present. *Note:* Organic voice tremor may occur as an isolated sign, which is prone to misinterpretation as being psychogenic.
PSYCHIATRIC/PSYCHOLOGICAL	Many patients report onset of voice, head, or hand tremor following an emotionally stressful life event. There is a danger of interpreting such events as proof that the tremor is psychogenic.

SOURCE: Aronson AE: *Clinical Voice Disorders*, p. 103. Thieme, New York, 1990.

TABLE 7.32. Vagus nerve lesions: effects on phonation and resonation.*

| | EFFECT ON VOCAL FOLDS | | EFFECT ON PHONATION | |
Level of lesion	Unilateral lesion	Bilateral lesions	Unilateral lesion	Bilateral lesions
I. Above origin of pharyngeal, superior laryngeal, and recurrent laryngeal nerves	One vocal fold fixed in abducted position.	Both vocal folds fixed in abducted position.	Breathy, moderate, reduced loudness and pitch.	Extremely breathy to whispered (aphonia).
II. Above origin of superior laryngeal and recurrent laryngeal nerves but below origin of pharyngeal nerve	Same as above.	Same as above.	Same as above.	Same as above.
III. Superior laryngeal nerve	Both vocal folds able to adduct, affected vocal fold shorter, asymmetric shift of epiglottis and anterior larynx toward intact side on phonation.	Absence of tilt of thyroid on cricoid cartilage, inability to view full length of vocal folds because of epiglottic overhang, vocal folds bowed.	Breathy, hoarse.	Breathy, hoarse, reduced loudness, restricted pitch range.
IV. Recurrent laryngeal nerve	One vocal fold fixed in paramethan position.	Both vocal folds fixed in paramethan position.	Breathy, hoarse, reduced loudness, diplophonia (not in all cases).	Breathy, hoarse, reduced loudness.
V. Myoneural junction (myasthenia gravis)	Not applicable.	Restriction of adductor–abductor movements.	Not applicable.	Breathy, hoarse, reduced loudness; symptoms worsen with sustained speaking.

(continued)

SOURCE: Aronson AE: *Clinical Voice Disorders*, pp. 78–79. Thieme, New York, 1990.
*Information in this table abstracted from Rontal M, Rontal E: Lesions of the Vague Nerve: Diagnosis, Treatment and Rehabilitation. *Laryngoscope* 87:72–86, 1977, and from Ward PH, Berci G, Calcaterra JC: Superior Laryngeal Nerve Paralysis: An Often Overlooked Entity. *Trans. Am. Aced. Ophthalmol. Otolaryngol.* 84: 78–89, 1977.

TABLE 7.32. (*continued*) **Vagus nerve lesions: effects on phonation and resonation*** (soft palate, nasal resonance, and associated signs)

Level of lesion	EFFECT ON SOFT PALATE		Effect on nasal resonation	Associated signs
	Unilateral lesion	*Bilateral lesions*		
I. Above origin of pharyngeal, superior laryngeal, and recurrent laryngeal nerves	One side low, immobile	Both sides low, immobile	Hypernasality, nasal emission	Glottal coup and cough absent, weak, or mushy; difficulty in swallowing; nasal regurgitation of food; aspiration of secretions; pharyngeal paralysis.
II. Above origin of superior laryngeal and recurrent laryngeal nerves but below origin of pharyngeal nerve	None	None	None	Same as above, except no pharyngeal paralysis or difficulty in swallowing.
III. Superior laryngeal nerve	None	None	None	None
IV. Recurrent laryngeal nerve	None	None	None	Unilateral: Marginal airway, weak cough. Bilateral: Severe difficulty on inhaling for life purposes, inhalatory stridor, tracheostomy often necessary.
V. Myoneural junction (myasthenia gravis)	Not applicable	Both sides low, immobile	Hypernasality, nasal emission; symptoms worsen with sustained speaking.	Difficulty in swallowing, nasal regurgitation of food, inhalatory stridor, articulation defects.

SOURCE: Aronson AE: *Clinical Voice Disorders*, pp. 78–79. Thieme, New York, 1990.
*Information in this table abstracted from Rontal M, Rontal E: Lesions of the Vague Nerve: Diagnosis, Treatment and Rehabilitation. *Laryngoscope* 87:72–86, 1977, and from Ward PH, Berci G, Calcaterra JC: Superior Laryngeal Nerve Paralysis: An Often Overlooked Entity. *Trans. Am. Aced. Ophthalmol. Otolaryngol.* 84: 78–89, 1977.

TABLE 7.33. Voice attributes: definitions and rating criteria.

Name of Attribute	Definition of Attribute
Tremor[a]	Rapidly occurring fluctuations in pitch and/or loudness, giving an impression of a tremulous voice.
Waver[a]	Consistent pattern of slow, gradual, rise–fall fluctuations in pitch and/or loudness resulting in a rhythmic modulation, which is slower than that seen for tremor.
Rough–fry[a]	A rough or unpleasant voice quality in low-pitched phonations. May or may not be associated with a rhythmic beating or crackling phenomenon of glottal fry.
Wet–hoarse[a]	A wet, liquid-sounding, unpleasant, and rough voice quality.
Harsh–shrill[a]	A rough or unpleasant, strident, metallic, or grating voice quality occurring in relatively high-pitched phonations, sometimes associated with a hard glottal attack.
Breathy[a]	Audible escape of air resulting in a thin, weak phonation, related to a functional inability to firmly adduct the vocal folds.
Strain–strangle[a]	Phonation gives the impression of an effortful squeezing of the voice through the glottis.
Pitch level[b]	Overall pitch level of phonation as compared to a synthesized vowel phonation appropriate for individual's age and sex.
Loudness level[b]	Overall loudness level of phonation as compared to a synthesized vowel presented at 80 dBC SPL (re: 20 micropascals).
Pitch breaks[c]	Voice shows an abrupt break in phonation. This break may involve an upward or downward shift in voice register or a momentary voice stoppage.
Nasality[d]	Amount of perceived nasal cavity resonance associated with vowel phonation.
Pitch stability[e]	The amount of pitch variation occurring within the vowel phonation.
Loudness stability[e]	The amount of loudness variation occurring within the vowel phonation.

a. Rating criteria
 1. Dimension is absent.
 2. Dimension is noticeably present but occurs to a mild degree in]el, than 25% of phonation duration.
 3. Dimension is present to a mild or moderate degree in over 25% of the phonation duration.
 4. Dimension is present to a severe degree in over 25% of the phonation duration.
b. Rating criteria
 1. Severely low pitch or soft loudness level associated with 25% or more of phonation duration.
 2. Mild or moderately lowered pitch or loudness in 25% or more of phonation.
 3. Inconsistent and/or slightly lowered pitch or loudness.
 4. Pitch or loudness is identical to the synthesized vowel.
 5. Pitch or loudness slightly higher than synthesized vowel in less than 25% of phonation duration.
 6. Mild to moderately raised pitch or loudness in more than 25% of phonation duration.
 7. Severely raised pitch or loudness associated with more than 25% of phonation duration.

(continued)

TABLE 7.33. (*continued*)

---

c. Rating criteria
  1. No pitch breaks occur during phonation.
  2. One pitch break occurs.
  3. Two or three pitch breaks occur.
  4. Four or more pitch breaks occur.
d. Rating criteria
  1. Normal amount of nasal resonance.
  2. Inconsistent (< 25% of phonation duration and mildly excessive amount of nasal cavity resonance.
  3. Consistent (> 25% of phonation duration) and mildly excessive amount of nasal cavity resonance.
  4. Consistent and severe degree of nasal resonance associated with phonation.
e. Rating criteria
  1. Pitch (loudness) falling steadily throughout more than 25% of the phonation duration.
  2. Slight fall in pitch (loudness) occurring in less than 25% of the phonation duration.
  3. Pitch (loudness) has inconsistent, mild rise–fall fluctuation or remains relatively stable throughout phonation.
  4. A slight rise in pitch (loudness) occurring in over 25% of phonation duration.
  5. Pitch (loudness) consistently (> 25%) rises to a moderate degree over the duration of vowel phonation.

SOURCE: With permission from Bassich CJ, Ludlow CL: The Use of Perceptual Methods for Assessing Voice Quality. *Journal of Speech and Hearing Disorders* 1986; 51:133.

TABLE 7.34. Voice disorders: behavioral and organic classifications.

Behavioural	Organic
1. *Excessive muscular tension* No changes in laryngeal mucosa	1. *Structural abnormalities* Laryngeal web Cleft palate Nasal obstruction Trauma
2. *Excessive muscular tension—* *changes in laryngeal mucosa* Vocal nodules Chronic laryngitis Oedema Polyps Contact ulcers	2. *Neurological conditions* Recurrent laryngeal nerve paralysis Pseudobulbar palsy Bulbar palsy Cerebellar ataxia Tremor Parkinsonism Chorea Athetosis Apraxia Multiple lesions (eg, motor neuron disease, multiple sclerosis)
3. *Psychogenic* Anxiety state Neurosis Conversion symptoms Delayed pubertal voice change (puberphonia) Transsexual conflict	3. *Endocrinological disorders* Thyrotoxicosis Myxoedema Male sexual mutational retardation Female virilization due to adverse hormone therapy Adverse drug therapy
	4. *Laryngeal disease* Tumor—benign/malignant Hyperkeratosis Papillomatosis Cyst Laryngitis—acute/chronic Cricoarytenoid arthritis Granuloma Fungal infection

SOURCE: With permission from Fawcus M: The Causes and Classification of Voice Disorders. In Fawcus M (ed): *Voice Disorders and Their Management*, p. 34. Singular Publishing Group, Inc., San Diego, 1992.

TABLE 7.35. Voice pathology: definition of terms.

Aperiodic: vibrations occurring at irregular periods.

Diplophonia: phonation at two different pitch levels due to asynchronous vibration of the vocal folds.

Elasticity: tendency to return to original shape after deformation under stress.

Formant: vocal tract resonance; formants are displayed in a spectrogram as broad bands of energy.

Frequency: cycles per second; acoustic correlate of pitch.

Fundamental frequency: the lowest frequency component of a complex tone.

Glottal attack: a mode of initiation of voicing in which the vocal folds are abruptly and tightly adducted at onset.

Harmonic: an oscillation whose frequency is an integral multiple of the fundamental.

Intensity: magnitude of sound expressed in power or pressure; acoustic correlate of loudness.

Periodic: vibrations recurring at equal intervals of time.

Vocal break: abrupt involuntary shift of voice to a higher or lower pitch.

Vocal registers: distinctive ranges of phonation, including pulse (lowest down to glottal fry), modal (normally used in speaking and singing), and loft (highest including falsetto).

Voice quality types: breathy (weak, airy voice due to glottal incompetence), harsh (strained voice produced with excessive vocal fold tension), hoarse (harsh and breathy voice due to combination of aperiodic vocal fold vibration and excessive air escape).

SOURCE: Kay MH, Hicks DM: Voice Pathology. In Tucker HM (ed): *The Larynx*, 2nd ed., p. 136. Thieme, New York, 1993.

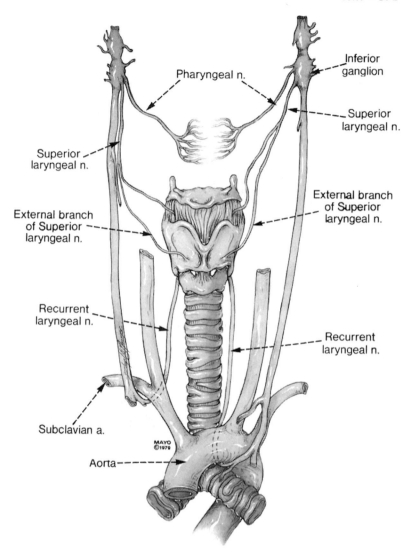

FIGURE 7.18. Recurrent laryngeal nerves: asymmetric pathways left and right.
Source: Aronson AE: *Clinical Voice Disorders,* p. 74. Thieme, New York, 1990.

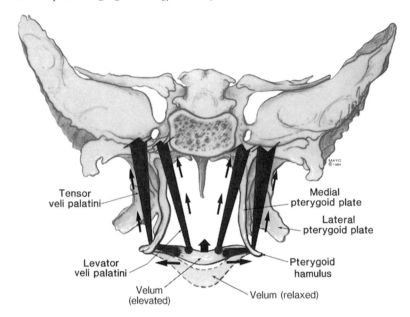

FIGURE 7.19. Sphenoid bone and schematic drawing of levator and tensor veli palatini muscles: posterior view.
SOURCE: Aronson AE: *Clinical Voice Disorders,* p. 203. Thieme, New York, 1990.

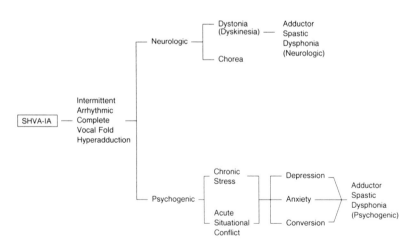

FIGURE 7.20. Strained hoarse voice arrest (intermittent *arrhythmic*): analysis schema.
SOURCE: Aronson AE: *Clinical Voice Disorders,* p. 286. Thieme, New York, 1990.

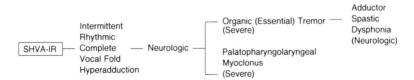

FIGURE 7.21. Strained hoarse voice arrest (intermittent rhythmic): analysis schema.
SOURCE: Aronson AE: *Clinical Voice Disorders,* p. 297. Thieme, New York, 1990.

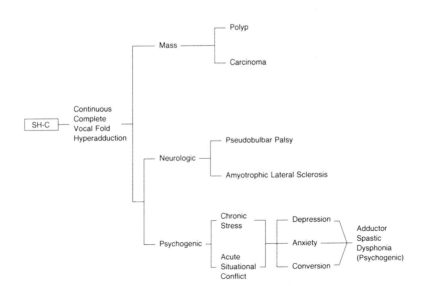

FIGURE 7.22. Strained hoarse voice arrest (continuous): analysis schema.
SOURCE: Aronson AE: *Clinical Voice Disorders,* p. 283. Thieme, New York, 1990.

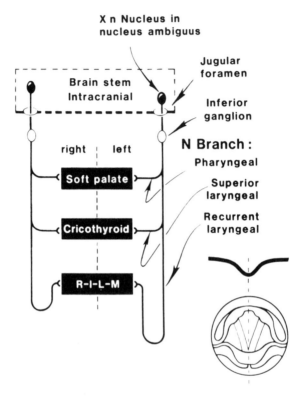

FIGURE 7.23. Vagus nerve pathway from brain stem to larynx (without lesion). R-I-L-M: remaining intrinsic laryngeal muscles.

SOURCE: Aronson AE: *Clinical Voice Disorders,* p. 73. Thieme, New York, 1990.

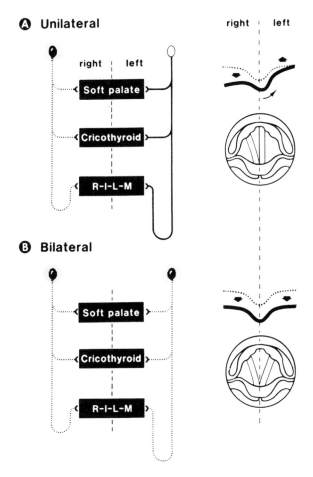

FIGURE 7.24. Vagus nerve (level I) unilateral and bilateral lesions (see corresponding information Table 7.32).

A: Unilateral lesion of vagus nerve (nucleus), above origin of pharyngeal, superior laryngeal, and recurrent laryngeal nerves. The right vocal fold is fixed in an abducted position, whereas the left adducts to the midline on phonation. The soft palate is paralyzed on the right, is resting low, and pulls to the left on phonation. B: Bilateral lesion. Both vocal folds are fixed in an abducted position on phonation. The soft palate is bilaterally paralyzed, is resting low, and does not move on phonation. R-I-L-M: remaining intrinsic laryngeal musculature.

SOURCE: Aronson AE: *Clinical Voice Disorders*, p. 76. Thieme, New York, 1990.

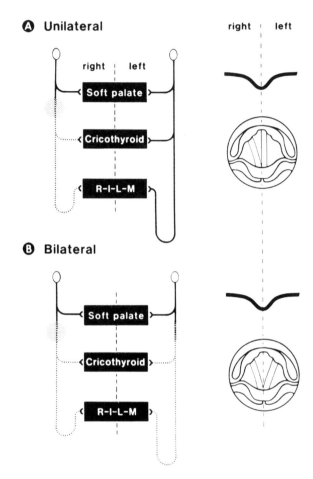

FIGURE 7.25. Vagus nerve (level II) unilateral and bilateral lesions (see corresponding information Table 7.32).

A: Unilateral lesion of vagus nerve above origin of superior laryngeal and recurrent laryngeal nerves, but below bifurcation of pharyngeal nerve. Same effect on vocal folds as 7.24A, but soft palate functions normally. B: Bilateral lesion. Same effects on vocal folds as 7-24B, but soft palate functions normally.

SOURCE: Aronson AE: *Clinical Voice Disorders,* p. 77. Thieme, New York, 1990.

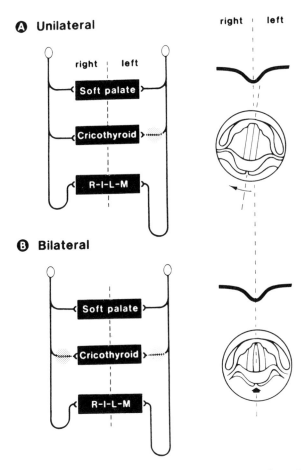

FIGURE 7.26. Vagus nerve (level III) superior laryngeal nerve unilateral and bilateral lesions (see corresponding information Table 7.32.

A: Unilateral lesion of superior laryngeal nerve. Both vocal folds adduct, but the anterior larynx twists toward the intact side on phonation. The soft palate is normal. B: Bilateral lesion. Both vocal folds adduct but are partially obscured by epiglottic overhang. Vocal folds are bowed. The soft palate is normal.

SOURCE: Aronson AE: *Clinical Voice Disorders,* p. 80. Thieme, New York, 1990.

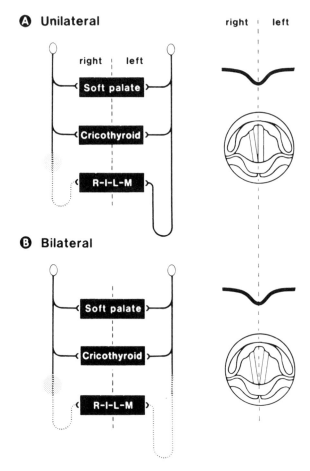

Ⓐ Unilateral

Ⓑ Bilateral

FIGURE 7.27. **Vagus nerve (level IV) recurrent laryngeal nerve (level IV) unilateral and bilateral lesions (see corresponding information Table 7.32).**

A: Unilateral lesion of recurrent laryngeal nerve. One vocal fold is fixed in a paramedian position on phonation, whereas the other adducts to the midline. The soft palate is normal. B: Bilateral lesion. Both vocal folds are fixed in a paramedian position on phonation. The soft palate is normal.

SOURCE: Aronson AE: *Clinical Voice Disorders,* p. 81. Thieme, New York, 1990.

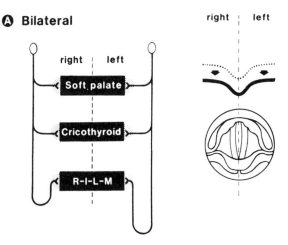

FIGURE 7.28. Vagus nerve (level V) myoneural junction bilateral lesions (see corresponding information Table 7.32).

There is bilateral paresis or paralysis of both abductor and abductor vocal fold movements on phonation and reduced or absent soft palate function.

SOURCE: Aronson AE: *Clinical Voice Disorders,* p. 81. Thieme, New York, 1990.

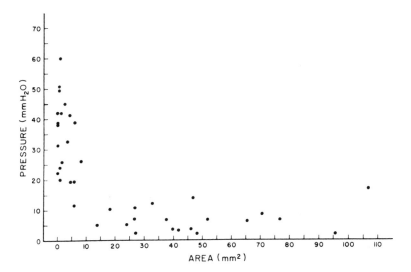

FIGURE 7.29. Velopharyngeal orifice size and intraoral pressure during consonant productions.

SOURCE: Aronson AE: *Clinical Voice Disorders,* p. 208. Thieme, New York, 1990.

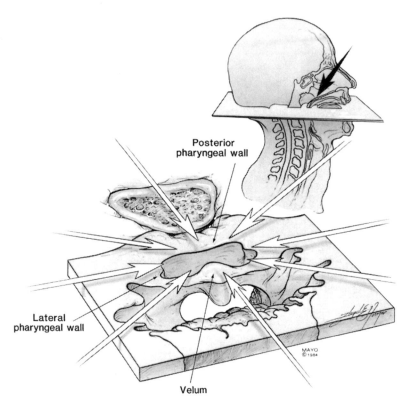

FIGURE 7.30. Velopharyngeal port: three-dimensional view of section.
SOURCE: Aronson AE: *Clinical Voice Disorders,* p. 201. Thieme, New York, 1990.

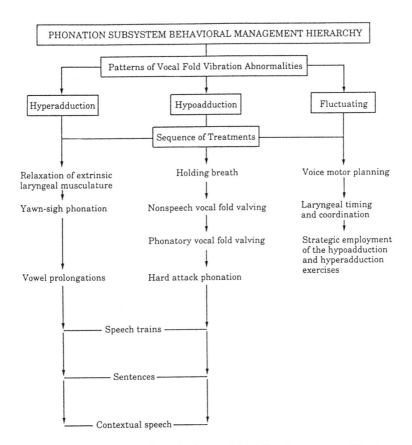

FIGURE 7.31. Voice therapy hierarchy for vocal fold vibration abnormalities: hyperadduction, hypoadduction, and fluctuation.
SOURCE: With permission from Dworkin JP: *Motor Speech Disorders: A Treatment Guide*, p. 183. Mosby Year Book, St. Louis, 1991.

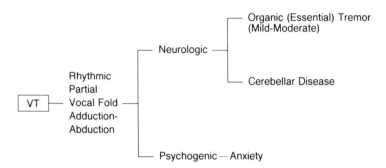

FIGURE 7.32. Voice tremor analysis schema.
SOURCE: Aronson AE: *Clinical Voice Disorders,* p. 299. Thieme, New York, 1990.

TABLE 7.36. **Voice Rating Scale.**

GRABS Voice Rating Scale

GRADE: degree of hoarseness or voice abnormality

0	1	2	3
Normal	Slight	Moderate	Extreme

ROUGH: auditory/acoustic impression of irregularity of vibration (jitter and shimmer)

0	1	2	3
Normal	Slight	Moderate	Extreme

BREATH: auditory/acoustic impression of degree of air leakage (related to turbulence)

0	1	2	3
Normal	Slight	Moderate	Extreme

ASTHENIC: weakness or lack of power (related to vocal intensity and energy in higher harmonics)

0	1	2	3
Normal	Slight	Moderate	Extreme

STRAINED: auditory/acoustic impression of hyperfunction (related to fundamental frequency, noise in high-frequency range, and energy in higher harmonics)

0	1	2	3
Normal	Slight	Moderate	Extreme

Check for presence of the following:

[   ] tremor   [   ] pitch variation   [   ] loudness variation
[   ] voice interruption   [   ] other: specify _____

SOURCE: Kent RD: The Perceptual Sensorimotor Examination for Motor Speech Disorders. In McNeil MR (ed): *Clinical Management of Sensorimotor Disorders,* p. 46. Thieme, New York, 1997.

TABLE 7.37. **Zoo passage.**

Look at this book with us. It's a story about a zoo. That is where bears go. Today it's very cold out of doors, but we see a cloud overhead that's a pretty, white fluffy shape. We hear straw covers the floor of cages to keep the chill away; yet a deer walks through the trees with her head high. They feed seeds to birds so they're able to fly.

SOURCE: With permission from Fletcher SG: *Diagnosing Speech Disorders from Cleft Palate,* Appendix B. W.B. Saunders, 1978.

8

Oralfacial Structure and Function

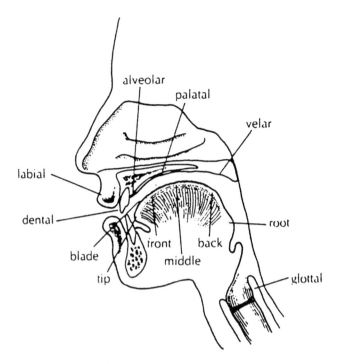

FIGURE 8.1. Articulatory places of constriction or contact.

SOURCE: From Creaghead NA, Newman PW, Secord WA: *Assessment and Remediation of Articulatory and Phonological Disorders,* 2nd ed. Copyright © 1989 by Allyn and Bacon. Reprinted/adapted by permission.

TABLE 8.1. **Dentition eruption sequence and average age of eruption.**

Tooth	Age of Eruption
Deciduous	
Lower central incisors (2)	6 months
Upper central incisors (2)	7 months
Lower lateral incisors (2)	7 months
Upper lateral incisors (2)	8 months
Lower first molars (2)	12 months
Upper first molars (2)	14 months
Lower canines (2)	16 months
Upper canines (2)	18 months
Lower second molars (2)	20 months
Upper first molars (2)	22 months
Permanent	
Lower first molars (2)	6 years
Upper first molars (2)	6 years
Lower central incisors (2)	6 years
Upper central incisors (2)	7 years
Lower lateral incisors (2)	7 years
Upper lateral incisors (2)	8 years
Lower 2st and 2nd premolars (4)	10–11 years
Upper 1st and 2nd premolars (4)	10–11 years
Lower 2nd molars	12 years
Upper 2nd molars	12 years
Lower and upper 3rd molars	17–25 years

SOURCE: Moller KT: Dental-Occlusal and Other Oral Conditions and speech. In Bernthal JE, Bankson NW (eds): *Child Phonology: Characteristics, Assessment, and Intervention with Special Populations,* p. 6. Thieme, New York, 1994.

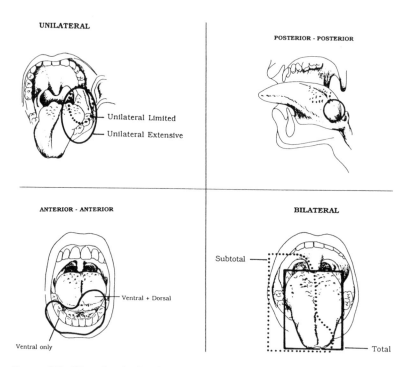

FIGURE 8.2. Glossal and related resection: major categories with approximate site and extent for each indicated in marked areas.

SOURCE: Leonard RJ: Characteristics of Speech in Speakers with Glossectomy and Other Oral/Oropharyngeal Ablation. In Bernthal JE, Bankson NW (eds): *Child Phonology: Characteristics, Assessment, and Intervention with Special Populations,* p. 62. Thieme, New York, 1994.

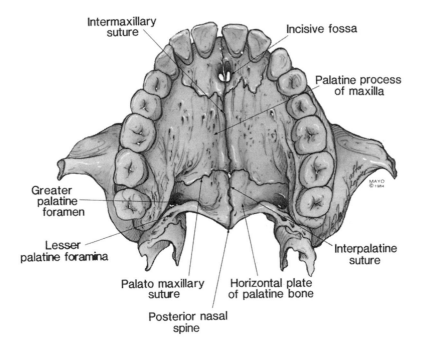

FIGURE 8.3. Hard palate: inferior view.
SOURCE: Aronson AE: *Clinical Voice Disorders,* p. 203. Thieme, New York, 1990.

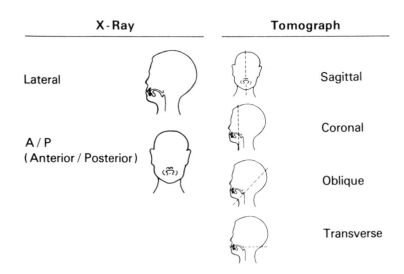

X - Ray	Tomograph

Lateral — Sagittal

A / P (Anterior / Posterior) — Coronal

Oblique

Transverse

FIGURE 8.4. Imaging techniques: tomographic imaging planes.
SOURCE: Sonies BC, Stone M: Speech Imaging. In McNeil MR (ed): *Clinical Management of Sensorimotor Disorders,* p. 179. Thieme, New York, 1997.

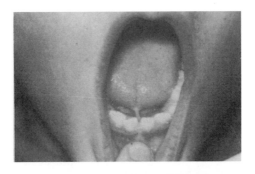
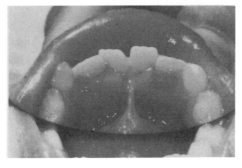

FIGURE 8.5. **Lingual frenum attached to the tongue tip (above) and gum (gingival) tissue behind the lower central incisors (below).**

SOURCE: Moller KT: Dental-Occlusal and Other Oral Conditions and Speech. In Bernthal JE, Bankson NW (eds): *Child Phonology: Characteristics, Assessment, and Intervention with Special Populations,* p. 19. Thieme, New York, 1994.

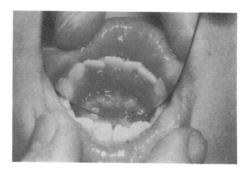

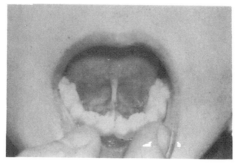

FIGURE 8.6. Lingual frenum following a frenectomy (above, lower attachment; below, under surface of tongue).

SOURCE: Moller KT: Dental-Occlusal and Other Oral Conditions and Speech. In Bernthal JE, Bankson NW (eds): *Child Phonology: Characteristics, Assessment, and Intervention with Special Populations*, p. 20. Thieme, New York, 1994.

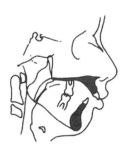
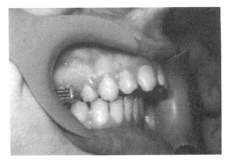

FIGURE 8.7. Malocclusion, class II: lateral diagrammatic and clinical view (note that the upper molar is excessively anterior to the lower molar and the anterior upper teeth are excessively anterior to the lower teeth; overjet).

SOURCE: Moller KT: Dental-Occlusal and Other Oral Conditions and Speech. In Bernthal JE, Bankson NW (eds): *Child Phonology: Characteristics, Assessment, and Intervention with Special Populations,* p. 7. Thieme, New York, 1994.

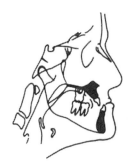
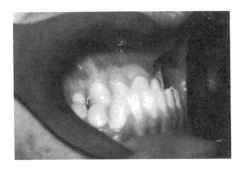

FIGURE 8.8. Malocclusion, class III: lateral diagrammatic and clinical view (note that the upper molar is excessively posterior to the lower molar and the anterior teeth are posterior to the lower teeth, creating negative overjet; anterior cross-bite).

SOURCE: Moller KT: Dental-Occlusal and Other Oral Conditions and Speech. In Bernthal JE, Bankson NW (eds): *Child Phonology: Characteristics, Assessment, and Intervention with Special Populations,* p. 8. Thieme, New York, 1994.

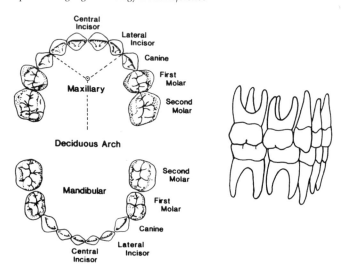

FIGURE 8.9. Normal occlusion (dental bite) or deciduous (primary) dentition.
SOURCE: Moller KT: Dental-Occlusal and Other Oral Conditions and Speech. In Bernthal JE, Bankson NW (eds): *Child Phonology: Characteristics, Assessment, and Intervention with Special Populations*, p. 5. Thieme, New York, 1994.

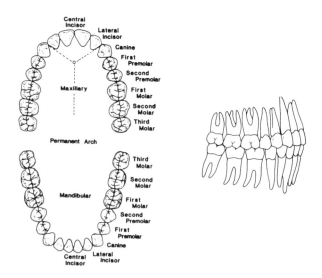

FIGURE 8.10. Normal occlusion (dental bite) of permanent (secondary) dentition.
SOURCE: Moller KT: Dental-Occlusal and Other Oral Conditions and Speech. In Bernthal JE, Bankson NW (eds): *Child Phonology: Characteristics, Assessment, and Intervention with Special Populations*, p. 5. Thieme, New York, 1994.

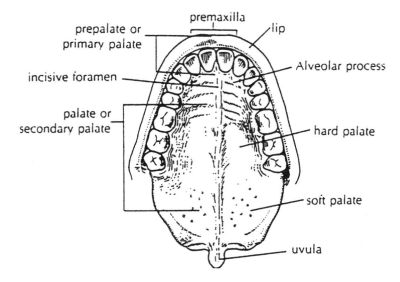

FIGURE 8.11. Normal palate: schematic diagram.

SOURCE: From Air DH, Wood AS, Neils JR: Considerations for Organic Disorders. In Creaghead NA, Newman PW, Secord WA (eds), *Assessment and Remediation of Articulatory and Phonological Disorders,* p. 290. Copyright © 1989 by Allyn and Bacon. Reprinted/adapted by permission.

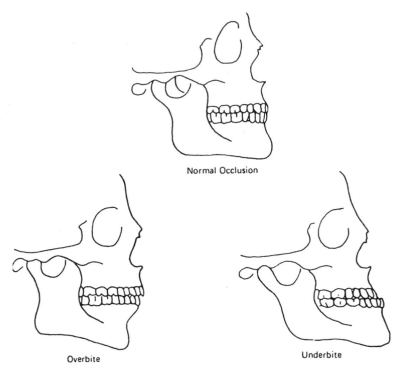

FIGURE 8.12. Occlusion types and examples.

SOURCE: From Bernthal JE, Bankson NW: *Articulation and Phonological Disorders,* 3rd ed., p. 178. Copyright © 1993 by Allyn & Bacon. Reprinted/adapted by permission.

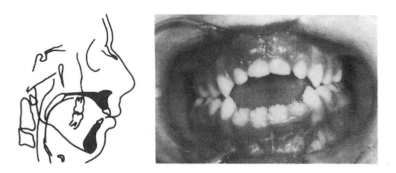

FIGURE 8.13. Openbite, anterior: lateral diagrammatic and clinical view (note that the upper front teeth do not overlap the lower front teeth).

SOURCE: Moller KT: Dental-Occlusal and Other Oral Conditions and Speech. In Bernthal JE, Bankson NW (eds): *Child Phonology: Characteristics, Assessment, and Intervention with Special Populations,* p. 8. Thieme, New York, 1994.

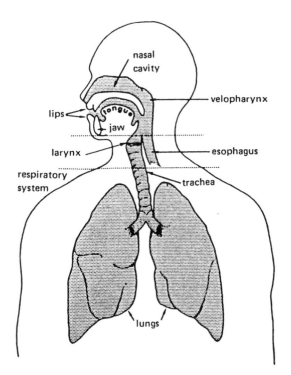

FIGURE 8.14. Organs of speech production.

SOURCE: From Kent R: Normal Aspects of Articulation. In Bernthal JE, Bankson NW, *Articulation and Phonological Disorders,* 3rd ed., p. 10. Copyright © 1993 by Allyn & Bacon. Reprinted/adapted by permission.

TABLE 8.2. Orofacial examination checklist.

Client name: _____ Age: _____ Date: _____

Examiner: _____

I. Facial Characteristics

A. General appearance: normal color _____; normal symmetry _____; adenoid facies _____; other _____

B. Frontal view

1. eye spacing: normal (one eye apart) _____; hypertelorism _____; other _____

2. zygomatic bones: _____; hypoplasia _____; other _____

3. nasal area: septum (straight) _____; or deviated _____; nares _____; columella _____; septum/turbinate _____ relationship _____; turbinate color _____; other notations _____

4. vertical facial dimensions:

   a. upper (40% of face) _____; other notations _____

   b. lower (60% of face) _____; other notations _____

5. lips: cupids bow present _____; muscular union _____; neuromuscular functioning —/i/ _____; /u/ _____; /p-p-p/ _____; other notations _____

C. Profile

1. normal (straight or convex) linear relationship between bridge of nose, to base of nose, to chin _____;

   retrusion $\Big\{$ maxilla _____; protrusion $\Big\{$ maxilla _____; mandible _____; mandible _____;

2. mandibular plane: normal _____; steep _____; flat _____;

D. General notations:

II. Intraoral Characteristics

A. Dentition

1. general hygiene: good _____; needs improvement ooooo; caries _____; gingival hyperplasia or recession _____

2. occlusal relationships ("bite on your back teeth" and separate cheek from teeth with tongue depressor)

   a. first molar contacts:

      Class I — normal molar occlusion (mandibular molar is one-half tooth ahead of maxillary molar) _____

      Class I malocclusion (normal molar relationship with variations in other areas of dentition) _____

      Class II malocclusion (maxillary ahead of mandibular first molar) _____

      Class III malocclusion (mandibular molar more than one-half tooth ahead of maxillary molar) _____

II. Intraoral Characteristics (continued)

b. biting surfaces: normal vertical overlap (overbite) _____; excessive vertical overlap A _____ / P _____; normal horizontal overlap (overjet) _____; excessive horizontal overlap A _____ / P _____; crossbite (mandibular tooth or teeth outside or wider than maxillary counterpart, or maxillary tooth or teeth inside mandibular counterpart) _____; notation of teeth involved _____; open bite (gap between biting surfaces) A _____ / P _____

c. sibilant production with teeth in occlusion: normal /s/ _____; /z/ _____; /f/ _____; /v/ _____

B. Hard palate ("extend your head backward")

1. midline coloration: normal (pink and white) _____; abnormal (blue tint) _____
2. lateral coloration: normal _____; torus palatinus (blue tint surrounding a raised midline bony growth) _____
3. posterior border and nasal spine: normal _____; short _____
4. general bony framework: normal _____; submucous cleft _____; cleft _____; repaired cleft _____; other _____
5. palatal vault: normal relationship between maxillary arch/vault _____; narrow maxillary arch/high vault _____; wide maxillary arch/flat vault _____; other _____
6. general notations _____

C. Soft palate or velum (Examiner's eye level should be client's mouth level. Client's head erect, mouth three-fourths open, and tongue not extended out of mouth.)

1. midline muscle union (say "ah"): normal (whitish-pinkish tissue line) _____; submucous cleft (blue tint with A-type configuration during phonation) _____; cleft _____; repaired cleft _____
2. length: effective (closure of nasopharyngeal port possible during phonation) _____; ineffective (hyperna [nsality noted) _____
3. velar dimple (where elevated soft palate buckles during phonation): normal 80% of total velar length (or 3–5 mm above tip of uvula) _____; other notations _____
4. velar elevation: normal (up to plane of hard palate) _____; reduced _____; other _____
5. range of velar excursion (up and back stretching during phonation): excellent _____; moderate _____; minimal _____
6. presence of hypernasality during counting: 60s _____; 70s _____; 80s _____; 90s _____
7. general notations: regarding air loss of unphonated sounds (nasal emission) and nasal resonance on phonated sounds _____

D. Uvula

1. shape: normal _____; bifid _____; other _____
2. position: midline _____; lateral _____

TABLE 8.2. (*continued*)

II. Intraoral Characteristics (continued)

E. Fauces
  1. open isthmus _____; tonsillar obstruction of isthmus _____
  2. tonsil coloration: normal (pinkish) _____; inflamed _____

F. Pharynx
  1. depth between velar dimple and pharyngeal wall on "ah": normal _____; deep _____; other _____
  2. Passavant's pad: present during physiologic activity?
  3. adenoidal surgery (ask client); intact _____; removed _____; date of tonsil/adenoid removal _____
  4. gag response: positive _____; negative _____; weak _____
  5. general notations: _____

G. Tongue
  1. size: normal _____; macroglossia (rare) _____; microglossia _____
  2. diadochokinetic rate — an estimate of neuromotor maturation for speech (observe consistency and pattern of rapid movements during the 15-repetition sequence)
     a. normal movement patterns: tuh _____; luh _____; kuh _____; puh-tuh-kuh _____; describe variations _____
     b. mandibular assist: normal (until age 7½) _____; possible neuromotor delay for speech (after 7½) _____
  3. lingual frenum: normal (tongue tip to alveolar ridge when mouth is one-half open) _____; short _____
  4. general notations: _____

III. General Observations and Other Findings

SOURCE: With permission from Mason N, Simon C: Orofacial Examinations Checklist. *Language, Speech and Hearing Services in Schools* 1977; 8:161–163.

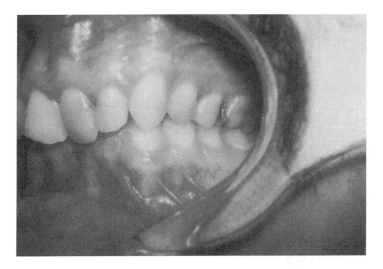

FIGURE 8.15. Overbite, excessive: clinical view (note that the upper front teeth excessively overlap the lower front teeth).

SOURCE: Moller KT: Dental-Occlusal and Other Oral Conditions and Speech. In Bernthal JE, Bankson NW (eds): *Child Phonology: Characteristics, Assessment, and Intervention with Special Populations,* p. 9. Thieme, New York, 1994.

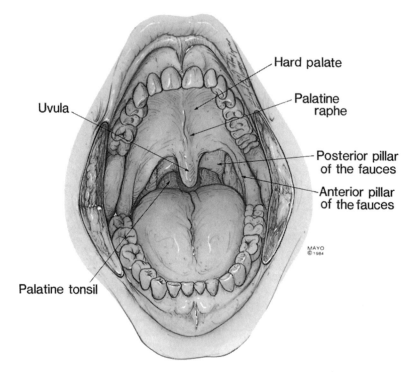

FIGURE 8.16. Soft palate and surrounding structures seen during peroral examination.

SOURCE: Aronson AE: *Clinical Voice Disorders,* p. 202. Thieme, New York, 1990.

TABLE 8.3. Speech imaging procedures: summary of advantages and limits.

X-Ray
1. Ionizing radiation
2. Video format for real-time studies
3. Limited repeatability
4. Poor soft-tissue resolution
5. Good resolution of bony skeleton

Computerized Tomography
1. Ionizing radiation
2. Static images
3. Clear definition of structures, especially bone
4. Static images
5. Slow speed of acquisition of images
6. Good ability to detect vascular lesions and small tumors
7. Positional discomfort during speech acquisition studies

Magnetic Resonance Imaging
1. Nonionizing radiation
2. Easy multiplanar views
3. Excellent tissue definition
4. Slow speed of acquisition of images
5. Image slices too thick
6. Claustrophobic responses
7. Magnetic field problems for metal objects
8. Likely to show continued technological advances

Ultrasound
1. No bioeffects
2. Totally noninvasive
3. Normal acquisition postures for speech
4. No limits on repeatability of studies
5. Real-time imaging
6. Excellent soft tissue definition
7. Bones not imaged
8. 140° sector with variable depth functions
9. Good tongue surface imaging
10. Rapid speech acquisition
11. Video format for playback and analysis

The clinician or investigator who desires to examine speech production in normal or impaired speakers should be able to select from among the various imaging systems. No single existing system is yet that "perfect, self-contained" system needed to analyze speech. Therefore, knowledge of many advanced technologies is imperative to capture the complexities of human communication.

SOURCE: Sonies BC, Stone M: Speech Imaging. In McNeil MR (ed): *Clinical Management of Sensorimotor Disorders,* p. 181. Thieme, New York, 1997.

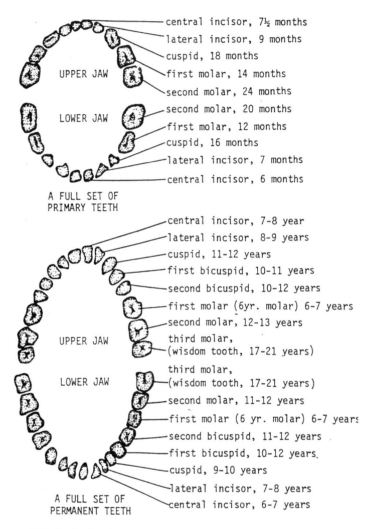

central incisor, 7½ months
lateral incisor, 9 months
cuspid, 18 months
first molar, 14 months
second molar, 24 months
second molar, 20 months
first molar, 12 months
cuspid, 16 months
lateral incisor, 7 months
central incisor, 6 months

UPPER JAW

LOWER JAW

A FULL SET OF
PRIMARY TEETH

central incisor, 7-8 year
lateral incisor, 8-9 years
cuspid, 11-12 years
first bicuspid, 10-11 years
second bicuspid, 10-12 years
first molar (6yr. molar) 6-7 years
second molar, 12-13 years
third molar,
(wisdom tooth, 17-21 years)
third molar,
(wisdom tooth, 17-21 years)
second molar, 11-12 years
first molar (6 yr. molar) 6-7 years
second bicuspid, 11-12 years
first bicuspid, 10-12 years.
cuspid, 9-10 years
lateral incisor, 7-8 years
central incisor, 6-7 years

UPPER JAW

LOWER JAW

A FULL SET OF
PERMANENT TEETH

FIGURE 8.17. Teeth: developmental eruption sequence of primary and permanent sets.

SOURCE: With permission from Schneiderman CR: *Basic Anatomy and Physiology in Speech and Hearing,* p. 98. College-Hill Press, San Diego, 1984.

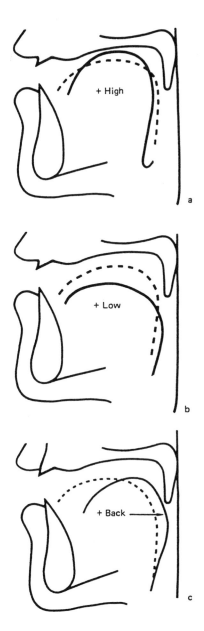

FIGURE 8.18. Tongue body features (a, high; b, low; c, back) relative to the neutral tongue position (broken line).

SOURCE: From Kent R: Normal Aspects of Articulation. In Bernthal JE, Bankson NW, *Articulation and Phonological Disorders,* 3rd ed., p. 19. Copyright © 1993 by Allyn & Bacon. Reprinted/adapted by permission.

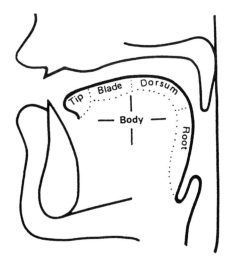

FIGURE 8.19. Tongue divisions: five functional parts for speech articulation.

SOURCE: Kent R: Normal Aspects of Articulation. In Bernthal JE, Bankson NW, *Articulation and Phonological Disorders,* 3rd ed., p. 11. Copyright © 1993 by Allyn & Bacon. Reprinted adapted by permission.

9

Dysphagia

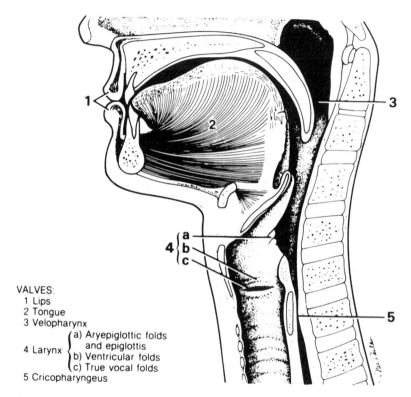

VALVES:
1 Lips
2 Tongue
3 Velopharynx
4 Larynx
 (a) Aryepiglottic folds
  and epiglottis
 (b) Ventricular folds
 (c) True vocal folds
5 Cricopharyngeus

FIGURE 9.1. Aerodigestive tract: upper view as a five-valve system.

SOURCE: Robin J: The Impact of Oral Motor Dysfunction on Swallowing: From Beginning to End. *Seminars in Speech and Language*; 13:58. Thieme, New York, 1992.

TABLE **9.1. Anoxia, meningitis, and encephalitis in infants and children: general characteristics and related feeding characteristics.**

Lack of blood flow to the brain may result in brain damage. **Anoxia/ hypoxia** may be caused by a variety of conditions, including

- perinatal trauma
- near-drowning
- cardiac complications
- pulmonary complications
- traumatic brain injury
- aneurism

Swallowing disorders are often secondary to reduced levels of alertness and responsiveness. Concomitant problems related to other facets of the injury may cause more specific feeding and swallowing problems. **Meningitis** is an inflammation of the meninges surrounding the brain and spinal cord, often caused by bacterial, viral, or fungal source. **Encephalitis** is an inflammation of the brain matter generally caused by viral infection, bacterial abscess, or inflammation. The general characteristic of these are similar. Specific feeding and swallowing problems will vary, but most are secondary to behavioral characteristics and general tone abnormalities.

General characteristics	*Related feeding characteristics*
• Increased agitation • Decreased cognition • Abnormal tone	• Weak suck • Poor coordination of breathing and swallowing • Delayed or absent initiation of the pharyngeal swallow

---

SOURCE: With permission from Boner MM, Perlin WS: Oral-Motor and Swallowing Skills in the Infant and Child: An Overview. In Cherney LR: *Clinical Management of Dysphagia in Adults and Children* (2nd edition), pp. 41–42. © 1994, Aspen Publishers, Inc.

TABLE 9.2. **Brain tumors in infants and children: general characteristics and related feeding characteristics.**

Swallowing problems are rarely a predominant characteristic of children who have brain tumors. However, swallowing problems may develop secondary to displacement of the pharyngeal and laryngeal structures, pressure on the brain stem associated with size and location of the tumor, or as a result of the radiation process sometimes used in treatment (Ravindarnath & Cushing, 1982). Gliomas are the most frequently occurring type of brain tumor in children. Medulloblastomas are the second most commonly occurring (Finlay, 1986). Brain stem gliomas are also seen in children. Children with brain stem gliomas are more likely to have oral motor or swallowing problems than children with other types of tumors (Frank, Schwartz, Epstein, & Beresford, 1989).

General characteristics	*Related feeding characteristics*
• Hypersensitivity secondary to radiation	• Changes in taste sensation
• Increased agitation	• Oral hypersensitivity
• Cerebellar mutism	• Poor suck response in infants secondary
• Ataxia (Albright, Price, & Guthkelch, 1983; Frank et al., 1989)	to cranial nerve involvement (Albright et al., 1983)
• Diplopia (Albright et al., 1983)	• Delay in the pharyngeal swallow
• Headache (Albright et al., 1983)	• Backflow secondary to decreased tone in
• Multiple cranial nerve palsies (Albright et al., 1983)	lower esophageal sphincter (Frank et al., 1989)
• Vertigo (Albright et al., 1983)	• Dysarthria
• Irritability and lethargy (Frank et al., 1989)	• Vomiting (Albright et al., 1983)
	• Possible reduced salivary gland function

SOURCE: With permission from Boner MM, Perlin WS: Oral-Motor and Swallowing Skills in the Infant and Child: An Overview. In Cherney LR: *Clinical Management of Dysphagia in Adults and Children* (2nd edition), pp. 42–43. © 1994, Aspen Publishers, Inc.

TABLE 9.3. **Cerebral palsy: general characteristics and related feeding characteristics.**

General characteristics	Related feeding characteristics
1. SPASTIC CEREBRAL PALSY	
• Increased tone • Decreased range of motion • Shallow respiration/decreased ribcage mobility (McGee, 1987) • Compensatory posturing • Cognitive deficits (Levitt, 1982) • Perceptual problems (Levitt, 1982) • Seizure disorder (Levitt, 1982)	• Loss of food/liquid secondary to poor lip closure and poor lingual control (Griggs et al., 1989) • Flattened, retracted tongue • Retracted lips • Decreased bolus formation • Decreased control of bolus secondary to poor lingual mobility (Griggs et al., 1989) • Increased oral transit time • Difficulty managing very thick or very thin textures • Inadequate velopharyngeal closure • Possible structural abnormalities (high-arched palate) • Inability to breathe through nose while sucking • Poor jaw control • Delay in pharyngeal swallow (Logemann, 1983) • Reduced pharyngeal peristalsis (Griggs et al., 1989) • Compensatory posturing during feeding • Drooling • Lower respiratory infections secondary to aspiration (Griggs et al., 1989; Jones, 1989)
2. ATHETOID CEREBRAL PALSY	
• Fluctuating tone • Inconsistent breathing patterns • Poor head control • Difficulty maintaining optimal positioning (McGee, 1987) • Involuntary movement patterns (Levitt, 1982) • Writhing/athetoid movements • Difficulty isolating eye movements from head movement (Connor, Williamson, & Siepp, 1978) • Possible cognitive deficits	• Loss of food or liquid secondary to poor lip closure • Retraction of lower lip (McGee, 1987) • Facial grimace • Poor coordination of lip and tongue movement • Inability to coordinate breathing and sucking • Poor manipulation of bolus • Drooling

(continued)

TABLE 9.3. (*continued*)

General characteristics	General characteristics
3. ATAXIC CEREBRAL PALSY	

General characteristics	General characteristics
• Generally decreased tone (Connor et al., 1978) • Imprecise direction of movement • Over- and undershooting movements • May have athetoid and/or spastic components (McGee, 1987) • Poor balance and coordination (Connor et al., 1978) • Postural fixation • Nystagmus (Levitt, 1982) • Possible cognitive deficits (Levitt, 1982) • Perceptual deficits (Levitt, 1982)	• Loss of food/liquid secondary to poor lip closure • Inconsistent poor coordination of breathing and eating/drinking • May present with any combination of feeding patterns listed under spastic or athetoid cerebral palsy (McGee, 1987) • Drooling

SOURCE: With permission from Boner MM, Perlin WS: Oral-Motor and Swallowing Skills in the Infant and Child: An Overview. In Cherney LR: *Clinical Management of Dysphagia in Adults and Children* (2nd edition), pp. 37–39. © 1994, Aspen Publishers, Inc.

TABLE 9.4. **Cocaine-dependent mothers' infants and children: general characteristics and related feeding characteristics.**

Use of cocaine by a pregnant woman may result in neurologic damage, medical complications, and physical abnormalities in the developing fetus. Postnatally, poor maternal bonding, inadequate nutrition, and prolonged hospitalization further impede normal development.

Cocaine is not evident in an adult's urine after 24 hours. However, its presence may be noted in a pregnant woman's urine and the urine of a newborn for 4 to 7 days (Bingol et al., 1987; Chasnoff, 1987).

General characteristics	Related feeding characteristics
• Increased agitation • Irritability (Chasnoff, Burns, & Burns, 1987) • Lower Apgar scores (MacGregor et al., 1987) • Lower birth weight (MacGregor et al., 1987) • Small for gestational age (MacGregor et al., 1987)	• Feeding intolerance (Cherukuri et al., 1988) • Poor coordination of suck and swallow (Lewis, Bennett, & Schmeder, 1989) • Inability to stabilize tongue in midline (Lewis et al., 1989) • Tremors in tongue (Lewis et al., 1989)

SOURCE: With permission from Boner MM, Perlin WS: Oral-Motor and Swallowing Skills in the Infant and Child: An Overview. In Cherney LR: *Clinical Management of Dysphagia in Adults and Children* (2nd edition), pp. 43–44. © 1994, Aspen Publishers, Inc..

TABLE 9.5. **Down syndrome in children: general characteristics and related feeding characteristics.**

Most children who have Down syndrome present with global developmental delays. Accordingly, feeding and swallowing skills also develop at a later date (Pueschel, 1984). There are three phenotypes associated with Down syndrome: trisomy 21, translocation, or mosaicism. Trisomy 21 is most common, accounting for 95 percent of individuals with Down syndrome (Jung, 1989).

General characteristics	*Related feeding characteristics*
• General developmental delay • Hypotonia • Hearing loss (Jung, 1989) • Delayed tooth eruption (Jung, 1989)	• Increased drooling (Palmer & Ekvall, 1978) • Tongue protrusion (Palmer & Ekvall, 1978) • Poor sucking and swallowing (Calvert, Vivian, & Calvert, 1976; Palmer & Ekvall, 1978) • Reduced chewing (Calvert et al., 1976; Palmer & Ekvall, 1978) • Shortened buccal cavity (Stoel-Gammon, 1982) • Small oral cavity (Stoel-Gammon, 1981) • High palate (Stoel-Gammon, 1981) • Obstruction of nasal passages (Stoel-Gammon, 1981) • Velopharyngeal dysfunction (Jung, 1989) • Small mandible (Ardran, Marker, & Kemp, 1972) • Abnormal dental bite (Jung, 1989) • Unusually high pharynx (Stoel-Gammon, 1981)

SOURCE: With permission from Boner MM, Perlin WS: Oral-Motor and Swallowing Skills in the Infant and Child: An Overview. In Cherney LR: *Clinical Management of Dysphagia in Adults and Children* (2nd edition), p. 44. © 1994, Aspen Publishers, Inc.

TABLE 9.6. **Dysphagic problems related to neurological damage: oral phase, pharyngeal phase, esophageal phase.**

Problem	Effect
ORAL PHASE	
Reduced labial closure	Food or liquid may leak from the mouth.
Reduced lateral and vertical range of tongue movement	Reduced ability to manipulate food in the mouth during mastication, to form and hold the bolus, and to propel the food posteriorly. This results in separation of food throughout the oral cavity; particles may fall over the base of the tongue into the pharynx and be partially aspirated *before* the initiation of the pharyngeal swallow.
Reduced buccal tension	Food may fall into the lateral sulcus during mastication and may be difficult to retrieve.
Reduced oral sensitivity	Material that lodges in areas of reduced sensitivity may not be felt; food particles may fall over the base of the tongue and be aspirated *before* the initiation of the pharyngeal swallow.
PHARYNGEAL PHASE	
Delayed/absent pharyngeal swallow	Pooling in the valleculae or pyriform sinuses may occur, with overflow into the airway and aspiration *before* the pharyngeal swallow is initiated.
Inadequate velopharyngeal closure	Material may enter the nasal cavity, resulting in possible nasal regurgitation.
Reduced laryngeal closure	Airway protection is compromised with aspiration occurring *during* the swallow.
Reduced pharyngeal peristalsis	Residue may remain in the valleculae and pyriform sinuses; if particles fall into the airway, aspiration may occur *after* the pharyngeal swallow.
Reduced laryngeal elevation	Some material may remain on top of the larynx; aspiration may occur *after* the swallow when the larynx opens to restore respiration.
Upper esophageal sphincter dysfunction	If the cricopharyngeus does not relax, or if the sphincter opens too late or closes too soon, material may collect in the pyriform sinuses, with overflow into the airway, and aspiration evident *after* the swallow.
ESOPHAGEAL PHASE	
Lax cricopharyngeus	A bolus of material that has entered the esophagus may reflux back into the pharynx and spill into the airway, causing aspiration *after* the swallow.
Reduced peristalsis	Material may remain in the esophagus because of reduced movement of the bolus.

SOURCE: With permission from Cherney LR: Dysphagia in Adults with Neurologic Disorders: An Overview. In Cherney LR: *Clinical Management of Dysphagia in Adults and Children* (2nd edition), pp. 14–15. © 1994, Aspen Publishers, Inc.

TABLE 9.7. **HIV/AIDS in infants and children: general characteristics and related feeding characteristics.**

The greatest percent of infants with human immunodeficiency virus (HIV) are infected *in vitro* from HIV-positive or acquired immune deficiency syndrome (AIDS)-infected mothers (Pressman & Morrison, 1988). The incidence of AIDS is expected to rise as a leading cause of death as more infants are born to HIV-positive women (*Early Intervention Quarterly Newsletter,* 1989). Children who display symptoms before 24 months of age have poor outcome, with many dying within 12 months of diagnosis (*Early Intervention Quarterly Newsletter,* 1989). Medical complications are numerous and include brain tumors and encephalopathy, which, in turn, lead to severe dysphagia (Pressman & Morrison, 1988).

General characteristics	*Related feeding characteristics*
• Bacterial and lung infections (*Early Intervention Quarterly Newsletter,* 1989)	• Pain with swallowing/odynophagia (Pressman & Morrison, 1988)
• Developmental delays (*Early Intervention Quarterly Newsletter,* 1989; Pressman & Morrison, 1988)	• Malnutrition leading to muscle wasting (Pressman & Morrison, 1988)
• Failure to thrive (Pressman & Morrison, 1988)	• Poor appetite (Pressman & Morrison, 1988)
• Progressive neurologic deterioration (Pressman & Morrison, 1988)	• Dysphagia secondary to thrush and candida (Pressman & Morrison, 1988)
• Hypoxia (Pressman & Morrison, 1988)	• Poor dentition (Pressman & Morrison, 1988)
• Cardiomyopathy (Pressman & Morrison, 1988)	

SOURCE: With permission from Boner MM, Perlin WS: Oral-Motor and Swallowing Skills in the Infant and Child: An Overview. In Cherney LR: *Clinical Management of Dysphagia in Adults and Children* (2nd edition), p. 43. © 1994, Aspen Publishers, Inc.

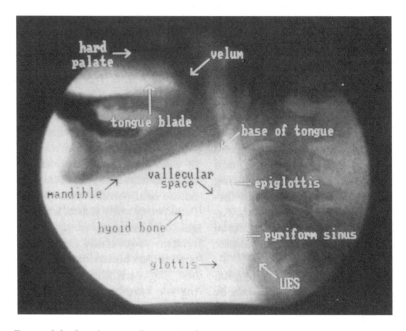

FIGURE 9.2. Oropharynx: fluorogram from a videofluoroscopic swallow study.
SOURCE: Robin J: The Impact of Oral Motor Dysfunction on Swallowing: From Beginning to End. *Seminars in Speech and Language*; 13:58. Thieme, New York, 1992.

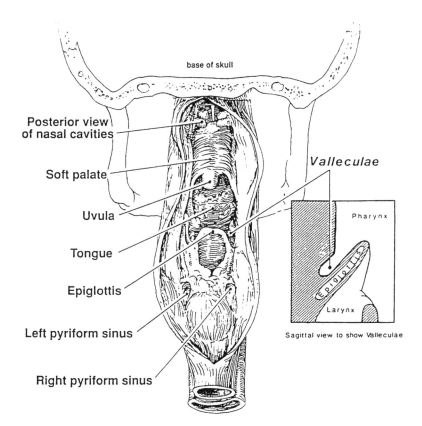

FIGURE 9.3. Pharynx: schematic drawing of anterior structures (posterior view with pharyngeal constrictors dissected away).

SOURCE: With permission from Cherney LR: Dysphagia in Adults with Neurologic Disorders: An Overview. In Cherney LR: *Clinical Management of Dysphagia in Adults and children,* p. 7. ©1994 by Aspen Publishers, Gaithersburg, MD.

TABLE 9.8. **Prematurity of birth/low birth weight: general characteristics and related feeding characteristics.**

General characteristics	Related feeding characteristics
• Low birth weight (Hill, 1975) • Hydrocephalus (McCormick, 1989) • Cerebral palsy (Babson et al., 1966; McCormick, 1989) • Seizure disorder (McCormick, 1989) • Sensorineural impairment (McCormick, 1989) • Developmental delay (McCormick, 1989) • Low Apgar scores (McCormick, 1989) • Cardiac failure (Babson et al., 1966) • Hyperirritability (Babson et al., 1966) • Lethargy (Babson et al., 1966) • Hypotonia (Babson et al., 1966) • Increased or decreased head growth (Babson et al., 1966) • Bowel obstruction (Babson et al., 1966) • Strabismus and retrolental fibroplasia (Babson et al., 1966)	• Intrauterine aspiration (Babson et al., 1966) • Hypyersensitivity • Difficulty coordinating sucking and breathing (Morris, 1989) • Hyperextension of head/neck secondary to positioning in the Neonatal Intensive Care Unit to increase the diameter of the pharynx for more efficient respiration (Morris, 1989) • Increased incidence of apnea and bradycardia secondary to feeding problems (Mathew, 1988) • Poor tolerance for fat in cow's milk (Hill, 1975)

SOURCE: With permission from Boner MM, Perlin WS: Oral-Motor and Swallowing Skills in the Infant and Child: An Overview. In Cherney LR: *Clinical Management of Dysphagia in Adults and Children* (2nd edition), p. 41. © 1994, Aspen Publishers, Inc.

TABLE **9.9.** **Strokes in children: general characteristics and related feeding characteristics.**

Strokes in childhood are primarily seen in children with sickle cell disease (Powers, Wilson, Imbus, Pegelow, & Allen, 1978) but also may be secondary to congenital malformations or may accompany syndromes such as Moya Moya (Rogers & Coleman, 1992; Takashita, Kagawa, Izawa, & Kitamura, 1986). In one study, 46.2 percent of juvenile hemorrhagic strokes were caused by primary hemorrhage, 38.5 percent were due to arteriovenous malformations, 5.7 percent were related to intracranial aneurysm, and Moya Moya syndrome accounted for 5.7 percent (Takashita et al., 1986).

   Characteristics will vary according to site and size of lesion, developmental level at the time of stroke, and history of strokes. Some of the deficits are directly related to the site of lesion. Other behaviors/patterns are secondary factors that interfere. There is limited research regarding disorders of feeding and swallowing with children who have had strokes.

General characteristics	Related feeding characteristics
• Possible hemiplegia • Seizure disorder (Powers et al., 1978) • Cognitive deficits • Language deficits	• Unilateral or bilateral facial weakness • Unilateral or bilateral oral/motor dysfunction possibly impeding labial and lingual movement • Loss of liquid/food • Decreased tongue lateralization • Decreased bolus formation • Decreased bolus manipulation • Decreased rotary chew • Delay in pharyngeal swallow

SOURCE: With permission from Boner MM, Perlin WS: Oral-Motor and Swallowing Skills in the Infant and Child: An Overview. In Cherney LR: *Clinical Management of Dysphagia in Adults and Children* (2nd edition), p. 45. © 1994, Aspen Publishers, Inc.

TABLE **9.10. Traumatic brain injury in children: general characteristics and related feeding characteristics.**

The following characteristics are typical of children who have sustained a traumatic brain injury. Characteristics vary widely depending on the stage of recovery and the site(s) of injury. Some direct effect on feeding skills may be seen, such as dysarthria and swallowing problems.

However, many of the problems are secondary to decreased cognition, orientation, alertness, attention, and abnormal muscle tone.

General characteristics	*Related feeding characteristics*
• Increased agitation • Abnormal sensation; hyper- and hyposensitivity (Ylvisaker & Logemann, 1985) • Poor initiation (Logemann, 1989) • Poor memory (Ewing-Cobbs, Fletcher, & Levin, 1985; Pang, 1985; Szekeres, Ylvisaker, & Holland, 1985) • Reduced orientation (Haarbauer-Krupa, Moser, Smith, Sullivan, & Szekeres, 1985) • Reduced attention (Adamovich, Henderson, & Auerbach, 1985; Szekeres et al., 1985) • Impulsivity (Ylvisaker & Weinstein, 1989) • Reduced alertness and awareness (Brink, Imbus, & Woo-San, 1980) • Confusion • Reduced visual perception skills (Szekeres et al., 1985) • Language and cognitive deficits (Ewing-Cobbs et al., 1985) • Reduced organization, reasoning, problem solving, and judgment skills (Szekeres et al., 1985) • Emotional lability (Pang, 1985) • Presence of primitive reflexes (Ylvisaker & Logemann, 1985) • Abnormal muscle tone (Jaffe, Mastrilli, Molitor, & Valko, 1985; Pang, 1985)	• Slow initiation of voluntary movement, including mouth opening and posterior propulsion of the bolus (Logemann, 1989) • Immature feeding and swallowing patterns (Ylvisaker & Logemann, 1985) • Oral hypersensitivity • Bite reflex • Absent or delayed initiation of pharyngeal swallow (Lazarus & Logemann, 1987; Ylvisaker & Logemann, 1985; Ylvisaker & Weinstein, 1989)

SOURCE: With permission from Boner MM, Perlin WS: Oral-Motor and Swallowing Skills in the Infant and Child: An Overview. In Cherney LR: *Clinical Management of Dysphagia in Adults and Children* (2nd edition), pp. 39–40. © 1994, Aspen Publishers, Inc.

10

Multicultural
Issues

TABLE 10.1. **African American English and standard American English: phonemic contrasts.**

	POSITION IN WORD		
SAE phonemes	*Initial*	*Medial*	*Final**
/p/		Unaspirated /p/	Unaspirated /p/
/n/			Reliance on preceding nasalized vowel
/w/	Omitted in specific words (*l'as, too!*)		
/b/		Unreleased /b/	Unreleased /b/
/g/		Unreleased /g/	Unreleased /g/
/k/		Unaspirated /k/	Unaspirated /k/
/d/	Omitted in specific words (*l'ont know*)	Unreleased /d/	Unreleased /d/
/ŋ/		/n/	/n/
/t/		Unaspirated /t/	Unaspirated /t/
/l/		Omitted before labial consonants (*help—hep*)	"uh" following a vowel (*Bill—Biuh*)
/ɹ/		Omitted or /ə/	Omitted or prolonged vowel or glide
/θ/	Unaspirated /t/ of /f/	Unaspirated /t/ of /f/ between vowels	Unaspirated /t/ of /f/ (*bath—baf*)
/v/	Sometimes /b/	/b/ before /m/ and /n/	Sometimes /b/
/ð/	/d/	/d/ or /v/ between vowels	/d/, /v/, /f/
/z/		Omitted or replaced by /d/ before nasal sound (*wasn't—wud'n*)	

Blends

/stɹ/ becomes /skɹ/
/ʃɹ/ becomes /stɹ/
/θɹ/ becomes /θ/
/pɹ/ becomes /p/
/bɹ/ becomes /b/
/kɹ/ becomes /k/
/gɹ/ becomes /g/

Final consonant clusters
(second consonant omitted when these clusters occur at the end of a word)

/sk/	/nd/	/sp/
/ft/	/ld/	/dʒ d/
/st/	/ɹd/	/nt/

SOURCE: From Owens RE: *Language Development: An Introduction,* 4th ed., p. 407. © 1996 by Allyn & Bacon. Reprinted/adapted by permission.
*Note weakening of final consonants.

TABLE 10.2. African American English and standard American English: grammatical contrasts.

AAE grammatical structure	SAE grammatical structure
Possessive -'s Nonobligatory where word position expresses possession Get *mother* coat. It *be* mother's.	Obligatory regardless of position. Get *mother's* coat. It's *mother's*.
Plural -s Nonobligatory with numerical quantifier He got ten *dollar*. Look at the *cats*.	Obligatory regardless of numerical quantifier. He has ten *dollars*. Look at the *cats*.
Regular past -ed Nonobligatory, reduced as consonant cluster Yesterday, I *walk* to school.	Obligatory Yesterday, I *walked* to school.
Irregular past Case by case, some verbs inflected, others not I *see* him last week.	All regular verbs inflected I *saw* him last week.
Regular present-tense third-person singular -s Nonobligatory She *eat* too much.	Obligatory She *eats* too much.
Irregular present-tense third-person singular -s Nonobligatory He *do* my job.	Obligatory He *does* my job.
Indefinite an Use of indefinite *a*. He ride in *a* airplane.	Use of *an* before nouns beginning with a vowel He rode in *an* airplane.
Pronouns Pronominal apposition: pronoun immediately follows noun Momma *she* mad. She . . .	Pronoun used elsewhere in sentence or in other sentence: not in apposition Momma *is* mad. She . . .
Future tense More frequent use of *be going to (gonna)* I be going to dance tonight. I *gonna* dance tonight. Omit *will* preceding *be* I *be* home later.	More frequent use of *will* I will dance tonight. I *am* going to dance tonight. Obligatory use of *will* I *will* (I'll) *be* home later.
Negation Triple negative Nobody *don't never* like me. Use of *ain't* I *ain't* going.	Absence of triple negative *No one ever* likes me. *Ain't* is unacceptable form. *I'm not* going.

(continued)

TABLE 10.2. (*continued*)

AAE grammatical structure	SAE grammatical structure

Modals
Double modals for such forms as *might*, *could*, and *should*
  I might could go.
	Single modal use
	  I might be able to go.

Questions
Same form for direct and indirect
  What *it is?*
  Do you know what *it is?*
	Different forms for direct and indirect
	  What *is it?*
	  Do you know what *it is?*

Relative pronouns
Nonobligatory in most cases
  He the one stole it.
  It the one you like.
	Nonobligatory with *that* only
	  He's the one *who* stole it.
	  It's the one (*that*) you like.

Conditional if
Use of *do* for conditional *if*
  I ask *did* she go.
	Use of *if*
	  I asked *if* she went.

Perfect construction
Been used for action in the distant past
  He *been* gone.
	Been not used
	  He left a long time ago.

Copula
Nonobligatory when contractible
  He sick.
	Obligatory in contractible and uncontractible forms
	  He's sick.

Habitual or general state
Marked with uninflected *be*
  She *be* workin'.
	Nonuse of *be:* verb inflected
	  She's *working* now.

SOURCE: From Owens RE: *Language Development: An Introduction,* 4th ed., pp. 408–409. © 1996 by Allyn & Bacon. Reprinted/adapted by permission.

TABLE 10.3. African American idioms: selected examples and definitions.

Idiom	Definition and example
All that	Excellent, fantastic, superb, all that it seems to be, as in "She bad, she definitely *all that*."
Amen corner	Place where older individuals usually sit in traditional African American church.
Barefoot as a river duck	Not wearing shows, as in "It too cold for you be runnin' around *barefoot as a river duck*."
Crack on	To insult seriously or in fun, as in "He jus' *crackin on* you."
Eagle-flyin' day	Pay day.
Old head	Older and wiser person.
On it	In control of the situation, as in "Don't worry, I *on it*."
That how you livin'?	Why are you acting like that?
Word	Affirmative response to an action or statement. "Right on, *word up!*"

SOURCE: From Owens RE: *Language Development: An Introduction,* 4th ed., p. 410. © 1996 by Allyn and Bacon. Reprinted/adapted by permission.

TABLE 10.4. Asian English and standard American English: grammatical contrasts.

AAE grammatical structure	*SAE grammatical structure*
Plural *-s*	
Not used with numerical adjective: *three cat*	Used regardless of numerical adjective: *three cats*
Used with irregular plural: *three sheeps*	Not used with irregular plural: *three sheep*
Auxiliaries *to be and to do*	
Omission: *I going home. She not want eat*	Obligatory and inflected in the present
Uninflected: *I is going. She do not want eat.*	progressive form: *I am going home. She does not want to eat.*
Verb *have*	
Omission	Obligatory and inflected: *You have been*
You been here.	*here. He has one.*
Uninflected	
He have one.	
Past-tense *-ed*	
Omission: *He talk yesterday*	Obligatory, nonovergeneralization, and
Overgeneralization: *I eated yesterday.*	single marking: *He talked yesterday.*
Double marking: *She didn't ate.*	*I ate yesterday. She didn't eat.*
Interrogative	
Nonreversal: *You are late?*	Reversal and obligatory auxiliary: *Are you*
Omitted auxiliary: *You like ice cream?*	*late? Do you like ice cream?*
Perfect marker	
Omission: *I have write letter.*	Obligatory: *I have written a letter.*
Verb–noun agreement	
Nonagreement: *He go to school. You goes to school.*	Agreement: *He goes to school. You go to school.*
Article	
Omission: *Please give gift.*	Obligatory with certain nouns: *Please give*
Overgeneralization: *She go the school.*	*the gift. She went to school.*
Preposition	
Misuse: I am in home.	Obligatory specific use: *I am at home. He*
Omission: *He go bus.*	*goes by bus.*
Pronoun	
Subjective/objective confusion: *Him go quickly.*	Subjective/objective distinction: *He gave it to her.*
Possessive confusion: *It him book.*	Possessive distinction: *It's his book.*
Demonstrative	
Confusion: I *like those horse.*	Singular/distinction: *I like that horse.*
Conjunction	
Omission: *You I go together.*	Obligatory use between last two items a series: *You and I are going together. Mary, John, and Carol went.*

(continued)

TABLE **10.4.** (*continued*)

AAE grammatical structure	SAE grammatical structure
Negation	
Double marking: *I didn't see nobody.* Simplified form: *He no come.*	Single obligatory marking: *I didn't see anybody. He didn't come.*
Word order	
Adjective following noun (Vietnamese): *clothes new.* Possessive following noun (Vietnamese): *dress her.* Omission of object with transitive verb: *I want.*	Most noun modifiers precede noun: *new clothes.* Possessive precedes noun: *her dress.* Use of direct object with most transitive verbs: *I want it.*

SOURCE: From Owens RE: *Language Development: An Introduction,* 4th ed., pp. 417–418. © 1996 by Allyn & Bacon. Reprinted/adapted by permission.

TABLE 10.5. **Asian English and standard American English: phonemic contrasts**

	POSITION IN WORD		
SAE phonemes	*Initial*	*Medial*	*Final**
/p/	/b/[4]	/b/[4]	Omission
/s/	Distortion[1]	Distortion[1]	Omission
/z/	/s/[2]	/s/[2]	Omission
/t/	Distortion[1]	Distortion[1]	Omission
/tʃ/	/ʃ/[4]	/ʃ/[4]	Omission
/ʃ/	/s/[2]	/s/[2]	Omission
/ɹ/, /l/	Confusion	Confusion[3]	Omission
/θ/	/s/	/s/	Omission
/dʒ/	/d/ or /z/[4]	/d/ or /z/[4]	Omission
/v/	/f/ɛ	/f/[3]	Omission
	/w/[2]	/w/[2]	Omission
/ð/	/z/[1]	/z/[1]	Omission
	/d/[4]	/d/[4]	Omission

Blends

Addition of /ə/ between consonants[3]
Omission of final consonant clusters[4]

Vowels

Shortening or lengthening of vowels (*seat—sit, it—eat*[1])
Difficulty with /I/, /ɔ/, and /æ/, and substitution of /ə/ for /æ/[2]
Difficulty with /I/, /æ/, /U/, and /ə/[4]

SOURCE: With permission from Owens RE: *Language Development: An Introduction*, 4th ed., pp. 417–418. © 1996 by Allyn & Bacon. Reprinted/adapted by permission.
[1]Mandarin dialect of Chinese only.
[2]Cantonese dialect of Chinese only.
[3]Mandarin, Cantonese, and Japanese
[4]Vietnamese only.

TABLE 10.6. **Asian/Pacific Islander region: languages spoken in the United States.** NEP/LEP (non-English-proficient and limited-English-proficient) students come from various language backgrounds, including the following:

Language	Description
Arabic	Southwest Semitic language; a variety of dialects are spoken in Arabia, Jordan, Syria, Palestine, Egypt, Iraq, and parts of northern Africa.
Bengali	Modern Indic language spoken in Bengal (East Bengal is Bangladesh; West Bengal is in Republic of India)
Chamorro	Language spoken in Guam, Saipan, and some Micronesian islands; belongs to the Austronesian language family
Chinese	One of a group of Sino-Tibetan languages and dialects spoken in China, including Mandarin, Cantonese, Amoy, Fukien, and Shanghai
Farsi	Language spoken in Southern Iran
French	Romance language spoken in France, Switzerland, southern Belgium, and other former French territories
German	West Germanic language spoken in Germany, Austria, and Switzerland and other former German territories
Hebrew	Semitic language of the ancient Hebrews
Hindi-Urdu	Hindustani language spoken in West Pakistan, where it is the principal language, and by Muslims in India
Hmong	Language spoken by the Hmong people from the mountain area of Laos
Ilokano (Ilocano)	Language spoken in the Philippines
Japanese	National language of Japan
Khmer	Mon-Khmer language of a people in Cambodia
Korean	Language of Korea, unclassified officially but containing many words of Chinese origin
Lao	Official language of Laos, a Tai language of a Buddhist people living in the area of the Mekong river in Laos and Thailand
Malay	Austronesian language of the Malays, a people inhabiting the Malay Peninsula, other parts of Malaysia, and Indonesia
Pilipino	National language of the Philippines
Portuguese	Romance language spoken in Portugal and Brazil and former territories
Punjabi	Indian language spoken in the Punjab, a region in northwest India
Samoan	National language of American Samoa, a region in the Pacific
Spanish	Romance language spoken in Spain, Central America, South America, and parts of the Caribbean
Tagalog	Austronesian language of a people native to the Philippines
Turkish	Turkic language of Turkey
Vietnamese	Language of Vietnam, belonging to the Mon-Khmer subfamily of Austro-Asiatic languages

SOURCE: With permission from Chong LL: Asian/Pacific Students and the Learning of English. In Bernthal JE, Bankson NW (eds): *Child Phonology: Characteristics, Assessment, and Intervention with Special Populations*, p. 257. Thieme, New York, 1994.

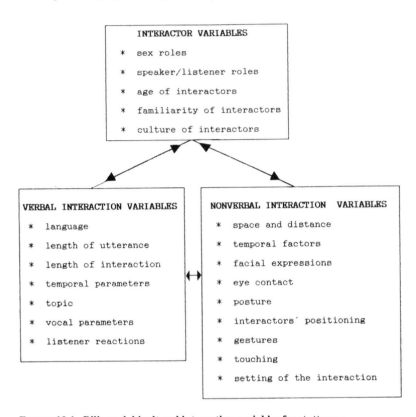

FIGURE 10.1. Bilingual–bicultural interaction variables for stutterers.
SOURCE: Watson JB, Kayser H: Assessment of Bilingual/Bicultural Children and Adults Who Stutter. *Seminars in Speech and Language*, 15:156. Thieme, New York, 1994.

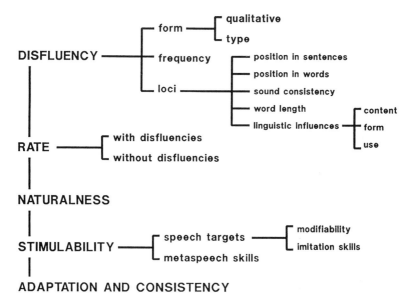

FIGURE 10.2. Bilingual–bicultural stutterers: behavioral analysis considerations.
SOURCE: Watson JB, Kayser H: Assessment of Bilingual/Bicultural Children and Adults Who Stutter. *Seminars in Speech and Language*, 15:157. Thieme, New York, 1994.

TABLE 10.7. **Black English speech characteristics: common productions compared to standard American English.**

CONSONANT CLUSTER CHANGES

1. Initial consonant clusters often delete [r] in conjunction with [p], [b], [k], [g], and [θ]
   Example: [p r e] becomes [p e], [grin] becomes [gin], or [θ r i] becomes [θ i]or [f i]
2. [str] changes to [s k r]
3. Simplification of final clusters occurs
   Example: [most] becomes [mos]

FRICATIVE CONSONANT CHANGES

1. Initial voiced dental [ð] often becomes stop [d]
   Example [ð o z] becomes [d o z]
2. Initial [θ] often becomes [f]
   Example: [θ ik] becomes [f I k]
3. Medial [ð] often becomes [d] or [v]
   Example: [m ʌ ð ɚ] becomes [m ʌ d ɚ]
4. Medial [θ] often becomes [f], [t], or [ʔ]
   Example: [h ɛ l θ I] become [h E l f I]
5. Final [θ] often becomes [f] or [t]
   Example: [b o θ] becomes [b o f] or [b æ θ] becomes [b æ t]
6. Final [ð] often becomes [v], [f], or [d]
   Example: [w l ð] becomes [w l f] or [s m U ð] becomes [s m U d]

LIQUID CHANGES

1. Deletion of intervocalic [r], final position [r], and [r] in a position preceding another consonant often occurs
   Example: [k a r] becomes [k a −]
2. Final position [l] often is omitted before [t], [d], and [p]
   Example: [d ɔ l] becomes [d ɔ −]

NASAL CONSONANT CHANGES

1. Final position nasals are often omitted
   Example: [m æ n] becomes [m æ]
2. Medial and final position alveolar [n] often replaces velar [ŋ]
   Example: [θ iŋ] becomes [θ in] or [s I ŋ I ŋ] often becomes [s I n I n]

STOP CONSONANT CHANGES

1. Final position voiced stops become devoiced
   Example: [b I g] becomes [b I k]
2. Final stops are often omitted or unreleased
   Example: [t a p] becomes [t a]

TABLE 10.8. **Black English vernacular: major phonological features distinguished from standard American English.**

- Deletion of / e r /, / r /, and / I /
  Example: [f a ð ə / substituted for / f a ð ɚ / (father); [b ɛ t] substitutes for / b E l t / (belt)
- Devoicing of final stops in words
  Example: [b I : k] substituted for / b I g / (big)
- Nasalization of preceding vowel with deletion of nasal consonant in the final position of words
  Example: [p æ] substituted for / p æn / (pan)
- Stopping of / θ / and / ð / in the initial position
  Example: [d æ t] substituted for / ð æ t / (that); [t ɔ t] substituted for / θ ɔ t / (thought)
- Substitution of the / I / vowel for / ɛ/ before nasala
  Example: [t I n] produced for / t ɛ n / (ten) and / t I n / (tin)
- Substitution of / f / for / θ / and / v / for / ð / in final position of words
  Example: [m au f] substituted for / m au θ / (mouth)
- Substitution of / f / for / θ / and / v / for / ð / in intervocalic position
  Example: [s ʌ m f I ŋ] substituted [s ʌ m θ I ŋ] (something) and [b e v I ŋ] substituted for [b e ð I ŋ] (bathing)
- Final position consonant cluster simplification, especially when alveolar consonants are present
  Example: [n ɛ s] substituted for / n ɛ s t / (nest)

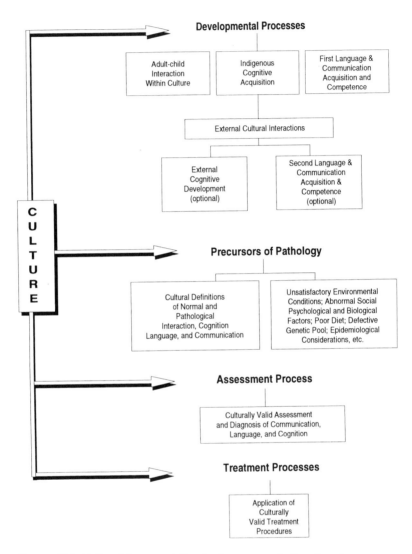

FIGURE 10.3. Cultural framework for viewing communication disorders.

SOURCE: Taylor OL, Clarke MG: Culture and Communication Disorders: A Theoretical Framework. *Seminars in Speech and Language*, 15:105. Thieme, New York, 1994.

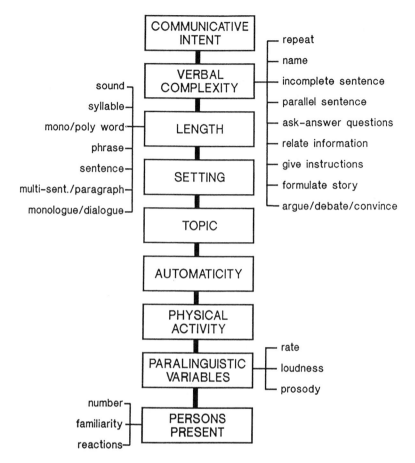

FIGURE 10.4. Cultural speaking context issues.

SOURCE: Watson JB, Kayser H: Assessment of Bilingual/Bicultural Children and Adults Who Stutter. *Seminars in Speech and Language*, 15:154. Thieme, New York, 1994.

TABLE **10.9.** **English as a second language: principles for establishing a language-learning environment.**

---

1. Expect and respect a silent period in which students listen actively, taken in language, and express themselves nonverbally or in their first language.
2. Expect errors in speech and celebrate approximations to correct form, but not at the expense of meaning.
3. As students talk, remember that their oral language proficiency in their second language does not necessarily reflect a level of cognitive functioning (thinking ability).
4. As students talk, pay attention to what they are saying (meaning) rather than how they say it (accent, grammar vocabulary).
5. Use instructional methodologies which focus on learning by doing and which require higher level thinking processes.
6. Develop nonverbal ways in which students can demonstrate their knowledge.
7. Celebrate the different languages and cultures represented by the students throughout the school year.
8. Arrange the environment so that all students can actively participate in and contribute to the success of the class regardless of language or culture.
9. Encourage high levels of interaction among students, and utilize experiences familiar to the students as part of the curriculum.

Additionally, by planning a general intervention program that addresses the following elements, an additive environment is typically established:

1. Plan goals and objectives tailored to naturalistic principles and relevancy.
2. Give the students as many opportunities as possible to read, write, talk, and listen in various group structures.
3. Allow the students to think and discuss options, make decisions, and establish accountability for what they do when working with you.
4. Immerse the students with print to build a literacy-rich environment.
5. Treat the students with respect and work to empower them as learners.
6. Utilize interesting and meaningful materials and activities.

SOURCE: Damico JS, Smith MD, Augustine LE: Multicultural Populations and Language Disorders. In Smith MD, Damico JS (eds): *Childhood Language Disorders,* p. 291. Thieme, New York, 1996.

TABLE 10.10. **Hispanic English and standard American English:
grammatical contrasts.**

HE grammatical structure	*SAE grammatical structure*
Possessive -*'s*	
Use postnoun modifier	Postnoun modifier used rarely
This is the homework of *my brother.*	This is *my brother's* homework.
Article used with body parts	Possessive pronoun used with body parts
I cut *the finger.*	I cut *my* finger.
Plural -*s*	
Nonobligatory	Obligatory, excluding exceptions
The *girl* are playing.	The *girls* are playing.
The *sheep* are playing.	The *sheep* are playing.
Regular past -*ed*	
Nonobligatory, especially when understood	Obligatory
I *talk* to her yesterday.	I *talked* to her yesterday.
Regular third-person-singular present-tense -*s*	
Nonobligatory	Obligatory
She *eat* too much.	She *eats* too much.
Articles	
Often omitted	Usually obligatory
I am going to store.	I am going to *the* store.
I am going to school.	I am going to school.
Subject pronouns	
Omitted when subject has been identified in the previous sentence.	Obligatory
Father is happy. Bought a new car.	Father is happy. He bought a new car.
Future tense	
Use go + to	Use be + *going to*
I *go to* dance.	I *am going to* the dance.
Negation	
Use no before the verb.	Use *not* (preceded by auxiliary verb where appropriate)
She *no* eat candy.	She does not eat candy.
Question	
Intonation: no noun–verb inversion	Noun–verb inversion usually
Maria is going?	*Is Maria* going?
Copula	
Occasional use of *have*	Use of *be*
I *have* ten years.	I *am* ten years old.
Negative imperatives	
No used for *don't*	*Don't* used
No throw stones.	*Don't* throw stones.

(continued)

TABLE **10.10.** (*continued*)

HE grammatical structure	SAE grammatical structure
Do insertion	
Nonobligatory in questions	Obligatory when no auxiliary verb
You like ice cream?	*Do* you like ice cream?
Comparatives	
More frequent use of longer form (*more*)	More frequent use of shorter *-er.*
He is *more* tall.	He *is taller.*

SOURCE: From Owens RE: *Language Development: An Introduction,* 4th ed., pp. 414–415. © 1996 by Allyn & Bacon. Reprinted/adapted by permission.

TABLE 10.11. **Hispanic English and standard American English: phonemic contrasts.**

	POSITION IN WORD		
SAE phonemes	*Initial*	*Medial*	*Final**
/p/	Unaspirated /p/		Omitted or weakened
/m/			Omitted
/w/	/hu/		Omitted
/b/			Omitted, distorted, or /p/
/g/			Omitted, distorted, or /k/
/k/	Unaspirated or /g/		Omitted, distorted, or /g/
/f/		Dentalized	Omitted, distorted, or /t/
/ŋ/	/n/	/d/	/n/ (*sing—sin*)
/j/	/dʒ/		
/t/			Omitted
/ʃ/	/tʃ/	/s/, /tʃ/	/tʃ/ (*wish—which*)
/tʃ/	/ʃ/ (*chair—share*)	/ʃ/	/ʃ/ (*watch—wash*)
/ɹ/	Distorted	Distorted	Distorted
/dʒ/	/d/	/j/	/ʃ/
/θ/	/t/, /s/ (*thin—tin, sin*)	Omitted	/ʃ/, /t/, /s/
/v/	/b/ (*vat—bat*)	/b/	Distorted
/z/	/s/ (*zip—sip*)	/s/ (*razor—racer*)	/s/
/ð/	/d/ (*then—den*)	/d/, /θ/, /v/ (*lather— ladder*)	/d/

Blends

/skw/ becomes /eskw/*
/sl/ becomes /esl/*
/st/ becomes /est/*

Vowels

/I/ becomes /i/ (bit—beet)
*Separates cluster into two syllables.

SOURCE: From Owens RE: *Language Development: An Introduction*, 4th ed., p. 413. © 1996 by Allyn & Bacon. Reprinted/adapted by permission.

TABLE 10.12. Mandarin initial consonants.

Manner of Articulation		BILABIAL	LABIODENTAL	APICODENTAL	ALVEOLAR	APICOPALATAL	LAMINOPALATAL	DORSOVELAR
		Upper lip	*Upper teeth*	*Lower teeth*	*Alveolar ridge*	*Hard palate*	*Hard palate*	*Velar*
		Lower lip	*Lower lip*	*Tongue tip*	*Tongue tip*	*Tongue tip*	*Tongue blade*	*Dorsum*
Stops	Voiceless Unasp.	p			t			k
	Asp.	p*			t*			k*
Affricates	Voiceless Unasp.			ts		tʂ	tɕ	
	Asp.			ts*		tʂ*	tɕ*	
Nasals	Voiced	m			n			(ŋ)
Lateral	Voiced			l				
Spirants	Voicless		f	s		ʂ	ɕ	x
	Voiced					ʐ		

SOURCE: Cheng LL: Asian/Pacific Students and the Learning of English. In Bernthal JE, Bankson NW (eds): *Child Phonology: Characteristics, Assessment, and Intervention with Special Populations,* p. 265. Thieme, New York, 1994.
Unasp., unaspiration; Asp., aspiration
*Occurs in the final position of a syllable only.

TABLE 10.13. **Multicultural areas to probe while obtaining stutterer's case history information.**

Reason left native country	Typical family size
Reason members of cultural gang settled in local community	Roles of individual family member
Generation first to move from homeland	Customs, values, beliefs, about children
Intentions to return to homeland	Child-rearing practices
Family members remaining in homeland	Medical practice
SES/occupation prior to moving to this country	Interpersonal relationships
Current SES/occupation	Concept of self
Cultural status of family (acculturation/ assimilation)	Social functions and leisure activities
Concept of majority and subculture	Cultural group's view of handicap and handicapped individual
Structure of the community	Cultural group's view of stuttering and stutterers

SOURCE: Watson JB, Kayser H: Assessment of Bilingual/Bicultural Children and Adults Who Stutter. *Seminars in Speech and Language*, 15:153. Thieme, New York, 1994.

TABLE 10.14. **Filipino vowels and diphthongs with English examples.**

	English		Filipino
/ɛ/	bed	/e/	eto (here it is)
/i/	meet	/i/	ibn (bird)
/I/	bit		
/aɪ/	bite	/ay/	kamay (hand)
/eɪ/	bait	/ey/	reyna (queen)
/æ/	bat		
/ə/	but		
	lesson, bonus, normal		
/ɚ/	later, author, sugar, fur, fir, her		
/o/	hot		
/a/	car, father	/a/	araw (sun, day)
/ô/	or	/o/	oo (yes)
/o/	no		
/u/	pool	/u/	ulo (head)
/U/	pull		
/au/	now	/aw/	ilaw (light)
/oɪ/	toy	/oy/	baboy (pig)
		/uy/	aruy (ouch!)
		/iw/	paksiw (a food cooked with vinegar)

SOURCE: Cheng LL: Asian/Pacific Students and the Learning of English. In Bernthal JE, Bankson NW (eds): *Child Phonology: Characteristics, Assessment, and Intervention with Special Populations*, p. 268. Thieme, New York, 1994.

TABLE 10.15. **Spanish consonants acquisition (number [n] of subjects who responded to each item at each grade level and the percent correct among the responding subjects).**

	UPPER LIMITS OF AGE LEVELS																
	3:3		3:7		3:11		4:3		4:7		4:11		5:3		5:7		Total
Sound	N	%	N	%	N	%	N	%	N	%	N	%	N	%	N	%	tested
p–	15	100	15	100	15	100	15	100	15	100	15	100	15	100	15	100	120
–p–	15	100	15	100	15	100	15	93	15	100	15	100	15	100	15	100	120
b–	14	100	15	100	15	100	15	100	15	100	15	93	15	100	15	100	119
ɸ	15	100	15	100	15	100	15	100	15	100	15	100	15	100	15	100	120
t–	15	80	15	93	15	93	15	100	15	100	15	93	15	100	15	100	120
–t–	15	100	15	100	15	100	15	100	15	100	15	100	15	100	15	100	120
d–	15	53	15	80	15	100	15	80	15	100	15	93	15	100	15	93	120
ɖ	15	80	15	93	15	100	15	87	15	100	15	100	15	100	15	93	120
k–	15	87	15	100	15	100	15	100	15	100	15	100	15	100	15	100	120
–k–	15	87	15	100	15	100	15	100	15	100	15	100	15	100	15	100	120
g–	15	60	15	67	15	53	15	73	15	93	15	87	15	93	15	100	120
g	15	67	15	87	15	93	15	67	15	87	15	93	15	100	15	100	120
f–	15	67	14	79	15	80	15	100	15	93	15	100	15	100	15	100	119
–f–	14	93	15	93	15	87	15	100	15	100	15	100	15	100	15	93	119
s–	15	33	15	73	15	80	15	87	15	87	15	87	15	87	15	93	120
–s–	15	67	15	60	15	93	15	87	15	100	15	87	15	73	15	93	120
s	14	53	15	67	15	80	15	93	15	87	15	93	15	80	15	80	119
x–	15	29	15	73	15	80	15	73	15	73	15	100	15	87	15	100	120
–x–	15	80	15	100	15	100	15	100	15	100	15	100	15	100	15	100	119
j–	15	60	14	86	15	87	15	93	15	100	15	100	15	87	15	100	120
–j–	15	93	15	93	15	100	15	100	15	100	15	100	15	100	14	100	119
w–	15	87	15	100	15	100	15	100	15	100	15	100	15	93	15	100	120
–w–	15	87	15	100	15	100	15	100	15	100	15	100	15	100	15	100	120

	%	n	%	n	%	n	%	n	%	n	%	n	%	n	%	n	Total
l–	40	15	80	15	87	15	80	15	100	15	100	15	93	15	100	15	120
–l–	60	15	93	15	93	15	100	15	100	15	100	15	100	15	93	15	120
–l	80	15	93	15	93	15	100	15	100	15	100	15	100	15	93	15	120
ř–	40	14	71	15	93	15	73	15	93	15	100	15	100	15	100	15	119
–ř–	47	15	60	15	73	15	80	15	73	15	53	15	53	15	100	15	120
r̄–	7	15	13	15	20	15	40	15	73	15	67	15	67	15	73	15	120
–r̄–	13	15	20	15	40	15	47	15	100	15	93	15	100	15	80	15	120
tʃ–	93	15	93	15	93	15	87	15	93	15	100	15	100	15	100	15	120
–tʃ–	73	15	80	15	100	15	87	15	100	15	100	15	100	15	100	15	120
m–	67	15	93	15	100	15	100	15	100	15	100	15	100	15	100	15	120
–m–	87	15	100	15	93	15	100	15	100	15	100	15	100	15	100	15	120
n–	67	15	80	15	100	15	100	93	100	15	100	15	100	15	100	15	120
–n–	80	15	100	15	100	15	100	15	100	15	100	15	100	15	100	15	120
–n	87	15	93	15	100	15	100	15	100	15	100	15	100	15	100	15	120
–ñ–	47	15	87	15	100	15	100	15	87	15	93	15	93	15	93	15	120

SOURCE: With permission from Jiminez B: Acquisition of Spanish Consonants in Children Aged 3–5 Years, 7 Months. *Language, Speech and Hearing Services in Schools* 1987; 18:363.

TABLE 10.16. **Spanish consonant production: stimulus items for initial, medial, and final positions.**

	SOUND		
Word	*I*	*M*	*F*
pato	p		
zapato		p	
vela	b		
escoda		b	
tasa	t		
gato		t	
diente(s)	d		
nido		d	
caballo	k		
boca		k	
guitarra	g		
bigote		g	
falda	f		
elefante		f	
sombrero	s		
payaso		s	
nariz			s
jirafa	x		
ojo		x	
lluvia	j		
cepillo		j	
heuso	w		
agua		w	—
lumbre	l		
pantalones		l	
sol			l
corazón		r̃	
doctor			r̃
rey	r̃		
burro		r̃	
chile	tʃ		
cuchillo		tʃ	
martillo	m		
limón		m	
nube	n		
canasta		n	
avión			n
bañera		ñ	

SOURCE: With permission from Jimenez B: Acquisition of Spanish Consonants in Children Aged 3–5 Years, 7 Months. *Language, Speech and Hearing Services in Schools* 1987; 18:363.

TABLE 10.17. **Spanish-influenced English compared to general American English: phonological differences.**

Phonological processes	Examples	GAE	Spanish-influenced English
SYLLABLE STRUCTURE PROCESSES			
Unstressed syllable deletion	Explain	/ɛkspleIn/	/spleIn/
Final consonant deletion	Girls, house	/gɝ̩z/, /haUs/	/gɝ̩l/, /haU/
Cluster reduction	Stairs, best	/stɛrz/, /bɛst/	/tɛrz/, /bɛs/
Epenthesis	Spain, stamp	/speIn/, /stæmp/	/ɛseIn/, /ɛstæmp/
Glottal omission	Hat, hand	/haæt/, /hænd/	/æt/, /ænd/
SUBSTITUTION PROCESSES			
Stopping of fricatives	Thumb, they	/θʌm/, /ðeI/	/tʌm/, /deI/[1]
Deaffrication	Chop, match	/tSap/, /mætS/	/Sap/, /maS/
Affrication	Shop, ship	/Sap/, /SIp/	/tSap/, /tSIp/[2]
Affrication of glide	You, yard	/ju/, /jard/	/dʒu/, /dʒard/,[3] or /ʒard/[4]
ASSIMILATION PROCESSES			
Dentalization	Two, do	/tu/, /du/	/tu/, /du/[5]
Labial assimilation	Very, voice	/vɛrI/, /vɔIs/	/bɛrI/, /bɔIs/
Prevocalic voicing	Sip, sink	/sIp/, /sIŋk/	/zIp/, /zIŋk/
Postvocalic devoicing	Chairs, cars	/tSɛrz/, /karz/	/tSɛrs/, /kars/[6]
OTHER PROCESSES			
Trilling	Around	/əraUnd/	/əɾUnd/, or /əř aUnd/, or /əRaUnd/[7]
Intrusive /h/	And, it	/ænd/, /It/	/hænd/, /hit/

SOURCE: Perez E: Phonological Differences among Speakers of Spanish-Influenced English. In Bernthal JE, Bankson NW (eds): *Child Phonology: Characteristics, Assessment, and Intervention with Special Populations,* p. 250. Thieme, New York, 1994.

[1]The /θ/ and /ð/ are not found in Spanish, although the /θ/ is substituted for the /s/ in Castilian Spanish.

[2]Occurs in Mexican and Chicano Spanish due to contact with English.

[3]May be used in some countries in South America, such as Venezuela and Peru.

[4]May be used in some countries in South America, such as Argentina and Chile.

[5]The /t/ and /d/ are both dentalized and unreleased in Spanish.

[6]The /z/ doe snot occur in Spanish.

[7]May be used by some variety of Puerto Rican English.

TABLE 10.18. **Spanish-influenced English vowel substitutions compared to general American English.**

Phonological processes	Examples	GAE	Spanish-influenced English
FRONT VOWELS			
I/i	Eat, feet, bee	/it/, /fit/, /bi/	/ɪt/, /fɪt/, /bɪ/
i/I	Is, sit	/ɪz/, /sɪt/	/iz/, /sit/
e/eI	Ace, bake, pay	/eɪs/, /beɪk/, /peɪ/	/es/, /bek/, /pe/
æ/ɛ	Excuse, head	/ɛkskjus/, /hɛd/	/ækskjuz/, /hæd/
eI/ɛ	Present	/prɛzənt/	/preɪzənt/
ɛ/æ	At, ham	/æt/ /hæm/	/ɛt/, /hɛm/
BACK VOWELS			
U/u	Ooze, food, to	/uz/, /fud/, tu/	/Uz/, /fUd/, /tU/
u/U	Should, foot	/Sud/, /fUt/	/Sud/, /fut/
o/oU	Oat, coat, so	/oUt/, /koUt/, /soU/	/ot/, /kot/, /so
o/ŋ	All, ball	/ŋl/, /bŋl/	/ol/, /bol/
CENTRAL VOWELS			
a/ʌ	Up, color	/ʌp/, /kʌlɚ/	/ap/, /kalɚ/
ɛr/ʒ̂	Early, bird, sir	/ʒ̂lI/, /bʒ̂d/, /sʒ̂/	/ɛrlI/, /bɛrd/, /sɛr/

SOURCE: Perez E: Phonological Difference among Speakers of Spanish Influenced English. In Bernthal JE, Bankson NW (eds): *Child Phonology: Characteristics, Assessment and Intervention with Special Populations,* p. 248. Thieme, New York, 1994.

TABLE 10.19. Spanish materials commercially available.

Title: Actividades Reparativas de Comunicacion (A.R.C.)
(Manual for high school age and adults—cognitive retraining and language therapy)
Publisher: Language Pathways
 2949 Los Amigos Ct., F.
 Las Cruces, NM 88011
 (505) 522–4950

Title: Bilingual Aphasia Test
(Examines phonemic, morphological, syntactic, semantic tasks involving comprehension, speaking, reading, and writing)
Publisher: Lawrence Erlbaum Associates
 10 Industrial Avenue
 Mahwah, NJ 07430-2262
 (201) 236–9500

Title: Ejercicios Orales
(Oral-motor exercises with illustrations)
Publisher: Ambi-Lingual Associates, Inc.
 4445 West 16th Avenue #500
 Hialeah, FL 33012
 (305) 556–1021

Title: Ejercicios para las Destrezas de Comunicacion (EDC)
(Manual of activities for vocabulary, speech, reading, and spelling)
Publisher: P. and R. Publications
 P.O. Box 46
 Escondido, CA 92025

Title: El Habla Despues de una Embolia
("Speech after Stroke"—activities to improve comprehension, vocabulary, reading, and writing)
Publisher: Stryker Illustrations
 1688 Meridian Avenue
 Suite 307
 Miami Beach, FL 33139
 (305) 534–3676

Title: Examen de Afasia Multilingue
(Multilingual Aphasia Examine Spanish Version)
Publisher: AJA Associates, Inc.
 504 Manor Drive
 PO Box 8740
 Iowa City, IA 52240-8740

Title: Examenes para Diagnosticar Impedimentos de Afasia
(Aphasia Language Performance Scales Spanish Version)
Publisher: Pinnacle Press
 PO Box 1122
 Murfreesboro, TN 37130

Title: Manual Terapeutico para el Adulto con Dificultades del Habla y Lenguaje
(Volume I Spanish Version of basic speech/language, listening/reading comprehension, writing/number skills)
Publisher: Visiting Nurses Service, Inc.
 1200 McArthur Drive
 Akron, OH 44320
 (216) 745–1601

(continued)

TABLE 10.19. (*continued*)

Title: Marketing to Multicultural Audiences (SLP)
(Spanish marketing kit for use with Hispanic population)
Publisher: ASHA Fulfillment Operations
    10801 Rockville Pike
    Rockville, MD 20852-3279
    (301) 897–5700

Title: Palabras Y Mas
(Pocket sized book of pictures, expressions, and terms of common categories)
Publisher: Primas Amigas Publishing, Inc.
    7000 S.W. 107th Street
    Miami, FL 33156
    (305) 666–8832

Title: Places and Things: Household Items
(Spanish terms and pictures of household items)
Publisher: Modern Education Corporation
    PO Box 721
    Tulsa, OK 74101

Title: Spanish Phrasing for Dysphagia and Dysarthria Drills
(Manual of words, phrases, and sentences with English translations)
Publisher: Language Pathways
    2949 Los Amigos, CT.F.
    Las Cruces, NM 88011
    (505) 522–4950

Title: Teaching Spanish Speech Sounds
(Child and adult consonant drills—reproducible)
Publisher: Academic Comm. Associates
    4149 Avenida de la Plata
    Dept. 205, PO Box 586249
    Oceanside, CA 92058-6249
    (619) 758–9593

Title: Tragando con Cuidado
(Spanish/English swallowing guide—one page including recommendations and precautions)
Publisher: Amvi-Lingual Associates, Inc.
    4445 West 16th Avenue #500
    Hialeah, FL 33012
    (305) 556–1021

Title: Tres Cosas Lindas hay en la Vida
(Spanish booklet explaining cause, prevention, and treatment of stroke)
Publisher: University of Arizona
    National Center for Neurogenic Communication Disorders
    Tuscon, AZ 85721
    (800) 926–2444

(Multiple materials for various speech-language areas)
Publisher: Bilingual Speech Source
    425 Circle Avenue
    Forest Prk, IL 60130-1733
    (800) 825–7133

TABLE 10.20. **Spanish phonemes and allophones with positions in words.**

Written symbol	Phoneme	Allophone	Word Position
p	p	p	initial, medial
b or v	b	b βv	initial, medial
t	t	t	initial, medial
d	d	d ð	initial, medial, final
qu or k	k	k	initial, medial
g	g	g ɣ	initial, medial
f	f	f ɸ	initial, medial
j	h	h	initial, medial
s or c	s	s	initial, medial, final
hu, gu	w	w u gw	initial, medial
hi, y	j	j i dʒ	initial, medial
ch	t	t	initial, medial
l	l	l	initial, medial, final
r	ɾ	ɾ	initial, medial, final
rr r	r	rR	initial, medial
m	m	m	initial, medial
n	n	n	initial, medial, final
ñ	ñ	ñ	initial, medial

TABLE **10.21.** **Vietnamese consonants.**

Sounds (IPA symbols)	Spelling	Key words		Initial	Final
				DISTRIBUTION	
p	p		dep (pretty)		x
b	b	ba (three)		x	
t	t	tai (ear)	hát (sing)	x	x (Northern)
t	th	thu' (letter)		x	
d	d	den (black)		x	
ʈ	tr	tre (bamboo)		x	
c	ch	cha (father)	sách (book)	x	x (Southern
				x	and Central)
k	c, k	ca (sing)	bác (uncle)	x	x
		ký (sign)			
kp̂	c		hoc (study)		x
g	g, gh	gan (liver)			
		ghét (hate)			
m	m	ma (ghost)	im (silent)	x	x
n	n	nó (he/she)	lan (orchid)	x	x (Northern)
ɲ	nh	nhà (house)	lính (soldier)	x	x (Southern
					and Central)
ŋ	ng, ngh	ngà (ivory)	làng (village)	x	x
		nghe (hear)	lông (hair)		x
ŋ m	ng	x		x	
f	ph	phi (waste)		x	
v	v	v´ê (go back)		x	
			(not in Southern)		
s	x	xa (far)		x	
z	d, gi, r	rong (seaweed)		x	
		da (skin)	(in Northern only)		
		già (old)			
ʃ	s	sai (wrong)		x	
			(not in Northern)		
ʒ	r	r´ông (dragon)		x	
			(not in Northern)		
j	d, gi	da (skin)		x	
		già (old)	(not in Northern)		
x	kh	khen (praise)		x	
h	h	hè (summer)		x	
l	l	lê (pear)		x	
r	r	ru´ôi (fly)		x	
			(in some dialects		
w	u, o	oà (burst out	only)	x	medial x
		crying)			
		hao (flower)			
		guý (precious)			
y	i	hai (two)		x	x

SOURCE: Cheng LL: Asian/Pacific Students and the Learning of English. In Bernthal JE, Bankson NW (eds): *Child Phonology: Characteristics, Assessment, and Intervention with Special Populations*, p. 266. Thieme, New York, 1994.

11

Audiology/Hearing Disorders

TABLE 11.1. **Articulation and phonological disorders in hearing-impaired school-aged children: factors accounting for range and complexity.**

1. Age of onset of hearing loss (prelingual, postlingual).
2. Age at detection of hearing loss.
3. Type of hearing loss (permanent sensorineural, acquired permanent sensorineural, intermittent conductive loss).
4. Degree of loss of hearing sensitivity (mild, moderate [conductive or sensorineural]severe, profound, total sensorineural).
5. Age at fitting and full-time use of amplification.
6. Individual response to the use of residual hearing.
7. Other concomitant organic factors (visual impairment and illness, e.g., meningitis, rubella, cerebral palsy).
8. Individual ability to exploit sensory input: use of residual hearing (where available), vision, and touch.
9. Method and quality of early intervention program.
10. Age at initiation of intervention.
11. Parental ability to cope, involvement in early education, and style of interaction.
12. Consistency and appropriateness of individual educational planning and treatment.
13. nowledge and skill of the professionals in the integration of knowledge of audition, amplification, communication, speech, and language development.
14. Child's cognitive and sociologic abilities and learning style.

SOURCE: Paterson MM: Articulation and Phonological Disorders in Hearing-Impaired School-Aged Children with Severe and Profound Sensorineural Losses. In Bernthal JE, Bankson NW (eds): *Child Phonology: Characteristics, Assessment, and Intervention with Special Populations,* p. 200. Thieme, New York, 1994.

TABLE 11.2. **Audiograms—pure tone descriptions.**

Term	Description	Audiometric configuration
Sloping	As frequency increases, the degree of loss increases.	
Rising	As frequency increases, the degree of loss decreases.	
Flat	There is little or no change in thresholds (±20 dB) across frequencies.	
High frequency	The hearing loss is limited to the frequencies above the speech range (2000–3000 Hz).	
4000–6000 Hz notch	Hearing is within normal limits through 3000 Hz and there is a sharp drop in the 4000–6000 Hz range, with improved thresholds at 8000 Hz.	
Scoop or trough shape	The greatest hearing loss is present in the midfrequencies, and hearing sensitivity is better in the low and high frequencies.	
Precipitous	There is a very sharp increase in the loss between one or two octaves.	
Inverted scoop or trough shape	The greatest hearing loss is in the low and high frequencies, and hearing sensitivity is better in the midfrequencies.	
Fragmentary	Thresholds are recorded only for low frequencies, and they are in the severe to profound range.	

TABLE 11.3. **Audiological evaluation procedures for infants and children: summary.**

Name of test	Explanation of technique	Indications for use	Advantages/disadvantages
Behavioral Observation Audiometry (BOA)	*Conditioning:* None A variety of test signals are presented through loudspeaker(s). Minimal Intensity is determined where behavioral changes are observed (e.g., sterling, scanning, cessation of activity, or change in sucking during testing). *Reinforcement:* None	Infants under 6 months and older youngsters with severe developmental delays. *Alternative:* Auditory evoked responses (particularly if test findings suggest a significant hearing loss).	*Advantages:* Can be used with unconditionable children. *Disadvantages:* 1. Rapid habituation of unconditioned behavior. 2. Unilateral losses may be missed. 3. Can only rule out severe and profound losses since relatively high intensities are required to elicit unconditioned responses even in normal hearing infants.
Conditioned Orientation Reflex Audiometry (COR) Visual Reinforcement Audiometry (VRA)	*Conditioning:* Establish bond between auditory signal and flashing lighted toy. *Reinforcement:* Lighted toy as well as social praise during test phase.	Toddlers from 6 to 24 months and many older children with developmental delays. *Alternative:* Auditory evoked responses.	*Advantages:* 1. Stimuli can be presented by earphones, bone conduction, or loudspeaker. 2. Does not require voluntary response. 3. Capitalizes on heightened visual alertness of hearing impaired children. *Disadvantages:* 1. Approximately 35% of infants under 12 months of age cannot be conditioned. 2. Many toddlers will not accept earphones initially. 3. If stimuli are presented in the sound field, a unilateral hearing loss may be missed.

| Tangible Reinforcement Operant Conditioning Audiometry (TROCA) | *Conditioning:* Connection is established between auditory stimuli and "button-pressing." *Reinforcement:* A tangible reinforcement (such as cereal) that is automatically dispensed following a correct response. | Preschoolers, especially those with short attention spans and those who work best with structure. Also many older mentally retarded children. *Alternative:* VRA (auditory evoked responses). | *Advantages:*
 1. Stimuli can be presented by earphones, bone conduction, or loudspeakers.
 2. Can be used in conjunction with frequency-specific measures.
 Disadvantages:
 1. Time-consuming and requires repeated sessions to establish conditioning.
 2. Children will often insist upon eating the reinforcer between trials, thus increasing the length of the test session substantially. |

SOURCE: From Roeser RJ, Yellin W: Pure-Tone Tests with Preschool Children. In Martin F (ed): *Hearing Disorders in Children*, pp. 217–264. Copyright © 1987 by Allyn & Bacon. (Reprinted/adapted by permission.)

TABLE 11.4. **Auditory skill development sequence.**

Auditory skills	Child behaviors	Stimulation skills
1. Attending/detection	Child attends to environmental sounds and voices. Child attends to distinct speech sounds.	Use auditory clues, show child sources of sound and reinforce child's responses to sound.
2. Recognizing	Child recognizes objects and events from their sounds.	Point out sounds and reinforce child's recognition of sound sources. Allow sound to be child's first source of information.
3. Locating	Child locates sound sources in space.	Create localization opportunities and reinforce all child attempts to localize.
4. Distances and levels	Child locates sound sources at increased distances and above and below.	Create opportunities for child to hear sounds above and below and at distances; reinforce responses.
5. Environmental discrimination, identification and comprehension	Child discriminates, identifies, and comprehends environmental sounds.	Repeatedly stimulate the child with environmental sounds and reinforce child's discrimination, identification and comprehension of sounds.
6. Vocal discrimination, identification and comprehension	Child discriminates, identifies, and comprehends gross vocal sounds, words, and phrases.	Provide opportunities for child to discriminate, identify, and comprehend onomatopoeic sounds, words, and phrases.
7. Speech discrimination, identification and comprehension	Child discriminates, identifies, and comprehends fine speech sounds: vowels then consonants.	Provide stimulation of vowel, then consonant sounds in meaningful words. Create opportunities for child to demonstrate discrimination, identification and comprehension of these words.

SOURCE: From Nerbonne MA, Schow RL: Auditory Stimuli in Communication. In Schow RL, Nerbonne MA: *Introduction to Aural Rehabilitation,* 2nd Edition, p. 324. Copyright © 1989 by Allyn & Bacon. Reprinted/adapted by permission.

TABLE 11.5. Cochlear implants: criteria for selection and contraindications.

A. Criteria for Children
1. Ages 2 to 17 years.
2. Bilateral profound sensorineural deafness (electrophysiologic assessment must corroborate behavioral evaluation for younger children).
3. Little or no benefit from a hearing (or vibrotactile) aid for a minimum of 6 months with appropriate amplification.
4. Motivation and appropriate expectations of families if possible, candidates.

B. Criteria for Adults
1. Profound sensorineural deafness.
2. Little or no benefit from a hearing aid.
3. Postlingually deafened.
4. Psychological and motivational suitability.

C. Contraindications for Cochlear Implants
1. Deafness caused by lesions to the acoustic nerve or the central auditory pathway.
2. Active middle ear infections.
3. Cochlear ossification that prevents electrode insertion.
4. Tympanic membrane perforation.

TABLE **11.6.** **Communication between parents and their hearing-impaired child:
objectives and methods for establishment.**

Objectives	*Method*
Establish an effective communication setting	1. Keep background noises at a minimum when communicating with child. 2. child freedom to explore and play. Child must have chance to explore objects and learn what they are and do if he is to understand communication about them. 3. Serve as a "communication consultant." Place child near you so you can frequently communicate with him. 4. Use interactive turn-taking. Encourage child to "take turns" in a variety of activities and situations. 5. Get down on child's level, as close to him as possible. Speech is most intelligible 3–4 feet from child. 6. Occasionally provide *ad concham* stimulation (talk directly into child's ear). 7. Maintain eye contact and direct conversation to child.
Establish effective nonverbal communication	1. Use interesting, varied facial expressions. 2. Use varied intonation and rhythm patterns. 3. Use natural gestures. 4. Touch child in stimulating way while vocalizing.
Establish effective verbal communication	1. Regard child's cry as communicative and respond accordingly. 2. Imitate and expand child's babbling and vocal play. Imitate and expand child's motions and add vocalizations. Introduce a few new babbling sounds each week for the child to hear. 3. Identify and respond to child's verbal and nonverbal intents (vocalizing, pointing, tugging, stretching, looking, playing) with simple language. 4. Use conversational turn-taking (wait expectantly for a response, signal the child to take a turn, use prods, chains, questions, etc., to keep conversation going). 5. Talk about obvious objects and events. Talk about child's meaningful daily activities and emotional experiences. 6. Talk about fun topics that interest child. Take advantage of child's curiosity. 7. Use short, simple sentences and expressions rather than long, complicated ones. 8. Communicate to child in ways he can understand (match child's communication level). 9. When child is ready, encourage a more mature communication level.

SOURCE: Watkins S, Schow RL: Aural Rehabilitation for Children. In Schow RL, Nerbonne MA: *Introduction to Aural Rehabilitation,* 2nd ed., p. 326. Copyright © 1989 by Allyn & Bacon. Reprinted/adapted by permission.

TABLE 11.7. **Deafness in infants and children: ABC high-risk factors.**

Asphyxia
Bacterial meningitis
Congenital perinatal infections
    Toxoplasmosis
    Other bacterial infections (i.e., syphilis)
    Rubella virus
    Cytomegalovirus
    Herpes simplex virus
Defects of the head and neck
Elevated bilirubin
Family history
Gram birthweight less than 1500 grams (3.3 lbs)

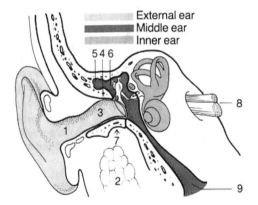

FIGURE 11.1. **Relations of the external auditory meatus.**
1, cartilaginous part; **2,** parotid gland; **3,** bony meatus; **4,** lateral attic wall; **5,** mastoid antrum; **6,** attic; **7,** temporomandibular joint; **8,** facial, vestibular and auditory nerves; **9,** Eustachian tube.

SOURCE: Becker W, Naumann HH, Pfaltz CR: *Ear, Nose, and Throat Diseases: A Pocket Reference,* 2nd rev. ed., p. 4. Thieme, New York, 1994.

TABLE 11.8. **Familiar sound intensity-level examples.**

Sources (measured operator/ listener distance from source)	Aural effect	Sound level in decibels
Shotgun blast	Human ear pain threshold	140
Jet plane at take-off		
Firecrackers, exploding		
Rock music (amplified)	Uncomfortably loud	120
Hockey game crowd		
Thunder, severe		
Pneumatic jackhammer		
Powered lawnmower	Extremely loud	100
Tractor, farm type		
Subway train (interior)		
Motorcycle		
Snowmobile		
Cocktail party (100 guests)		
Window air-conditioner	Moderately loud	80
Crowded restaurant		
Diesel-powered truck/tractor		
Singing birds	Quiet	60
Normal conversation		
Rustle of leaves	Very quiet	40
Faucet, dripping		
Light rainfall		
Whisper	Just audible	10

SOURCE: With permission from Olishifski JB, Harford ER: *Industrial Noise and Hearing Conservation*, p. 2. National Safety Council, Chicago, 1975. Used by permission of the National Safety Council, Itasca, Illinois.

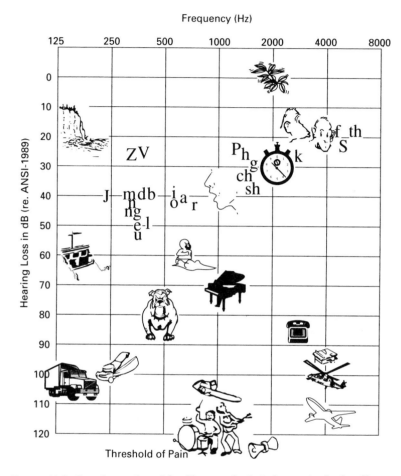

FIGURE 11.2. Speech sounds and familiar sounds plotted on a standard audiogram form.

SOURCE: With permission from Northern JL., Downs MP., *Hearing in Children,* 4th ed., page 17. Baltimore: Williams & Wilkins, 1991.

TABLE 11.9. Hearing loss: associated behaviors of children.

---

1. Frequently asks to have things repeated.
2. Turns one side of head toward speaker.
3. Talks too loudly or too softly.
4. Shows strain in trying to hear.
5. Watches and concentrates on teacher's lips.
6. Is inattentive in classroom discussion.
7. Makes frequent mistakes in following directions.
8. Makes unusual mistakes in taking dictation
9. Tends to isolate self
10. Tends to be passive.
11. Is tense.
12. Tires easily.
13. Has a speech problem.
14. Is not working up to apparent capacity.
15. Has academic failure following severe illness.

Physical symptoms may include:
1. Mouth breathing.
2. Draining ears.
3. Earaches.
4. Dizziness.
5. Reports of ringing, buzzing, or roaring in ears.

TABLE **11.10.** **Hearing loss: degrees and effects on communication abilities.**

Level of hearing loss based on PTA (500, 1000, 2000 Hz)	Degree of Hearing loss	Effects of hearing loss
26 to 40	Mild	Demonstrates difficulty understanding soft-spoken speech; needs preferential seating and may benefit from speechreading training: good candidate for a hearing aid.
41 to 55	Moderate	Demonstrates an understanding of speech at 3 to 5 feet; requires amplification, preferential seating, speechreading training, and speech therapy.
56 to 70	Moderate to Severe	Speech must be loud for auditory reception; difficulty in group and classroom discussion; may require special classes for hearing-impaired, plus all of the above needs.
71 to 90	Severe	Loud speech may be understood at 1 foot from ear; may distinguish vowels but not consonants; requires classroom for hearing-impaired and mainstreaming at a later date.
91+	Profound	Does not rely on audition as primary modality for communication; may work well with total communication approach; may eventually be mainstreamed at higher grade levels.

SOURCE: With permission from Goodman A: Reference Zero Levels for Pure Tone Audiometers. *ASHA* 1965;7:262–263.

TABLE 11.11. **Hearing loss identification at an early age: pros and cons of various approaches.**

Screening Approach	Pros	Cons
•**Public awareness campaigns**	Relatively inexpensive; easy to prepare and disseminate; provide broad coverage	Uncertain yield: parental suspicions often ignored or parents placated by primary care providers; uncertain population exposure/readership
•**High-Risk Registries (HRR)**		
Maternal Questionnaires	Relatively inexpensive; discrete referral criteria	Difficulty in maintaining high compliance; many infants lost to follow-up. Substantial percentage of children with confirmed hearing losses manifest no risk factors; no examples of long-term success
Birth certificate–based	Relatively inexpensive; discrete referral criteria; demonstrated success in identifying large numbers of children	Hospital coding of some variables suspect (e.g., family history): birth certificate protocol difficult to modify for risk factors; substantial percentage of children with confirmed hearing losses manifest no risk factors; many infants lost to follow-up
•**Behavioral screening**		
Behavioral Observation Audiometry (BOA)	Relatively inexpensive: time-efficient: straightforward equipment requiring little maintenance; tests frequency-specific, behavioral responses to hearing	High number of false-positive and false-negative results; subjective; requires a sound-treated room: requires trained personnel proficient in observation of very subtle physical responses to sound; unreliable
Home health visitors	Opportunity to assess hearing in natural setting. In countries where universal home visits are conducted, approach is economical and has resulted in reported ages of identification of between 7 and 10 months of age.	Cost prohibitive in the U.S.; difficulties in training personnel; difficulties in ensuring 100% coverage of population; children most at-risk least likely to be screened; complications regarding influence of otitis media in screen results
Crib-O-Gram (COG)	Automated, thereby easily operated; requires a minimum of personnel; does not require a sound-treated room; does not interrupt the nursery routine; objective	Many false-positive and false-negatives, particularly in NICU population: difficult to determine threshold vs. habituation: may miss mild, moderate, and unilateral hearing losses

•Auditory Brainstem Response (ABR)

Traditionally applied ABR

Valid auditory measure; objective measurement; ear-specific information; air vs. bone conduction; results independent of subject state and cerebral status; sound booth not required; measures peripheral auditory and neurological function

Costs with respect to personnel, time, and equipment; cannot detect losses below 1,000 Hz; subjective analysis of results; requires highly skilled personnel; not a test of behavioral responses to hearing; lack of longitudinal data on large samples of infants tested in both normal nurseries and NICUs

Automated ABR

ALGO-1 Plus: portability, battery power, artifact rejection; does not require highly-skilled personnel; less expensive than traditional ABR apparatus

Quite expensive, especially in small institutional settings and settings in which only at-risk newborns are screened; no longitudinal results in published literature following infants who passed automated ABR; not a diagnostic procedure—cannot determine degree and nature of hearing loss; not a test of behavioral responses to hearing

•Transient evoked Otocoustic Emissions (TEOAEs)

Simple; quick; noninvasive; objective; sensitive; cost-efficient; does not require highly-skilled personnel; yields frequency-specific data; demonstrated success in identifying large numbers of infants with impaired hearing

Does not measure activity of the auditory nerve or brainstem auditory nuclei; not a diagnostic procedure— cannot determine degree and nature of hearing loss; still considered "experimental" by some; not a measure of behavioral responses to hearing

SOURCE: Mauk GW, Behrens TR: Historical, Political, and Technological Context. *Seminars in Hearing* 1993; 14:9.

TABLE 11.12. Hearing loss in children: handicapping effects and probable needs.

Average threshold–level at 500 2000 Hz (ANSI)	Description	Common causes	What can be heard without amplification	Degree of handicap (if not treated in first year of life)	Probable needs
0–15 dB 16–25 dB	Normal range Slight hearing loss	Serous otitis, perforation, monomeric membrane, sensorineural loss, tympanosclerosis	All speech sounds Vowel sounds heard clearly, may miss unvoiced consonant sounds	None Possible mild or transitory auditory dysfunction Difficulty in perceiving some speech sounds	None Consideration of need for hearing aid Lip reading Auditory training Speech therapy Preferential seating Appropriate surgery
26–40 dB	Mild hearing loss	Serous otitis, perforation, tympanosclerosis, monomeric membrane, sensorineural loss	Hears only some of speech sounds–the louder voiced sounds	Auditory learning dysfunction Mild language retardation Mild speech problems Inattention	Hearing aid Lip reading Auditory training Speech therapy Appropriate surgery
41–65 dB	Moderate hearing loss	Chronic otitis, middle ear anomaly, sensorineural loss	Misses most speech sounds at normal conversational level	Speech problems Language retardation Learning dysfunction Inattention	All of the above plus consideration of special classroom situation
66–95 dB	Severe hearing loss	Sensorineural loss or mixed loss due to sensorineural loss plus middle ear disease	Hears no speech sound of normal conversations	Language retardation Learning dysfunction Inattention Severe speech problems	All of the above, probable assignment to special classes
96+ dB	Profound hearing loss	Sensorineural loss or mixed	Hears no speech or other sounds	Language retardation Learning dysfunction Inattention Severe speech problems	All of the above; probable assignment to special classes

SOURCE: With permission from Northern JL, Downs MP: *Hearing in Children*, 4th ed., p. 99. Williams & Wilkins, Baltimore, MD, 1991.

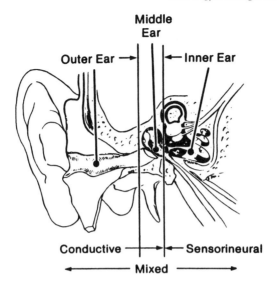

FIGURE 11.3. Hearing loss: three types classified according to anatomic site involved.
SOURCE: Roeser RJ: Audiometric and Immittance Measures: Principles and Interpretation, p. 31. In Roeser RJ, Downs MP: *Auditory Disorders in Schoolchildren,* 3rd ed. Thieme, New York, 1995.

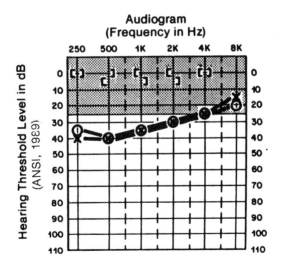

FIGURE 11.4. Hearing loss: conductive—Pure-tone and bone-conduction audiogram pattern.
SOURCE: Roeser RJ: Audiometric and Immittance Measures: Principles and Interpretation, p. 31. In Roeser RJ, Downs MP: *Auditory Disorders in Schoolchildren,* 3rd ed. Thieme, New York, 1995.

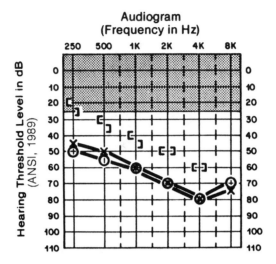

FIGURE 11.5. Hearing loss: mixed—pure-tone air and bone-conduction audiogram pattern.

SOURCE: Roeser RJ: Audiometric and Immittance Measures: Principles and Interpretation, p. 32. In Roeser RJ, Downs MP: *Auditory Disorders in Schoolchildren,* 3rd ed. Thieme, New York, 1995.

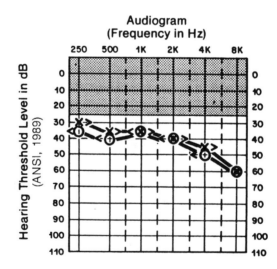

FIGURE 11.6. Hearing loss: sensorineural—pure-tone and bone-conduction audiogram pattern.

SOURCE: Roeser RJ: Audiometric and Immittance Measures: Principles and Interpretation, p. 32. In Roeser RJ, Downs MP: *Auditory Disorders in Schoolchildren,* 3rd ed. Thieme, New York, 1995.

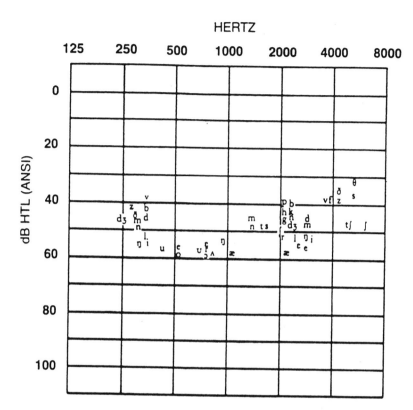

FIGURE 11.7. Speech sounds in English: intensity and frequency distribution.

The values given should only be considered approximations and are based on data reported by Fletcher (1953) and Ling and Ling (1978). Sounds with more than one major component appear in the figure in more than one location.

SOURCE: From Schow RL, Nerbonne MA: *Introduction to Aural Rehabilitation.* Copyright ©1989 by Allyn & Bacon. Reprinted/adapted by permission.

TABLE 11.13. Hereditary deafness classifications.

I. CONGENITAL SENSORINEURAL HEARING LOSS DISORDERS

Craniofacial and Skeletal Disorders
Absence of tibia
Cleidocranial dysostosis
Diastrophic dwarfism
Hand–hearing syndrome
Klippel–Feil
Saddle nose and myopia
Split-hand and foot

Integumentary and Pigmentary Disorders
Albinism with blue irides
Congenital atopic dermatitis
Ectodermal dysplasia
Keratopachyderma
Lentigines
Onychodystrophy
Partial albinism
Piebaldness
Pili torti
Waardenburg's syndrome

Eye Disorders
Hallgren's
Laurence–Moon–Biedl–Bardet

Nervous System Disorders
Cerebral palsy
Muscular dystrophy

II. CONGENITAL CONDUCTIVE HEARING LOSS DISORDERS

Craniofacial and Skeletal Disorders
Apert's syndrome
Fanconi's anemia syndrome
Goldenhar's syndrome
Madelung's deformity
Malformed, low-set ears
Mohr's syndrome
Otopalatodigital
Preauricular appendages
Proximal symphalangism
Thickened ears
Treacher–Collins

Integumentary and Pigmentary Disorders
Forney's syndrome

Eye Disorders
Cryptophthalmos
Duane's syndrome

Renal Disorders
Nephrosis, urinary tract malformations
Renal–genital syndrome
Taylor's syndrome

III. DISORDERS OF CONGENITAL SENSORINEURAL AND/OR CONDUCTIVE HEARING LOSS

IV. PROGRESSIVE HEARING LOSS DISORDERS

Sensorineural Progressive Hearing Loss of Later Onset

Craniofacial and Skeletal Disorders
Roaf's syndrome
Van Buchem's syndrome

Eye Disorders
Alström's syndrome
Cockayne's syndrome
Fehr's corneal dystrophy
Flynn–Aird
Norrie's syndrome
Optic atrophy and diabetes mellitus
Refsum's syndrome

Nervous System Disorders
Acoustic neuromas
Friedreich's ataxia
Herrmann's syndrome
Myoclonic seizures
Sensory radicular neuropathy
Severe infantile muscular dystrophy

Endocrine and Metabolic Disorders
Alport's syndrome
Amyloidosis, nephritis, and urticaria
Hyperprolinemia 11
Hyperuricemia
Primary testicular insufficiency

Myoclonic epilepsy
Opticocochleodentate degeneration
Richards–Rundel

Cardiovascular System Disorders
Jervell and Lange–Nielsen

Endocrine and Metabolic Disorders
Goiter
Hyperprolinemia I
Iminoglycinuria
Pendred's

Miscellaneous Somatic Disorders
Trisomy 13–15
Trisomy 18

Craniofacial and Skeletal Disorders
Achondroplasia
Crouzon's syndrome
Marfan's syndrome
Pierre–Robin
Pyle's disease

Integumentary and Pigmentary Disorders
Knuckle pads and leukonychia

Eye Disorders
Möbius' syndrome

Miscellaneous Somatic Disorders
Turner's syndrome

Sensorineural or Conductive Progressive Hearing Loss
Craniofacial and Skeletal Disorders
Albers–Schönberg disease
Engelmann's syndrome
Osteogenesis imperfecta
Paget's disease
Endocrine and Metabolic Disorder
Hunter's syndrome
Hurler's syndrome

Progressive Conductive or Mixed Hearing Loss
Otosclerosis

SOURCE: With permission from Northern JL, Downs MP: *Hearing in Children*, 4th ed., p. 92. Williams & Wilkins, Baltimore, MD, 1991.

TABLE 11.14. **Immittance results summary.**

Tympanogram	Pressure peak	Location of Static compliance	Acoustic reflex
A	Normal (+50 to −100 dapa)	Normal (0.28–2.50 ml)	Present at normal levels Partial, elevated, or absent
A$_d$	Normal (+50 to −100$_{da.Pa}$)	Abnormally high (greater than 2.50 ml)	Present at normal levels Partial, elevated, or absent
A$_s$	Normal (+50 to −100$_{dapa}$)	Abnormally low (less than 0.28 ml)	Present at normal levels Partial, elevated, or absent
B	No peak (flat or rounded)	Abnormally low (less than 0.28 ml)	Present at normal levels Partial, elevated, or absent
C	Abnormally negative (more negative than −100 dapa)	Normal (0.28–2.50 cc), or low (less than 0.28 ml)	Present at normal levels Partial, elevated, or absent

SOURCE: Roeser RJ, Downs MP: *Auditory Disorders in Schoolchildren*, p. 28. Thieme, New York, 1988.

TABLE 11.15. Indicators associated with sensorineural or conductive hearing loss.*

A. *For use with neonates* (birth through age 28 days) when universal screening is not available.
   1. Family history of hereditary childhood sensorineural hearing loss
   2. In utero infection, such as cytomegalovirus, rubella, syphilis, herpes, and toxoplasmosis
   3. Craniofacial anomalies, including those with morphological abnormalities of the pinna and ear canal
   4. Birth weight less than 1,500 grams (3.3 lbs)
   5. Hyperbilirubinemia at a serum level requiring exchange transfusion
   6. Ototoxic medications, including but not limited to the aminoglycosides, used in multiple courses or in combination with loop diuretics
   7. Bacterial meningitis
   8. Apgar scores of 0–4 at 1 minute or 0–6 at 5 minutes
   9. Mechanical ventilation lasting 5 days or longer
   10. Stigmata or other findings associated with a syndrome known to include a sensorineural and or conductive hearing loss.

B. *For use with infants* (age 29 days through 2 years) when certain health conditions develop that require rescreening.
   1. Parent/caregiver concern regarding hearing, speech, language, and/or developmental delay
   2. Bacterial meningitis and other infections associated with sensorineural hearing loss
   3. Head trauma associated with loss of consciousness or skull fracture
   4. Stigmata or other findings associated with a syndrome known to include a sensorineural and/or conductive hearing loss
   5. Ototoxic medications, including but not limited to chemotherapeutic agents or aminoglycosides, used in multiple courses or in combination with loop diuretics
   6. Recurrent or persistent otitis media with effusion for at least 3 months

C. *For use with infants* (age 29 days through 3 years) who require periodic monitoring of hearing.

Some newborns and infants may pass initial hearing screening but require periodic monitoring of hearing to detect delayed-onset sensorineural and/or conductive hearing loss. Infants with these indicators require hearing evaluation at least every 6 months until age 3 years, and at appropriate intervals thereafter. Indicators associated with delayed onset sensorineural hearing loss include:

   1. Family history of hereditary childhood hearing loss
   2. In utero infection, such as cytomegalovirus, rubella, syphilis, herpes, or toxoplasmosis
   3. Neurofibromatosis Type II and neurodegenerative disorders

Indicators associated with conductive hearing loss include:

   1. Recurrent or persistent otitis media with effusion
   2. Anatomic deformities and other disorders that affect eustachian tube function
   3. Neurodegenerative disorders

---

*Joint Committee on Infant Hearing 1994 Position Statement.

TABLE 11.16. Infant Auditory Behavior Index: stimulus and level of response.*

Age	Noisemakers (approx. SPL)	Warbled pure tones (Re: dB HL)	Speech (Re: dB HL)	Expected response	Startle to speech (Re: dB HL)
0–6 wks	50–70 dB	78 dB	40–60 dB	Eye widening, eye blinking, stirring or arousal from sleep, startle	65 dB
6 wks–4 mo	50–60 dB	70 dB	47 dB	Eye widening, eye shift, eye blinking, quieting; beginning rudimentary head turn by 4 months	65 dB
4–7 mo	40–50 dB	51 dB	21 dB	Head-turn on lateral plane toward sound; listening attitude	65 dB
7–9 mo	30–40 dB	45 dB	15 dB	Direct localization of sounds to side, indirectly below ear level	65 dB
9–13 mo	25–35 dB	38 dB	8 dB	Direct localization of sounds to side, directly below, ear level, indirectly above ear level	65 dB
13–16 mo					
16–21 mo	25–30 dB	32 dB	5 dB	Direct localization of sound on side, above and below	65 dB
21–24 mo	25 dB	25 dB	5 dB	Direct localization of sound on side, above and below	65 dB
	25 dB	25 dB	3 dB	Direct localization of sound on side, above and below	65 dB

SOURCE: With permission from Northern JL, Downs MP: *Hearing in Children*, 3rd ed., p. 135. Williams & Wilkins, Baltimore, MD, 1984.

*Testing done in a sound room. (Modified with permission from F. McConnell and P. H. Ward: *Deafness in Childhood*, Nashville, Tenn., Vanderbilt University Press, 1967.)

TABLE 11.17. **Letter for children who fail pure-tone screening and/or immittance screening.**

Dear _____,

The results of your child's hearing screening at school indicate a need for further evaluation. It is recommended that your child receive:

_____ a rescreening in two weeks

_____ medical examination by an ear specialist and/or family physician

_____ a referral to an audiologist for a complete diagnostic evaluation

After your child's examination or diagnostic evaluation is completed, please return a copy of the report of the findings and recommendations to the school. Feel free to contact me if you have any questions or need assistance in obtaining services.

Sincerely,

_____
Date

School Nurse

_____ _____ _____
Name of Student   Grade   Teacher

SCHOOL PURE-TONE SCREENING RESULTS

Left Ear			
500	1000	2000	4000

Right Ear			
500	1000	2000	4000

_____ Immittance (tympanometer) screening results indicate possible middle ear problems.

REPORT TO SCHOOL

Findings and Recommendations _____

_____

_____

_____ _____
Date of Examination   Signature of Examiner and Credentials

TABLE 11.18. Middle-ear pathologies: tympanometric configuration examples.

Middle-ear disorder	SHAPE			
	Pressure peak	Amplitude	High-frequency probe tone	Low-frequency probe tone
Serous otitis acute	None–severe negative	None–shallow	Flat–slight rising	Flat–falling
Serous otitis resolving "glue" ear	Moderate–negative	Shallow–normal	Normal	Normal
	Moderate–severe negative	Flat–shallow	Flat	Flat–falling
Cholesteatoma	Normal–negative to absent	Nonshallow	Flattened	Lower at negative pressure
Acute otitis media	Positive	Normal	Normal	Normal
Blocked eustachian tube	Mild–moderate negative	Normal	Normal	Normal
Glomus turner	Nonnormal	Extremely shallow	Vascular perturbations	Vascular perturbations
Otosclerosis	Normal	Shallow	Normal	Normal
Malleoar fixation	Normal	Shallow	Normal	Normal
Incudostapedial interruption	Normal	Large	Peaked–normal	Deep notches, peaked and undulating
Crural interpretation	Normal	Large	Peaked–normal	Deep notches, peaked and undulating
Healed TM perforation	Normal	Large	Normal–peaked	Notch-peaked
Perforated TM	None	Elevated baseline	Flat	Flat
Stapedectomy	Normal	Large	Normal	Notched and undulating

(Converging)

SOURCE: With permission from Feldman AS, Wilber LA: *Acoustic Impedance and Admittance—The Measurement of Middle Ear Function.* William & Wilkins, Baltimore, MD, 1976.

TABLE 11.19. Milestones of an infant's hearing.

Birth to 3 months . . .
  Startles or jumps when there is a sudden loud sound.
  Stirs, wakes up or cries when someone talks or makes a noise.
  Recognizes your voice and quiets when you speak.
3 to 6 months . . .
  Turns eyes toward interesting sound.
  Appears to listen.
  Awakes easily to sounds.
6 to 12 months . . .
  Turns head toward soft sounds.
  Understands "no" and "bye-bye."
  Begins to imitate speech sounds.
12 months . . .
  Says first words such as "Da-Da," "Ma-Ma," or "bye-bye."

SOURCE: Reprinted by permission of American Academy of Audiology, Washington, DC.

TABLE 11.20. Nonspeech deficits associated with hearing loss.

A. Cognitive deficits
   1. Mental retardation
   2. Dementia
B. Behavioral disorder
C. Psychiatric disorder
D. Language delay and disorder
E. Learning disability
   1. Reading deficits
   2. Writing deficits
F. Nervous system disease
   1. Motor disturbances
   2. Seizures
   3. Glioma or neuroma
   4. Spina bifida
   5. Impaired taste and smell
   6. Vestibular disturbances
G. Eye disease
   1. Optic degeneration and atrophy
   2. Ocular lens abnormalities
   3. Retinitis pigmentosa
     a. Night blindness
     b. Tunnel vision
     c. Blindness
   4. Oculomotor disturbances
H. Renal disease
I. Musculoskeletal disease
   1. Head and neck abnormalities
     a. Abnormalities of the skull
     b. Malformations of the lip and palate
     c. Eyelid malformations
     d. Abnormal facial features
     e. Malformations of the outer ear
     f. Malformations of the middle ear
     g. and maxillary malformations
     h. Dental abnormalities
     i. Nasal abnormalities

   2. Digital anomalies
   3. Limb abnormalities
   4. Joint abnormalities
   5. Limb and joint pain
   6. Bone disease
   7. Growth retardation
   8. Vertebral abnormalities
   9. Shoulder abnormalities
   10. Winged scapula
J. Skin disease
   1. Pigmentary disorder
     a. Albinism
     b. White forelock
     c. Vitiligo
     d. Leukonychia
     e. Cafe-au-lait spots
     f. Axillary freckling
     g. Iris bicolor or heterochromia
     h. Salt and pepper retinal pigmentation
   2. Lichenfield skin eruptions
   3. Recurrent urticaria
   4. Keratosis
   5. Sun sensitivity
   6. Thick, coarse hair
   7. Abnormal whorl patterns on hands
   8. Malformed fingernails and toenails
K. Metabolic disease
   1. Diabetes
   2. Goiter
   3. Liver and spleen enlargement
   4. Impaired metabolism of carbohydrates
L. Cardiac and vascular disease
M. Urogenital malformations

SOURCE: McNeil MR, Robin DA, Schmidt RA: Apraxia of Speech: Definition, Differentiation, and Treatment. In McNeil MR (ed): *Clinical Management of Sensorimotor Disorders,* p. 356. Thieme, New York, 1997.

TABLE 11.21. (continued)

Disorder	Synonym(s)	Selected characteristics	Conductive	Sensorineural	CNS
Refsum syndrome	—	Eye disorder; ataxia; muscle atrophy; neuropathy	—	−/+	—
Richards–Rundel syndrome	Ataxia–hypogonadism syndrome	CNS disorder; ataxia: MR; arreflexia	—	−/+	—
Rubella	—	Numerous possible defects of heart, eyes, CNS, viscera	—	+	+
Saddle nose syndrome	Marshall syndrome	Facial abnormalities; eye defects	—	−/+	—
Schilder disease	—	Mental deterioration; encephalopathy	—	+	+
Small syndrome	—	MR; muscular atrophy; eye (retinal) defect	—	+	+
Treacher Collins syndrome	Mandibular dysostosis	Facial abnormalities; multiple ear anomalies	+	—	—
Trisomy 13–15	—	Multiple abnormalities; MR; heart defects	—	+	+
Trisomy 18	—	Microcephaly; heart defects; cleft lip/palate; MR	+	+	+
Turner syndrome	—	Multiple abnormalities; low hairline; oral–facial defects	+	+	—
Unverricht disease	—	Progressive myoclonic epilepsy; neurologic degeneration	—	−/+	+
Usher's syndrome	—	Progressive visual deficits; MR; epilepsy	—	+	+
Van Buchem's syndrome	—	Craniofacial & skeletal disorder; nerve palsies	+	−/+	+

TABLE 11.21. (continued)

Disorder	Synonym(s)	Selected characteristics	Conductive	Sensorineural	CNS
DeSanctis-Cacchione syndrome	—	Skin and neurological abnormalities	—	+	—
Diastrophic dwarfism	—	Craniofacial abnormalities; hand & foot defects	—	+	—
Down's syndrome	Trisomy 21; mongolism	MR; craniofacial and multiple structural abnormalities	+	+	+
Duane syndrome	Cervico-oculoacoustic dysplasia	Eye defect; oculomotor paralysis	—/+	+	—
Ectodermal dysplasia	Lobster-claw syndrome	Skin & pigment disorder, hand & foot abnormalities	—/+	—/+	—
Engelmann disease	Craniodiaphyseal dysplasia	Skeletal abnormality of long bones; skull base defect	—/+	—/+	—
Fanconi anemia syndrome	—	Renal impairment; retarded growth	—	—/+	—
Fehr's corneal dystrophy	Harboyan syndrome	Eye abnormality	—	—/+	—
First branchial arch syndrome	—	Hemifacial atrophy	+	—	—
Flynn–Aird syndrome	—	Eye defects; mental deterioration	+	—/+	—
Forney syndrome	—	Heart defects	+	—	—
Goldenhar syndrome	—	Craniofacial abnormalities	+	—	—
Gorlin–Hart syndrome	Frontometaphyseal dysplasia	Dysplasia of frontal ridges; facial abnormalities	+	+	—
Hallgren's syndrome	—	Eye abnormality; progressive ataxia; MR sometimes	—	+	+
Herrmann's syndrome	—	Diabetes mellitus; CNS abnormalities; renal disease	—	—/+	+
Hunter syndrome	Mucopolysaccharidosis II	Affects males; growth retarded; facial defects; death	+	+	+
Hurler syndrome	Mucopolysaccharidosis I	Corneal clouding; see Hunter syndrome; early death	+	—/+	+
Jervell–Lange–Nielsen syndrome	—	Cardiovascular defects; consanguinity factor; death	—	+	—

Syndrome	Alternate name	Description				
Klippel–Feil syndrome	Wildervanck syndrome	Craniofacial disorder; short neck; multiple abnormalities	+	+	+	+
Laurence–Moon–Biedl syndrome	—	MR; hand abnormalities; retinitis pigmentosa; obesity	—	+	+	+
Leopard syndrome	Multiple lentigines	Skin pigment & multiple bodily abnormalities	—	+	+	—
Long-arm 18-deletion	—	MR; microcephaly: multiple bodily abnormalities	+	+	+	+
Madelung deformity	Leri–Weill disease	Craniofacial & skeletal abnormality	+	—	+	—
Marfan syndrome	—	Craniofacial & skeletal abnormality; heart defects	—	+	+	—
Möbius syndrome	—	Craniofacial & CNS abnormalities; hand & foot defects	+	+	+	+
Muckle–Wells syndrome	Amyloidosis; nephritis	Urticaria; renal failure; endocrine disturbance	—	+	+	—
Norrie's syndrome	Oculoacousticocerebral degeneration	Progressive eye disorder; MR	—	—/+	—/+	+
Osteogenesis imperfecta	Van der Hoeve syndrome	Brittle bones; possible infant death; secondary defects	—/+	—/+	—/+	—
Otofacial cervical syndrome	—	Face is narrowed and midface is flattened	+	—	—	—
Otopalatodigital syndrome	—	Craniofacial & skeletal abnormalities; cleft palate	+	—	—	—
Paget disease	Hereditary hyperphosphatemia	Skeletal disorder; cranial nerve dysfunction; large head	—/+	—/+	—/+	—
Pendred's syndrome	—	Endocrine & metabolic disorder; goiter	—	+	+	—
Piebaldism	—	Skin & pigment disorder; MR; ataxia	—	+	+	+
Pierre Robin syndrome	—	Cleft palate; micrognathia; skeletal defects	+	+	+	—
Pyle's disease	Craniometaphyseal dysplasia	Craniofacial & skeletal disorder	—/+	—/+	—/+	—

(continued)

TABLE 11.21. (continued)

Disorder	Synonym(s)	Selected characteristics	Conductive	Sensorineural	CNS
Refsum syndrome	—	Eye disorder; ataxia; muscle atrophy; neuropathy	—	−/+	—
Richards–Rundel syndrome	Ataxia–hypogonadism syndrome	CNS disorder; ataxia; MR; arreflexia	—	−/+	—
Rubella	—	Numerous possible defects of heart, eyes, CNS, viscera	—	+	+
Saddle nose syndrome	Marshall syndrome	Facial abnormalities; eye defects	—	−/+	—
Schilder disease	—	Mental deterioration; encephalopathy	—	+	+
Small syndrome	—	MR; muscular atrophy: eye (retinal) defect	—	+	+
Treacher Collins syndrome	Mandibular dysostosis	Facial abnormalities; multiple ear anomalies	+	—	—
Trisomy 13–15	—	Multiple abnormalities; MR; heart defects	—	+	+
Trisomy 18	—	Microcephaly; heart defects; cleft lip/palate; MR	+	+	+
Turner syndrome	—	Multiple abnormalities; low hairline; oral–facial defects	+	+	—
Unverricht disease	—	Progressive myoclonic epilepsy; neurologic degeneration	—	−/+	+
Usher's syndrome	—	Progressive visual deficits; MR; epilepsy	—	+	+
Van Buchem's syndrome	—	Craniofacial & skeletal disorder; nerve palsies	+	−/+	+

Syndrome/Disease		Associated findings			
Waardenburg's syndrome	—	Skin abnormalities; white forelock; facial abnormalities	—	+	—
Wildervanck syndrome	—	Neck, hand, and foot abnormalities	+	+	—
Wilson disease	—	Hepatic pathology	—	+	—

*From Jaffe BF (Ed.) (1977). *Hearing Loss in Children*, 1977, Baltimore: University Park Press; and Northern JL, and Downs MP, *Hearing in Children*, 3rd ed., Baltimore: Williams & Wilkins, 1984. Adapted by permission.

[a]Mental retardation (MR)

SOURCE: With permission from Hall JW: *Handbook of Auditory Evoked Responses*, p. 363. Copyright © 1992 by Allyn & Bacon. Reprinted/adapted by permission.

TABLE 11.22. **Prelingual deafness: summary of known exogenous causes.**

PRECONCEPTION AND PRENATAL CAUSES
　Rubella
　CMV
　Ototoxic and other drugs, maternal alcoholism
　Hypoxia (and its possible causes: high altitude, general anesthetic, severe hemorrhage)
　Syphilis
　Toxemia, diabetes, and other severe systematic maternal illness
　Paternal irradiation
　Toxoplasmosis

PERINATAL CAUSES
　Hypoxia
　Traumatic delivery
　Maternal infection
　Ototoxic drugs
　Premature delivery

NEONATAL AND POSTNATAL CAUSES
　Hypoxia
　Infection
　Ototoxic drugs
　Erythroblastosis fetalis
　Infantile measles or mumps
　Otitis media (acute, chronic, serous)
　Noise-induced
　Meningitis
　Encephalitis

SOURCE: With permission from Northern JL, Downs MP: *Hearing in Children,* 4th ed., p. 89.
Williams & Wilkins, Baltimore, MD, 1991.

TABLE 11.23. **Screening guidelines: comparison of several recommended procedures.**

Source	Test frequencies	Intensity level (ANSI-1989)	Pass–fail criteria
American Speech and Hearing Association Committee on Identification Audiometry (1975)[a]	1000, 2000, and 4000 Hz	20 dB at 1000 and 2000 Hz 25 dB at 4000 Hz	Fail to respond to any frequency in either ear
American Speech Language Hearing Association (1985)[b]	1000, 2000, and 4000 Hz	20 dB	Fail to respond to 1 tone in either ear
Anderson[c]	000, 2000, and 4000 Hz	20 dB	Fail to respond to any 1 signal in any ear
Downs[d]	1000, 2000, 4000, and 6000 or 8000 Hz	15 dB	Fail to respond to either 1000 or 2000 Hz or to both 4000 and 6000–8000 Hz in either ear
National Conference on Identification Audiometry[e]	1000, 2000, 4000, and 6000 Hz	20 dB at 1000, 2000, and 6000 Hz 30 dB at 4000 Hz	Fail to hear any signals at these levels in either ear
Northern & Downs[f]	1000, 2000, 3000, and/or 4000 and 6000 Hz	25 dB	Fail to respond to 1 tone at 1000 or 2000 Hz; or Fail to respond to 2 of 3 tones at 3000, 4000, and 6000 Hz
State of Illinois Department of Public Health[g]	500, 1000, 2000, and 4000 Hz	25 or 35 dB	Fail to respond to 1 tone at 35 dB in either ear or respond to any 2 tones at 25 dB in the same ear

[a]American Speech and Hearing Association (ASHA) Committee on Audiometric Evaluation Guidelines for Identification Audiometry, *ASHA* 17, 1975:94–99.

[b]American Speech-Language Hearing Association (ASHA), "Guidelines for screening hearing impairment and middle ear disorders," *ASHA* 32 Suppl. 2, 1990; 17–24.

[c]Anderson CV: Conversation of hearing. In Katz J. (ed) *Handbook of Clinical Audiology,* 2nd ed., Baltimore: Williams & Wilkins,1978.

[d]Downs MP: Auditory Screening. *Otolaryngol. Clin North Am.* 11, 1968; 611–629.

[e]Darley FL: Identification Audiometry for School-Age Children: Basic Procedures, *J. Speech Hear. Dis. Suppl. 9,* 1962; 26–34.

[f]Northern JL, Downs MP: *Hearing in Children,* 4th ed., Baltimore: Williams & Wilkins, 1991.

[g]*A Manual for Audiometrists,* Springfield, Illinois Department of Public Health, 1974.

TABLE 11.24. **Speech sounds: examples of intensities produced at conversational levels.**

Phoneme	Intensity (dB SPL)
ɔ	65
ɛ	61
i	58
l	58
ʃ	56
n	52
t	50
h	48
s	45
θ	40

SOURCE: With permission from Levitt H: The Acoustics of Speech Production. In Ross M, Giolas TD (eds): *Auditory Management of Hearing-Impaired Children,* pp. 45–115. University Park Press, Baltimore, MD, 1978.

12

Professional Issues/Information

TABLE **12.1. Certificate of Clinical Competence: Outline of** *New* **Standards:*** **effective for Applications for Certification postmarked January 1, 1993, and thereafter.**

I. DEGREE: Applicants for either certificate must hold a master's or doctoral degree. Effective 1/1/94, all graduate coursework and clinical practicum required in the professional area for which the Certificate is sought must have been initiated and completed at an institution whose program was accredited by the ESB in the area for which the Certificate is sought.

II. ACADEMIC COURSEWORK: 75 semester credit hours (s.c.h.)

A. BASIC SCIENCE COURSEWORK: 27 s.c.h.
- 6 s.c.h. in biological/physical sciences and mathematics.
- 6 s.c.h. in behavioral and/or social sciences.
- 15 s.c.h. in basic human communication processes to include the anatomic and physiologic bases, the physical and psycholinguistic aspects.

B. PROFESSIONAL COURSEWORK: 36 s.c.h., 30 in courses for which graduate credit was received and 21 in the professional area for which the Certificate is sought.

CCC-SLP
- 30 s.c.h. in speech-language pathology.
  - 6 in speech disorders.[1]
  - 6 in language disorders.[1]
- 6 s.c.h. in audiology.
  - 3 in hearing disorders and hearing evaluation.[1]
  - 3 in habilitative/rehabilitative procedures.[1]

III. SUPERVISED CLINICAL OBSERVATION AND CLINICAL PRACTICUM: 375 clock hours (c.h.)

A. CLINICAL OBSERVATION: 25 c.h., prior to beginning initial clinical practicum.

B. CLINICAL PRACTICUM: 350 c.h. total.
- 250 c.h. at graduate level in the area in which the Certificate is sought.
- 50 c.h. in each of three types of clinical settings.

CCC-SLP
- 20 c.h. in each of the following 8 categories:
  1. Evaluation: Speech[2] disorders in children
  2. Evaluation: Speech[2] disorders in adults
  3. Evaluation: Language disorders in children
  4. Evaluation: Language disorders in adults
  5. Treatment: Speech[2] disorders in children
  6. Treatment: Speech[2] disorders in adults
  7. Treatment: Language disorders in children
  8. Treatment: Language disorders in adults
- Up to 20 c.h. in the major professional area may be in related disorders.
- 35 c.h. in audiology
  - 15 in evaluation/screening
  - 15 in habilitation/rehabilitation

TABLE **12.1.** (*continued*)

IV. NATIONAL EXAMINATIONS IN SPEECH-LANGUAGE PATHOLOGY
     AND AUDIOLOGY
 V. THE CLINICAL FELLOWSHIP

*Material excerpted from the full Standards document, which is available from ASHA. Standards are currently under revision. For complete information and updates, refer to "Certification Handbook," or ASHA's Certification Branch.

[1]Academic credit for clinical practicum may not be used to satisfy these minimum requirements. However, a maximum of 6 s.c.h. for practicum may be applied to the 36 s.c.h. minimum professional coursework.

[2]"Speech" disorders include disorders of articulation, voice, and fluency.

TABLE 12.2. **Code of Ethics (revised January 1, 1994): American Speech-Language-Hearing Association.**

PREAMBLE

The preservation of the highest standards of integrity and ethical principles is vital to the responsible discharge of obligations in the professions of speech-language pathology and audiology. This Code of Ethics sets forth the fundamental principles and rules considered essential to this purpose.

Every individual who is (a) a member of the American Speech-Language-Hearing Association, whether certified or not, (b) a nonmember holding the Certificate of clinical Competence from the Association, (c) an applicant for membership or certification, or (d) a Clinical Fellow seeking to fulfill standards for certification shall abide by this Code of Ethics.

Any action that violates the spirit and purpose of this Code shall be considered unethical. Failure to specify any particular responsibility or practice in this Code of Ethics shall not be construed as denial of the existence of such responsibilities or practices.

The fundamentals of ethical conduct are described by Principles of Ethics and by Rules of Ethics as they relate to responsibility to persons served, to the public, and to the professions of speech-language pathology and audiology.

Principles of Ethics, aspirational and inspiration in nature, form the underlying moral basis for the Code of Ethics. Individuals shall observe these principles as affirmative obligations under all conditions of professional activity.

Rules of Ethics are specific statements of minimally acceptable professional conduct or of prohibitions and are applicable to all individuals.

PRINCIPLE OF ETHICS I

Individuals shall honor their responsibility to hold paramount the welfare of persons they serve professionally.

Rules of Ethics

A. Individuals shall provide all services competently.

B. Individuals shall use every resource, including referral when appropriate, to ensure that high-quality service is provided.

C. Individuals shall not discriminate in the delivery of professional services on the basis of race or ethnicity, gender, age, national origin, sexual orientation, or disability.

D. Individuals shall fully inform the persons they serve of the nature and possible effects of services rendered and products dispensed.

E. Individuals shall evaluate the effectiveness of services rendered and of products dispensed and shall provide services or dispense products only when benefit can reasonably be expected.

F. Individuals shall not guarantee the results of any treatment or procedure, directly or by implication; however, they may make a reasonable statement of prognosis.

G. Individuals shall not evaluate or treat speech, language, or hearing disorders solely by correspondence.

H. Individuals shall maintain adequate records of professional services rendered and products dispensed and shall allow access to these records when appropriately authorized.

I. Individuals shall not reveal, without authorization, any professional or personal information about the person served professionally, unless required by law to do so, or unless doing so is necessary to protect the welfare of the person or of the community.

J. Individuals shall not charge for services not rendered, nor shall they misrepresent[1] in any fashion, services rendered or products dispensed.

TABLE 12.2. (*continued*)

K. Individuals shall use persons in research or as subjects of teaching demonstrations only with their informed consent.
L. Individuals whose professional services are adversely affected by substance abuse or other health-related conditions shall seek professional assistance and, where appropriate, withdraw from the affected areas of practice.

PRINCIPLES OF ETHICS II
Individuals shall honor their responsibility to achieve and maintain the highest level of professional competence.

Rules of Ethics
A. Individuals shall engage in the provision of clinical services only when they hold the appropriate Certificate of Clinical Competence or when they are in the certification process and are supervised by an individual who holds the appropriate Certificate of Clinical Competence.
B. Individuals shall engage in only those aspects of the professions that are within the scope of their competence, considering their level of education, training, and experience.
C. Individuals shall continue their professional development throughout their careers.
D. Individuals shall delegate the provision of clinical services only to persons who are certified or to persons in the education or certification process who are appropriately supervised. The provision of support services may be delegated to persons who are neither certified nor in the certification process only when a certificate holder provides appropriate supervision.
E. Individuals shall prohibit any of their professional staff from providing services that exceed the staff member's competence, considering the staff member's level of education, training, and experience.
F. Individuals shall ensure that all equipment used in the provision of services is in proper working order and is properly calibrated.

PRINCIPLE OF ETHICS III
Individuals shall honor their responsibility to the public by promoting public understanding of the professions, by supporting the development of services designed to fulfill the unmet needs of the public, and by providing accurate information in all communications involving any aspect of the professions.

Rules of Ethics
A. Individuals shall not misrepresent their credentials, competence, education, training, or experience.
B. Individuals shall not participate in professional activities that constitute a conflict of interest.
C. Individuals shall not misrepresent diagnostic information, services rendered, or products dispensed or engage in any scheme or artifice to defraud in connection with obtaining payment or reimbursement for such services or products.
D. Individuals' statements to the public shall provide accurate information about the nature and management of communication disorders, about the professions, and about professional services.
E. Individuals' statements to the public—advertising, announcing, and marketing their professional services, reporting research results, and promoting products—shall adhere to prevailing professional standards and shall not contain misrepresentation.

(*continued*)

TABLE 12.2. (*continued*)

PRINCIPLES OF ETHICS IV
    Individuals shall honor their responsibilities to the professions and their relationships with colleagues, students, and members of allied professions. Individuals shall uphold the dignity and autonomy of the professions, maintain harmonious interprofessional and intraprofessional relationships, and accept the professions' self-imposed standards.

Rules of Ethics
A. Individuals shall prohibit anyone under their supervision from engaging in any practice that violates the Code of Ethics.
B. Individuals shall not engage in dishonesty, fraud, deceit, misrepresentation, or any form of conduct that adversely reflects on the professions or on the individual's fitness to serve persons professionally.
C. Individuals shall assign credit only to those who have contributed to a publication, presentation, or product. Credit shall be assigned in proportion to the contribution and only with the contributor's consent.
D. Individuals' statements to colleagues about professional services, research results, and products shall adhere to prevailing professional standards and shall contain no misrepresentations.
E. Individuals shall not provide professional services without exercising independent professional judgment, regardless of referral source or prescription.
F. Individuals shall not discriminate in their relationships with colleagues, students, and members of allied professions on the basis or race or ethnicity, gender, age, religion, national origin, sexual orientation, or disability.
G. Individuals who have reason to believe that the Code of Ethics has been violated shall inform the Ethical Practice Board.
H. Individuals shall cooperate fully with the Ethical Practice Board in its investigation and adjudication of matters related to this Code of Ethics.

---

[1]For purposes of this Code of Ethics, misrepresentation includes any untrue statements or statements that are likely to mislead. Misrepresentation also includes the failure to state any information that is material and that ought, in fairness, to be considered.
American Speech-Language-Hearing Association (1994). Code of ethics. ASHA, 36 (March, Suppl. 13), pp. 1–2.

TABLE 12.3. **Scope of practice in speech-language pathology: Ad Hoc Committee on Scope of Practice in Speech-Language Pathology.**
This scope of practice in speech-language pathology statement is an official policy of the American Speech-Language-Hearing Association (ASHA). It was developed by the Ad Hoc Committee on Scope of Practice in Speech-Language Pathology: Sarah W. Blackstone, chair; Diane Paul-Brown, ex officio; David A. Brandt; Rhonda Friedlander; Luis F. Riquelme; and Mark Ylvisaker. Crystal S. Cooper, vice-president for professional practices in speech-language pathology, served as monitoring vice-president. The contributions of the editor, Jude Langsam, and select and widespread peer reviewers are gratefully acknowledged. This statement supersedes the Scope of Practice, Speech-Language Pathology and Audiology statement (LC 6-89), ASHA, April 1990, 1–2.

PREAMBLE

The purpose of this statement is to define the scope of practice of speech-language pathology in order to:

(1) delineate areas of services and supports provided by ASHA members and certificate holders in accordance with the ASHA Code of Ethics. Services refer to clinical services for individuals with speech, voice, language, communication, and swallowing disorders, aimed at the amelioration of difficulties stemming from such disorders. Supports refer to environmental modifications, assistive technology, and guidance for communication partners to help persons with these disorders;

(2) educate health care, education, and other professionals, consumers, payers, regulators, and members of the general public about treatment and other services and supports offered by speech-language pathologists as qualified providers;

(3) assist members and certificate holders in their efforts to provide appropriate and high quality speech-language pathology services and supports to persons across the life span with speech, voice, language, communication, and swallowing disabilities;

(4) establish a reference for curriculum review of education programs in speech-language pathology.

The scope of practice defined here and the areas specifically set forth are part of an effort to describe the broad range of services and supports offered within the profession. It is recognized, however, that levels of experience, skill, and proficiency with respect to the activities identified within this scope of practice vary among the individual providers. It may not be possible for speech-language pathologists to practice in all areas of the field. As the ASHA Code of Ethics specifies, individuals may only practice in areas where they are competent based on their education, training, and experience (American Speech-Language-Hearing Association 1994). However, nothing limits speech-language pathologists from expanding their current level of expertise. Certain clients or practice settings may necessitate that speech-language pathologists pursue additional education or training to expand their personal scope of practice.

This scope of practice statement does not supersede existing state licensure laws or affect the interpretation or implementation of such laws. It may serve, however, as a model for the development or modification of licensure laws.

Finally, it is recognized that speech-language pathology is a dynamic and continuously developing practice area. Listing specific areas within this scope of practice does not necessarily exclude other, new, or emerging areas. Indeed, changes in service delivery systems, the increasing numbers of persons who need communication services, and technological and scientific advances have mandated that a scope of practice for the profession of speech-language pathology be a dynamic statement. For these reasons this document will undergo periodic review and possible revision.

(continued)

TABLE 12.3. (*continued*)

STATEMENT

The goal of the profession of speech-language pathology and its members is provision of the highest quality treatment and other services consistent with the fundamental right of those served to participate in decisions that affect their lives.

Speech-language pathologists hold the master's or doctoral degree, the Certificate of Clinical Competence of the American Speech-Language-Hearing Association, and state licensure where applicable.

These professionals serve individuals, families, groups, and the general public through their involvement in a broad range of professional activities. They work to prevent speech, voice, language, communication, swallowing, and related disabilities. They screen, identify, assess, diagnose, refer, and provide treatment and intervention, including consultation and follow-up services, to persons of all ages with, or at risk for, speech, voice, language, communication, swallowing, and related disabilities. They counsel individuals with these disorders, as well as their families, caregivers, and other service providers, related to the disorders and their management. Speech-language pathologists select, prescribe, dispense, and provide services supporting the effective use of augmentative and alternative communication devices and other communication prostheses and assistive devices.

Speech-language pathologists also teach, supervise, and manage clinical and educational programs, and engage in program development, program oversight, and research activities related to communication sciences and disorders, swallowing, and related areas.

They measure treatment outcomes, evaluate the effectiveness of their practices, modify services in relation to their evaluations, and disseminate these findings. They also serve as case managers and expert witnesses. As an integral part of their practice, speech-language pathologists work to increase public awareness and advocate for the people they serve.

Speech-language pathologists provide services in settings that are deemed appropriate, including but not limited to health care, educational, community, vocational and home settings. Speech-language pathologists serve diverse populations. The client population includes persons of different race, age, gender, religion, national origin, and sexual orientation. Speech-language pathologists' caseloads include persons from diverse ethnic, cultural, or linguistic backgrounds, and persons with disabilities. Although speech-language pathologists are prohibited from discriminating in the provision of professional services based on these factors, in some cases such factors may be relevant to the development of an appropriate treatment plan. These factors may be considered in treatment plans only when firmly grounded in scientific and professional knowledge.

As primary care providers of communication treatment and other services, speech-language pathologists are autonomous professionals; that is, their services need not be prescribed by another. However, in most cases individuals are best served when speech-language pathologists work collaboratively with other professionals, individuals with disabilities, and their family members. Similarly, it is recognized that related fields and professions may have some knowledge, skills, and experience that could be applied to some areas within this scope of practice. Defining the scope of practice of speech-language pathologists is not meant to exclude members of other professions or related fields from rendering services in common practice areas.

The practice of speech-language pathology includes:

(1) Providing screening, identification, assessment, diagnosis, treatment, intervention (i.e., prevention, restoration, amelioration, compensation) and follow-up services for disorders of:

TABLE 12.3. (*continued*)

- speech: articulation, fluency, voice (including respiration, phonation, and resonance)
- language (involving the parameters of phonology, morphology, syntax, semantics, and pragmatics; and including disorders of receptive and expressive communication in oral, written, graphic, and manual modalities)
- oral, pharyngeal, cervical esophageal, and related functions (e.g., dysphagia, including disorders of swallowing and oral function for feeding; orofacial myofunctional disorders)
- cognitive aspects of communication (including communication disability and other functional disabilities associated with cognitive impairment)
- social aspects of communication (including challenging behavior, ineffective social skills, lack of communication opportunities);

(2) Providing consultation and counseling, and making referrals when appropriate;

(3) Training and supporting family members and other communication partners of individuals with speech, voice, language, communication, and swallowing disabilities;

(4) Developing and establishing effective augmentative and alternative communication techniques and strategies, including selecting, prescribing, and dispensing of aids and devices and training individuals, their families, and other communication partners in their use;

(5) Selecting, fitting, and establishing effective use of appropriate prosthetic/adaptive devices for speaking and swallowing (e.g., tracheoesophageal valves, electrolarynges, speaking valves);

(6) Using instrumental technology to diagnose and treat disorders of communication and swallowing (e.g., videofluoroscopy, nasendoscopy, ultrasonography, stroboscopy);

(7) Providing aural rehabilitation and related counseling services to individuals with hearing loss and to their families;

(8) Collaborating in the assessment of central auditory processing disorders in cases in which there is evidence of speech, language, and/or other cognitive-communication disorders; providing intervention for individuals with central auditory processing disorders.

(9) Conducting pure-tone air conduction hearing screening and screening tympanometry for the purpose of the initial identification and/or referral of individuals with other communication disorders or possible middle ear pathology.

(10) Enhancing speech and language proficiency and communication effectiveness, including but not limited to accent reduction, collaboration with teachers of English as a second language, and improvement of voice, performance, and singing;

(11) Training and supervising support personnel;

(12) Developing and managing academic and clinical programs in communication sciences and disorders;

(13) Conducting, disseminating, and applying research in communication sciences and disorders;

(14) Measuring outcomes of treatment and conducting continuous evaluation of the effectiveness of practices and programs to improve and maintain quality of services.

*American Speech-Language-Hearing Association. Scope of practice in speech-language pathology. *ASHA* 38 (Suppl. 16), 1996, pp. 16–20.

13

Periodicals and Professional Organizations

I. Periodicals in Speech-Language Pathology and Related Areas

The following lists titles of periodicals related to speech-language pathology; the name and address of the publisher and, when it was available, first year of publication are listed.

A.M.A. Archives of Otolaryngology
Publisher: American Medical
  Association
535 Dearborn Street
Chicago, IL 60610
Year: 1898

Acta Oto-Laryngologica
Publisher: Almqvist and Wiksell
  Periodical Company
Gamla Brogatan 26
P.O. Box 638
S-101 28 Stockholm, Sweden
Year: 1910

American Annals of the Deaf
Publisher: Conference of Educational
  Administrators of Schools and
  Programs for the Deaf
800 Florida Avenue, NE
Washington, DC 20002
Year: 1847

American Journal of Otolaryngology
Publisher: W. B. Saunders Company
The Curtis Center
Independence Square West
Philadelphia, PA 19106-3399

American Journal of Speech-Language Pathology
A Journal of Clinical Practice
Publisher: American Speech-Language Hearing Association
10801 Rockville Pike
Rockville, MD 20852-3279
Year: 1991

American Speech-Language Hearing Association
Publisher: ASHA
10801 Rockville Pike
Rockville, MD 20852-3279
Year: 1959

Annals of Otology, Rhinology, and Laryngology
Publisher: Annals Publishing Company
4507 Laclede Avenue
St. Louis, MO 63108
Year: 1891

Applied Psycholinguistics
Publisher: Cambridge University Press
40 West 20th Street
New York, NY 10011
Year: 1979

Archives of Otolaryngology—Head and Neck Surgery
Publisher: American Medical Association
535 North Dearborn Street
Chicago, IL 60610
Year: 1874

Augmentative and Alternative Communication
Publisher: Decker Periodicals
4 Hughson Street South
P.O. Box 620 LCD1
Hamilton, ON LN8 3K7
Year: 1984

Brain
Publisher: Oxford University Press
Academic Division
Oxford, Ox26DP, UK

Brain and Language
Publisher: Academic Press, Inc.
1 East First Street
Duluth, MN 55802
Year: 1975

Brain Behavior and Evolution
Publisher: Medical and Scientific Publishers
P.O. Box CH-4009
Basel, Switzerland
Year: 1968

Brain, A Journal of Neurology
Publisher: Oxford University Press
Pinkhill House
Southfield Road
Eynsham, Oxford OX8, 1JJ, UK
Year: 1878

British Journal of Disorders of Communication
Publisher: The College of Speech Therapists
Harold Poster House
6 Lechmere Road
London NW2 5BU, UK
Year: 1966

Child Development
Publisher: University of Chicago Press
Journals Division
P.O. Box 37005
Chicago, IL 60637
Year: 1930

Child Language Teaching and Therapy
Publisher: Edward Arnold Publishers, Ltd.
41 Bedford Square
London WC1B 3DQ, UK

Cleft Palate Journal
Publisher: American Cleft Palate Craniofacial Association
1218 Grandview Avenue
Pittsburgh, PA 15211
Year: 1963

Cleft Palate—Craniofacial Journal
Publisher: American Cleft Palate-
Craniofacial Association
1218 Grandview Ave.
Pittsburgh, PA 15211
Year: 1963

Clinical Linguistics and Phonetics
Publisher: Taylor and Francis Ltd.
4 John Street
London, WC1N 2ET, UK

Cortex
Publisher: Masson S.P.A.
Via Filli Bressan
2-20126
Milano, Italy
Year: 1964

Developmental Psychology
Publisher: American Psychological
Association
750 First Street, NE
Washington, DC 20002-4242
Year: 1969

Discourse Processes
Publisher: Ablex Publishing
Corporation
355 Chestnut Street
Norwood, NJ 07648
Year: 1978

Ear Nose and Throat Journal
Publisher: Medquest Communications
629 Euclid Avenue
Suite 500
Cleveland, OH 44114
Year: 1921

*European Journal of Disorders of
Communication: The Journal of the
College of Speech and Language
Therapists, London*
Allen Press, Inc.
Publisher: Whurr Publishers Ltd.
810 10th Street
Lawrence, KS 66044
Year: 1966

Exceptional Children
Publisher: The Council for Exceptional
Children
1920 Association Drive
Reston, VA 20191-1589
Year: 1933

*Exceptional Child Education
Resources*
Publisher: The Council for Exceptional
Children
1920 Association Drive
Reston, VA 20191-1589
Year: 1968

First Language
Publisher: Alpha Academic
Halfpenny Furze
Mill Lane
Chalfont St. Giles
Buckinghamshire, UK
Year: 1980

Folia Phonatrica
Publisher: Skarger Publishers, Inc.
79 Fifth Avenue
New York, NY 10003
Year: 1948

Hearing and Speech News
Publisher: National Association for
Hearing and Speech Action
814 Thayer Avenue
Silver Spring, MD 20910
Year: 1956

Human Communication Research
Publisher: International
Communication Association
8140 Burnet Road
Austin, TX 78758

*International Journal of Pediatric
Otorhinolaryngology*
Publisher: Elsevier Science Publishers
P.O. Box 221
1000 AM Asterdam
The Netherlands

Journal of Acoustical Society of America
Publisher: American Institute of Physics
335 East 45th Street
New York, NY 10017

Journal of Autism and Developmental Disorders
Publisher: Plenum Publishing Corporation
233 Spring Street
New York, NY 10013
Year: 1970

Journal of Child Language
Publisher: Cambridge University press
32 East 57th Street
New York, NY 10022
Year: 1974

Journal of Childhood Communication Disorders
Publisher: Council for Exceptional Children Division for Children with Communication Disorders
1920 Association Drive
Reston, VA 22091
Year: 1976

Journal of Communication Disorders
Publisher: Elsevier Science Publishing Co., Inc.
655 Avenue of the Americas
New York, NY 10032
Year: 1967

Journal of Fluency Disorders
Publisher: Elsevier Science Publishing Co., Inc.
655 Avenue of the Americas
New York, NY 10010
Year: 1976

Journal of Laryngology and Otology
Publisher: Headly Brothers Ltd.
109 Kingsway
London, WC 2 UK
Year: 1887

Journal of Learning Disabilities
Publisher: PRO-ED
8700 Shoal Creek Boulevard
Austin, TX 78757-6897
Year: 1968

Journal of Medical Speech Language Pathology
Publisher: Singular Publishing Group, Inc.
401 West A Street
Suite 325
San Diego, CA 92101-7904
Year: 1993

Journal of Memory and Language
Publisher: Academic Press, Inc.
1 East First Street
Duluth, MN 55802
Year: 1961

Journal of Neurolinguistics
Publisher: Elsevier Science Ltd.
P.O. Box 211
1000 AM Amsterdam
The Netherlands
Year: 1985

Journal of Phonetics
Publisher: Academic Press
24-28 Oval Road
London NW1 7DX, UK
Year: 1973

Journal of Pragmatics
Publisher: Elsevier Science Publishers B.V.
P.O. Box 1991
1000 BZ Amsterdam, The Netherlands
Year: 1977

Journal of Psycholinguistic Research
Publisher: Plenum Publishing Corporation
233 Spring Street
New York, NY 10013
Year: 1971

Journal of Speech and Hearing Disorders
Publisher: ASHA
10801 Rockville Pike
Rockville, MD 20852-3279
Year: 1935

Journal of Speech and Hearing Research
Publisher: ASHA
10801 Rockville Pike
Rockville, MD 20852-3279
Year: 1958

Journal of Speech Disorders
Publisher: Interstate Printers and Publishers, Inc.
19-27 North Jackson Street
Danville, IL 61832
Year: 1936

Journal of the American Deafness and Rehabilitation Association
Publisher: American Deafness and Rehabilitation Association
P.O. Box 251554
Little Rock, AR 72225
Year: 1967

Journal of Verbal Learning and Verbal Behavior
Publisher: Academic Press, Inc.
21 Congress Street
Salem, MA 01970
Year: 1962

Journal of Voice
c/o Raven Press, Ltd.
Publisher: The Voice Foundation
1185 Avenue of the Americas
New York, NY 10036
Year: 1986

Language
Publisher: Linguistic Society of America
428 East Preston Street
Baltimore, MD 21202
Year: 1925

Language and Cognitive Processes
Publisher: Dr. L. K. Tyler
Department of Experimental Psychology
University of Cambridge
Downing Street
Cambridge CB2 3EB, UK
Year: 1985

Language and Speech
Publisher: Kingston Press Services, Ltd.
28 High Street
Teddington, Middlesex TW 118EW, UK
Year: 1958

Language and Style
Publisher: Language and Style Editorial Services
Kiely Hall 1309
Queens College of the City University of New York
Flushing, NY 11367-0904
Year:

Language in Society
Publisher: Cambridge University Press
40 West 20th Street
New York, NY 10011

Language, Speech, and Hearing Services in Schools
Publisher: ASHA
10801 Rockville Pike
Rockville, MD 20852
Year: 1970

Laryngoscope
Publisher: The Laryngoscope
The Triological Foundation, Inc.
9216 Clayton Road
St. Louis, MO 63124-1561
Year: 1890

Linguistic Inquiry
Publisher: MIT Press
55 Hayward Street
Cambridge, MA 02142
Year: 1970

Linguistic Reporter
Publisher: Center for Applied Linguistics
1611 North Kent Street
Arlington, VA 22209
Year: 1957

Neuropsychologia
Publisher: Pergamon Press, Inc.
Maxwell House
660 White Plains Rd.
Tarrytown, NY 10591
Year: 1963

Otolaryngology Head and Neck Surgery
Publisher: C.V. Mosby Company
11830 Westline Industrial Drive
St. Louis, MO 63146
Year: 1892

Perception and Psychophysics
Publisher: Psychonomic Society, Inc.
1710 Fortview Road
Austin, TX 70704
Year: 1966

Perspectives for Teachers of the Hearing Impaired
Publisher: Precollege Programs of Gallaudet University
800 Florida Avenue, NE
KDES PAS-6
Washington, DC 20002
Year: 1981

Perspectives in Education and Deafness
Publisher: Precollege Programs of Gallaudet University
800 Florida Avenue, NE
Washington, DC 20002
Year: 1981

Phonetica
Publisher: S. Karger AG
P.O. Box CH-4009
Basel, Switzerland
Year: 1944

Phonology
Publisher: Cambridge University Press
The Edinburgh Building
Shaflesbury Road
Cambridge CB2 2RU, UK

Seminars in Speech and Language
Publisher: Thieme New York
333 Seventh Avenue
New York, NY 10001
Year: 1979

Sign Language Studies
Publisher: Linstok Press, Inc.
4020 Blackburn Lane
Burtonsville, MD 20866
Year: 1973

Speech Communication
Publisher: Elsevier Science B.V.
P.O. Box 521
1000 AM Amsterdam
The Netherlands
Year: 1981

Speech Pathology and Therapy
Publisher: Pitman Medical Publishing Co.
46 Charlotte Street
London W.1., UK
Year: 1958

Sprache–Stimme–Gehor
Publisher: Georg Thieme Verlag
P.O. Box 301120
D-70451 Stuttgart, Germany
Year: 1996

Status Report on Speech Research
Publisher: Haskins Laboratories
270 Crown Street
New Haven, CT 06511-6695
Year: 1940

International Journal of Orofacial Myology
Publisher: International Association of Orofacial Myology
P.O. Box 540
Green Forest, AR 72638
Year: 1974

Topics in Language Disorders
Publisher: Aspen Publishers, Inc.
7201 McKinney Circle
Fredrick, MD 21701
Year: 1980

Volta Review
Publisher: Alexander Graham Bell Association for the Deaf
3417 Volta Place, NW
Washington, DC 20007
Year: 1898

II. Professional Organizations Related to Speech-Language Pathology

The following are names of organizations related to speech-language pathology. Included are the most current address and, when available, telephone number, fax number, E-mail address, and World Wide Web home page. Asterisks (*) indicate that the information was verified through mail survey, telephone contact, or Internet search.

Alexander Graham Bell Association for the Deaf*
Volta Bureau
3417 Volta Place NW
Washington, DC 20007
Phone: 202–337–5220
TDD: 202–337–5220
E-mail: agbell2@aol.com
Fax: 202–337–8314
WWW Home Page:
http://www.agbel.org

ALS Association*
21021 Ventura Boulevard
Suite 321
Woodlandhills, CA 91364
Phone: 818–340–7500
Fax: 818–340–2060
WWW Home Page:
http://www.aan.com

American Academy of Cerebral Palsy and Developmental Medicine*
P.O. Box 11083
Richmond, VA 23230
Phone: 847–698–1635
Fax: 847–823–0536

American Academy of Otolaryngology Head and Neck Surgery
1 Prince Street
Alexandria, VA 22314
Phone: 703–836–4444

American Academy of Pediatrics*
141 NW Point Road
P.O. Box 927
Elk Grove Village, IL 60009-0927
Phone: 847–228–5005
Fax: 847–288–5097
E-mail: kidsdocs@aap.org
WWW Home Page:
http://www.aap.org

American Association for Advancement of Science
1200 New York Avenue NW
Washington, DC 20005
Phone: 202–326–6400

American Association on Mental Retardation*
444 North Capitol Street NW
Suite 846
Washington, DC 20001-1512
Phone: 800–424–3688
Fax: 202–387–2193
E-mail: aamr@access.digex.net

American Cleft Palate-Craniofacial Association*
1218 Grandview Avenue
Pittsburg, PA 15211
Phone: 412–481–1376
Fax: 412–481–0847

American Council of the Blind*
1155 15th Street, NW
Suite 720
Washington, DC 20005
Phone: 202–467–5081
Fax: 202–467–5085
WWW Home Page:
http://www.realtime.net

American Foundation for the Blind*
11 Penn Plaza
Suite 300
New York, NY 10001
Phone: 800–232–5463
E-mail: afbinfo@afb.org
WWW Home Page:
http://www.afb.org/afb

American Geriatrics Society, Inc.*
770 Lexington Avenue
Suite 300
New York, NY 10021
Phone: 800–247–4779
Fax: 212–832–8646
E-mail: agsync@soho.10s.com

American Medical Association*
515 N. State Street
Chicago, IL 60610
Phone: 312–464–4635
Fax: 312–464–5830
E-mail: Fred???Lenhoff@ama-assn.org
WWW Home Page: http://www.ama-assn.org

**American National Standards
Institute***
11 West 42nd Street
New York, NY 10036
Phone: 212–642–4900
Fax: 212–398–6023
WWW Home Page:
    http://www.ansi.org

**American Physical Therapy
Association**
1111 North Fairfax Street
Alexandria, VA 22314
Phone: 703–684–APTA

**American Speech-Language-Hearing
Association***
10801 Rockville Pike
Rockville, MD 20852
Phone: 301–897–5700
Fax: 301–571–0457
E-mail: webmaster@asha.org
WWW Home Page:
    http://www.asha.org

**American Speech-Language-Hearing
Foundation***
10801 Rockville Pike
Rockville, MD 20852-3279
Phone: 301–897–5700
Fax: 301–571–0457
E-mail: vsmolka@asha.org

**Association for the Care of Children's
Health***
Suite 300
Bethesda, MD 20814
Phone: 301–654–6549
Fax: 301–986–4553
E-mail: acch@clark.net
WWW Home Page:
    http://www.wsd.com/acch.org

Autism Services Center
605 9th Street
P.O. Box 507
Huntington, WV 25710
Phone: 304–525–8014
Fax: 304–525–8026

Autism Society of America*
7910 Woodmont Avenue
Suite 650
Bethesda, MD 20814-3015
Phone: 800–3Autism
Fax: 301–657–0869
WWW Home Page:
    http://www.autism???society.org

Bazelon Center*
1101 15th Street, NW
Suite 1212
Washington, DC 20005
Phone: 202–467–5730
E-mail: han1660@handsnet.org
WWW Home Page:
    http://www.bazelon.org

**Children with Attention Deficit
Disorders (CHADD)***
499 NW 70th Avenue
Suite 185
Plantation, FL 33317
Phone: 954–587–3700
Fax: 954–587–4599
WWW Home Page:
    http://www.chadd.org

**Cornelia de Lange Syndrome
Foundation***
60 Dyer Avenue
Collinsville, CT 06022
Phone: 302–693–0159
Fax: 860–693–6819
WWW Home Page:
    http://www.cdlsoutreach.org

Council for Exceptional Children*
1920 Association Boulevard
Reston, VA 22071
Phone: 707–620–3660
Fax: 703–264–9494
E-mail: cec@ece.sped.org
WWW Home Page:
    http://www.cec.sped.org

Council for Learning Disabilities*
P.O. Box 40303
Overland Park, KS 66204
Phone: 913–492–8755
Fax: 913–492–2546
WWW Home Page:
    http://www/.winthrop.edu/cld/

**Council of Graduate Programs
    in Communicative Sciences
    and Disorders**
P.O. Box 26532
Minneapolis, MN 55426
Phone: 612–920–0966
Fax: 612–920–6098
E-mail: cgp@cgpcsd.org

Epilepsy Foundation of America*
4351 Garden City Drive
Landover, MD 20785-2267
Phone: 301–459–3700
Fax: 301–577–2684
WWW Home Page:
    http://www.efa.org

**FACES—National Association for
    the Craniofacially Handicapped***
P.O. Box 11082
Chattanooga, TN 37401
Phone: 615–266–1632
Fax: 615–267–3124

Fetal Alcohol Education Program
School of Medicine, Boston University
7 Kent Street
Brookline, MA 12146
Phone: 617–739–1424

International Reading Association*
800 Barksdale Road
Box 8139
Newark, DE 19711
Phone: 302–731–1600 ext. 293
Fax: 302–731–1057
E-mail:
    74673.3646@compuserve.com
WWW Home Page: www.reading.org

Kids on the Block*
9385 C Gerwig Lane
Columbia, MD 21406
Phone: 410–290–9095
WWW Home Page:
    http://www.kotb.com

**Learning Disabilities Association
    of America***
4156 Library Road
Pittsburg, PA 15234
Phone: 412–341–1515
Fax: 412–344–0224
E-mail: Idanatl@usaor.net
WWW Home Page:
    http://www.ldanatl.org

Linguistic Society of America*
1325 18th Street, NW
Suite 211
Washington, DC 20036-6501
Phone: 202–835–1714
E-mail: zzlsa@gallua.bitnet
WWW Home Page:
    http://www.lsadc.org

March of Dimes Foundation
1275 Mamaroneck Avenue
White Plains, NY 10605
Phone: 914–428–7100

Muscular Dystrophy Association*
3300 East Sunrise Drive
Tuscon, AZ 85718
Phone: 800–572–1717
Fax: 520–529–5300
E-mail: publications@mdausa.org
WWW Home Page:
    http://www.mdausa.org

Myasthenia Gravis Foundation*
222 South Riverside Plaza
Suite 1540
Chicago, IL 60606
Phone: 312–258–0522
Fax: 312–258–0461
E-mail: mgfa@aol.com
WWW Home Page:
   http://www.med.unc.edu/mgfa/

National Association for Home Care*
228 Seventh Street, SE
Washington, DC 20003
Phone: 202–547–7424
Fax: 202–547–3540
E-mail: webmaster@nahc.org
WWW Home Page:
   http://www.nahc.org

National Association for the
   Education of Young Children*
1509 16th Street, NW
Washington, DC 20036
Phone: 202–232–8777
Fax: 202–328–1846
E-mail: naeyc@naeyc.org

National Association of Private
   Schools for Exceptional Children*
1522 K Street, NW
Suite 1032
Washington, DC 20005
Phone: 202–408–3338
Fax: 202–408–3340
E-mail: napes@aol.com
WWW Home Page:
   http://www.spedschools.com/napsec
   .html

National Association of the Deaf
814 Thayer Avenue
Silver Springs, MD 20910-4500
Phone: 301–587–1788
Fax: 301–587–1791

National Center for Stuttering*
200 E. 33rd Street
New York, NY 10016
Phone: 800–221–2483
E-mail:
   executivedirector@stuttering.com
WWW Home Page:
   http://www.stuttering.com

National Cued Speech Association*
Nazareth College
4245 East Avenue
Rochester, NY 14618
Phone: 716–389–2776
Fax: 716–586–2452
E-mail: ncsa@naz.edu

National Down Syndrome Congress*
1605 Chantilly Road
Suite 250
Atlanta, GA 30324
Phone: 800–232–NDSC
Fax: 404–633–3817
E-mail: ndsc@charitiesusa.com
WWW Home Page:
   http://www.carol.net/~ndsc/

National Down Syndrome Society*
666 Broadway
New York, NY 10012
Phone: 212–460–9330
Fax: 212–979–2873
WWW Home Page:
   http://www.ndss.org

National Easter Seal Society*
2800 13th Street, NW
Washington, DC 20009
Phone: 202–232–2342
Fax: 202–462–7379
WWW Home Page:
   http://www.seals.com

National Education Association
1201 16th Street, NW
Suite 317
Washington, DC 20036
Phone: 202–822–7015
Fax: 202–822–7997
E-mail: lhaynes@nea.org
WWW Home Page:
   http://www.nea.org

National Head Injury Foundation, Inc.
333 Turnpike Road
Shouthboro, MA 01722
Phone: 800–444–6443

National Information Center for Children and Youth with Disabilities*
P.O. Box 1492
Washington, DC 20013
Phone: 202–884–8200
Fax: 202–884–8441
E-mail: nichcy@aed.org
WWW Home Page:
http://www.nichcy.org

National Institute on Aging*
National Institute of Health
9000 Rockville Pike
Building 31, Room 2C-02
Bethesda, MD 20205
Phone: 301–496–1752
Fax: 301–496–1072
WWW Home Page:
http://www.nih.govlnia

National Multiple Sclerosis Society
733 3rd Avenue
New York, NY 10017
Phone: 800–344–4867
WWW Home Page:
http://www.nmss.org

National Organization on Fetal Alcohol Syndrome*
1819 H. Street, NW
Suite 750
Washington, DC 20006
Phone: 202–785–4585
Fax: 202–466–6456
E-mail: nofas@erols.com
WWW Home Page:
http://www.nofas.org

National Organization on Disability*
910 16th Street, NW
Suite 600
Washington, DC 20006
Phone: 202–293–5960
TDD: 202–293–5968
Fax: 202–293–7999
WWW Home Page:
http://www.nod.org

National Student Speech Language Hearing Association (NSSLHA)*
10801 Rockville Pike
Rockville, MD 20852-3279
Phone: 301–897–7350
Fax: 301–571–0457
E-mail: jmartinez@asha.org

Orton Dyslexia Society*
Chester Building, Suite 382
8600 La Salle Road
Baltimore, MD 21286-2044
Phone: 410–296–0232
Fax: 410–321–5069
E-mail: infor@ods.org

Parkinson's Disease Foundation
William Black Medical Research Building
640 West 168th Street
New York, NY 10032

Rehabilitation Research and Training Center*
Rancho Los Amigos Medical Center
7601 Imperial Highway
Downing, CA 90242
Phone: 310–401–7402
Fax: 310–401–7011

Sertoma Foundation*
P.O. Box 17003
Kansas City, MO 64123
Phone: 816–333–8300
Fax: 816–333–4320
E-mail: infosertoma@sertoma.org
WWW Home Page:
http://www.sertoma.org

Sibling Information Network
The University of Connecticut
AJ Pappanikou Center
249 Glenbrooke Road
Storrs, CT 06269-2064
Phone: 203–648–1205

Special Olympics*
1325 G. Street, NW
Suite 500
Washington, DC 20005-3104
Phone: 202–628–3630
Fax: 202–824–0200
E-mail: specialolympics@msn.com
WWW Home Page:
http://www.specialolympics.org

**Spina Bifida Association
of America***
4590 MacArthur Boulevard, NW
Suite 250
Washington, DC 20007-4226
Phone: 202–944–3285
Fax: 202–944–3295
E-mail: spinabifda@aol.com
WWW Home Page:
http://www.infohiway.com/
spinabifida

Stuttering Foundation of America*
3100 Walnut Grove Road
Suite 603
Memphis, TN 38111
Phone: 800–992–9392
Fax: 901–452–3931
E-mail: stuttersfa@aol.com

**TEACCH (Treatment and
Education of Autistic and Related
Communication Handicapped
Children and Adults)***
Division TEACCH, CB#7180
310 Medical School Wing E
Chapel Hill, NC 27599-7180
Phone: 919–966–2174
Fax: 919–966–4127
WWW Home Page:
http://www.unc.edu/depts/teacch

**The Association for Persons with
Severe Handicaps***
29 West Susquehanna Avenue
Suite 210
Baltimore, MD 21204
Phone: 410–828–8274
Fax: 410–828–6706
TDD: 410–828–1306
E-mail: info@tash.org
WWW Home Page:
http://www.tash.org

United Cerebral Palsy Association*
425 Eye Street, NW
Suite 141
Washington, DC 29001
Phone: 800–872–5827
Fax: 202–776–0414
TDD: 202–973–7197
WWW Home Page:
http://www.ucpa.org

INDEX